LIVING WITH ALZHEIMER'S

Living with Alzheimer's

Managing Memory Loss,
Identity, and Illness

Renée L. Beard

NEW YORK UNIVERSITY PRESS
New York and London

NEW YORK UNIVERSITY PRESS
New York and London
www.nyupress.org

References to Internet websites (URLs) were accurate at the time of writing. Neither the author nor New York University Press is responsible for URLs that may have expired or changed since the manuscript was prepared.

Library of Congress Cataloging-in-Publication Data
Names: Beard, Renée L., author.
Title: Living with Alzheimer's : managing memory loss, identity, and illness / Renée L. Beard.
Description: New York : New York University Press, [2016] | Includes bibliographical references and index.
Identifiers: LCCN 2015043570| ISBN 9781479800117 (cl : alk. paper) | ISBN 9781479889808 (pb : alk. paper)
Subjects: LCSH: Alzheimer's disease. | Alzheimer's disease—Patients—Care.
Classification: LCC RC523 .B396 2016 | DDC 616.8/31—dc23
LC record available at http://lccn.loc.gov/2015043570

New York University Press books are printed on acid-free paper, and their binding materials are chosen for strength and durability. We strive to use environmentally responsible suppliers and materials to the greatest extent possible in publishing our books.

Manufactured in the United States of America

10 9 8 7 6 5 4 3 2 1

Also available as an ebook

This book is dedicated to
Margarita Wheeler, Jenny Knauss, Richard Taylor,
and all of those who are currently being denied
meaningful human interaction because of
inaccurate assumptions that such exchanges
cannot be of any benefit to people with memory loss.
This is also for anyone who has seen a glimpse
of what I saw in Margarita in someone else
and took the time to join them.

CONTENTS

ACKNOWLEDGMENTS

This long process has been made significantly easier by numerous people, many of whom are unaware of their contributions. I owe the most thanks to my confidant and best friend, Adam, who is decidedly aware of his role in this book. Both his patience and ability to know how to help me get this done often exceeded my own. His parents Ellen and Jonathan, both academics themselves, no doubt socialized him well into the role—and for that and much else I am thankful to them also. I am especially grateful for my two sons, Ari and Asher, who made it impossible to retreat too far away emotionally or physically. There was no better excuse to take a break than playing with you two.

I thank my parents, Robert and Ruth Beard, who unselfishly gave me everything and told me that I could do anything; Grace Richardson who—in life and in death—showed me the beauty of aging and gave me the gift of what I now proudly think of as my "farming stock"; Jeanette Wilder, who called me "blueberry eyes" and had faith in me when I myself did not; and Harley Richardson, who taught me about the labor of love without even trying. I appreciate Robin and Richard Beard for giving me the richness of sibling life. I am indebted to Margarita Wheeler, the first person I ever met with what at the time was called Oldtimers, for sharing her world with me, encouraging me to join her where she was, inciting the passion behind all these years of study, and for unapologetically knowing me only as "Goldilocks." The motivation for this book, when I look back now, started with Margarita; a strong, proud, and witty woman who too few people in the nursing home where I had my first job—as a housecleaner—took the time to get to know.

I am deeply indebted to the seniors who allowed me to enter into one of the most private, vulnerable times in their lives and spoke honestly and openly with me about their experiences. I feel grateful to have heard their unique stories and for the honor of being present during an already taxing experience. I also could not have done this without the willingness and time of the many clinicians and Alzheimer's Association staff involved in this study. I admire your tenacity and heart-felt commitment to helping the deeply forgetful among us.

The intellectual support I got on this project at the University of California, San Francisco (UCSF) came first and foremost from Patrick Fox, who guided my research from the very first day we discovered our shared passion for Alzheimer's. An insightful, encouraging, and astute dissertation chair, you energized me every time we met. Carroll Estes was also an essential contributor to my intellectual persona. Your desire to expose the mistreatment of seniors and create meaningful social change has left a strong imprint. Sharon Kaufman pushed me longer and harder theoretically than I knew possible and remains one of my primary models of academic success. Special thanks to Carolyn Wiener, who encouraged me to continue this research when I was repeatedly told it was impossible to interview people with memory loss. As one of the last vestiges of what I imagine to be a distinctly Straussian mentoring style, your engagement with my data also greatly helped me tell the story. Jennie Kayser-Jones taught me the art of doing robust and meaningful ethnographic fieldwork. While being on your end-of-life study was one of the most challenging jobs I have ever had, the compassion and drive to improve the dying process I saw in you fuels my own work.

I also feel sincere gratitude to two other sociologists who have mentored me since my undergraduate days at Boston College. John Williamson has devoted endless hours teaching, advising, and supporting me in my choice to pursue a career in sociology. Your guidance and friendship are among the most valuable things in my academic life. David Karp taught me the art of qualitative methods. Being in your Research Methods class while you were writing *Speaking of Sadness*, and then later reading the book, was a formative experience personally and professionally. Your intellectual influence on this book is significant. John McKinlay at the New England Research Institute was the first self-proclaimed medical sociologist I ever met. I continue to admire your dedication to the field and willingness to say things the way they are. Sharon Tennstedt also supervised and trained me in conducting research with older people during my time at NERI.

Dale Rose and Chris Ganchoff were instrumental in providing insight, support, and motivation throughout this project and remain the most important aspect of my graduate experience at UCSF. Dale was especially helpful in holding me accountable for finishing the book once I set out to do so. At Holy Cross, Ara Francis provided me with the inspiration of a generalist sociologist, the support of a fellow interactionist, and a concrete model for how to get this book done. Kyle Carr also helped me manage the minutiae involved in assembling this book—saving me much time and stress. I appreciate that my students in the spring of 2014 Illness Narratives seminar gave honest and helpful input on the manuscript. My colleagues at Holy Cross have been incredibly supportive. I cannot imagine a better fit as a teacher scholar or as someone who aspires to having a balanced approach to work.

Ilene Kalish and three reviewers provided me insightful and apt suggestions for improving the book. The various NYU staff members who helped me with logistics also deserve accolades. I especially appreciate Ilene's confidence that this was a story worth telling and that I was the person to do so.

I hope I have done justice to the complexities of diagnosing, treating, serving, and experiencing memory loss. If this book begins to change, in whatever small way, how we view people with AD, then we will all be the better for it.

Prologue

Lost in Translation

I enter the small waiting room in the memory clinic just before 9 a.m. Shortly thereafter, Mr. and Mrs. R arrive to learn the results of the cognitive evaluation they had each undergone two weeks earlier. Mrs. R is 67 years old and Mr. R is 72 years old and they have both recently retired. As they begin talking about the groceries that they need to get at the Safeway on their way home, the ease with which they converse suggests a long and intimate relationship. They seem nonchalant about the information they have come to hear. Having observed their initial testing and learned from them at that time that they simply "came in to get a baseline" in the event of future memory troubles, their relaxed demeanor is as I would anticipate. When I first met them and observed their evaluations, it seemed clear to me that neither of them had any pathological memory difficulties. The following week, at the team conference, where cases are presented and diagnoses are determined at this clinic, I learned that Mr. R was very slightly below average and that Mrs. R was normal. No medical labels, as such, were used in reference to either of them.

Thirty minutes after their appointment time, Dr. K, a neuropsychiatrist, comes rushing into the waiting room, apologizes, and signals to them that they should follow her. She heads to her office at a pace quicker than Mr. and Mrs. R, and the three of us make small talk as I walk behind her with them. In the office, the doctor sits on one side of her rectangular desk, Mr. and Mrs. R sit on the other side, and I pull up a chair between them at the end of the desk. I imagine this will be a short and painless delivery. Honestly, at the time I could not help but feel that their family conference would not provide much by way of data for my research on how people experience memory loss.

Dr. K hands Mrs. R a packet and begins, "I'm going to start with you, Mrs. R, since yours is the clearest. Basically, you did very well. You are fine." The doctor goes over her tests and reports that she did "average or above" on all of them. Not five minutes after initiating the conversation with Mrs. R, Dr. K says, "You have no cognitive impairment at this time. Do you have any questions?" Mrs. R expresses her satisfaction and doesn't ask any questions.

Turning away from Mrs. R, the doctor says, "Yours was really easy and quick." As Dr. K turns her head toward Mr. R, she continues, "Now I'll move to Mr. R's," and I felt the customary weight in my stomach when watching someone receive an Alzheimer's diagnosis. The doctor's severe tone told me that this gentleman was about to get bad news. I was confused. Speaking to Mrs. R, she says, "Now I will go over his results." Dr. K draws a picture of the brain [shrinking][1] and talks about what happens when someone has dementia. She is drawing it in front of Mrs. R and Mr. R cranes his neck to see it.

Mrs. R asks what causes it and the clinician dismissively replies, "That's what I was going to tell you." Mrs. R apologizes and looking at Mrs. R, the doctor continues, "It can be [caused by] shrinkage from early Alzheimer's disease or increased fluid. I don't think it's hydrocephalitis [fluid on the brain], though, I think there's some atrophy. In terms of testing, he had some troubles, especially with memory. Basically, he did worse on the [neurocognitive] testing with [the research assistant]. Counting backwards from 100 and the blocks . . . he was very slow on those. On recalling animals, he also scored low. He did not do terribly, terribly well. It's not dementia but mild cognitive impairment. There are changes in his level of functioning. The reason, we think, is early Alzheimer's disease. Now, we don't know for sure, but there's been no stroke, so we think it could be early AD. It's not a problem demanding major attention but we should do close follow-up."

Dr. K continues, now addressing Mr. R, "You will need services in the future. Let's go over the legal and financial issues. I think anyone with memory problems needs to talk about a DPA [durable power of attorney] with health or medical conditions and finances. It takes a long time to go through it all. [Nursing home] Placement is not needed at this point but I would call Family Caregiver Alliance [a local nonprofit devoted to supporting long-term care providers] if you need that in the future. There are also support groups. I don't think you need it yet but in case you want to later, call the Alzheimer's Association. Regarding your PCP, see him 1–2 times a year. You need to be watched and periodically tested to see if you can dial

911. . . . People with conditions like this need to be checked." Looking at Mrs. R, Dr. K nods her head and raises her eyebrows to ascertain agreement. She pauses, nods again, and then turns back to Mr. R and says, "You should be tested to see if you can complete a list of things. These things are not for now, if you follow our recommendations, you can live a long, long time well. Day care is not significant for you now [but] . . . Keep active socially and be stimulated intellectually."

Dr. K concludes, "So, having told you all of this, do you have any questions for me?" Both Mr. and Mrs. R are silent as they indicate no with a shake of their heads, depicting the look of bewilderment I've come to recognize as the typical affect of people being diagnosed. Mr. R glances down at his feet and in a deflated tone says, "I guess you've covered it all." The entire meeting for both cases has taken less than 20 minutes. They get up to leave the office, solemnly thanking the doctor on their way out, and I follow behind them. Mr. and Mrs. R walk, very slowly, back to the office where they are to be asked if they consent to be participants in research. They seem not to notice me trailing behind and I overhear Mr. R say, "Well, you know, it's not as bad as it could've been," and I detect the sound of his voice shaking as he chokes up.

* * *

About two weeks later, I scheduled an interview to meet with Mr. and Mrs. R. When I arrived at their home and told him that I wanted to talk about their experiences at the memory clinic, Mr. R paused and then said, "I remember it very well." I asked him what the doctor had told him was going on and, without hesitation, he said, "Alzheimer's." In fact, they both thought that he had been diagnosed with early Alzheimer's disease [AD]. When I mentioned mild cognitive impairment [MCI], neither Mr. R nor Mrs. R recalled ever having heard of it and certainly did not think of these words as a diagnosis. The following excerpt summarizes their impressions of the exchange:

> RB: What stands out the most about your experience at the memory clinic?

> MR. R: It was like she was reading a death notice to me.

Mrs. R: But she was making it to me, like I was a caregiver of his, which I'm definitely not. I may be some day, or he may be a caregiver of me, but . . .

Mr. R: You better not be a caregiver right now, we've got too many plans! (Laughter).

RB: What were you told was wrong, was causing this?

Mr. R: She said that I was going into Alzheimer's. She talked as though I am in the late stages with nursing homes, power-of-attorney, and things. I mean, give me some hope!

Mrs. R: And that was the feeling that I had too. I wondered, "What in the world is going on here? She's acting like he's not a person anymore."

Mr. R: I left thinking, "This is the beginning of a quick end. I just hope I make it to the check-up next year."

A few months later, Mr. and Mrs. R would narrate a decidedly different anticipated future than the one suggested here. Shortly after this exchange, they sought a second opinion from Mr. R's primary care doctor. When I visited with them a month later, Mr. R was almost giddy as he told me that his PCP had assured them that nothing was wrong with him and that his memory loss was the result of normal aging. Mr. and Mrs. R consciously chose to dismiss the news rendered by Dr. K, the specialist clinician. Of course, very few people ultimately seek second opinions after seeing a specialist.

1

The Meaning of Memory Loss

Illness, Identity, and Biography

The first case of Alzheimer's disease (AD) was observed by German psychiatrist Alois Alzheimer in 1906. Alzheimer's is a progressive brain disease that affects memory and other functions of daily living. The leading cause of dementia, AD is currently constructed as a problem of epidemic proportion. Historically, such perceptions were not the case. Scientific debate about the qualitative difference between age-related memory loss and Alzheimer's persists,[1] as does skepticism regarding the efficacy of treatment alternatives.[2] Yet the overwhelming majority of research efforts and monies remain narrowly focused on cause and cure. Together with the related focus on prevention, while laudable for its potential long-term benefits, the everyday lived experiences of AD are erased for those *currently* diagnosed and their family members alike. Contemporary epidemiological projections engender a crisis rhetoric, or "apocalyptic demography,"[3] that may contribute to mis-/overdiagnoses of Alzheimer's and its potential precursor,[4] and/or the conflation of memory loss and AD, as suggested in the prologue.

It's hard to believe that in the 1980s, when I had my first job in a nursing home, people with memory loss were said to have "Oldtimers"; something so common that while certainly undesirable, it was a far cry from the death sentence it is today. Most people that I have talked to about my research over the past two decades have either known someone with Alzheimer's or vehemently declared that they themselves had it. Why the relatively recent preoccupation with a condition that was discovered over a hundred years ago? And why do Americans assume that people with AD and their families warrant such pity? How did we get to a place where Alzheimer's is assumed to render meaningful interactions and moments impossible? Who tells us this and why?

While Alzheimer's is seemingly ubiquitous in contemporary American society, it unfortunately reveals itself far less through the life stories of real people with the condition than the rapidly escalating appearances in the public media, Hollywood movies, or on television programs and best-selling book lists that reinforce an almost universally pejorative view of the condition. Where are the real-life stories of people with Alzheimer's? And what can they add to the cultural dialogue that so influences their experiences? This chapter addresses what it means to be ill in a general sense in a health-obsessed society, what it feels like to be seen as old in a youth culture, how social perceptions of dementia shape notions of self-worth in what bioethicist Stephen Post calls a hypercognitive society, and how the story we tell about ourselves is threatened if we are presumed incompetent by others.

Although Alzheimer's disease was discovered well over a century ago, only since the 1980s has it been a topic of global health interest. In large part, the relatively recent surge of attention has been the result of clinical expansions—initiated by the National Institute on Aging (NIA) and the U.S. Alzheimer's Association in the late 1970s—to include what was previously called senile dementia (colloquially known as Oldtimers) under the rubric of Alzheimer's. This historical shift in the biomedical conceptualization of AD transformed *senility*, formerly viewed as a common component of aging, into *dementia*. The processes through which AD became identified as a distinct entity and attempts were made to categorize it as dementia generated both the widespread popularization of AD and a subsequently massive increase in research monies (including the notable 1974 establishment of a National Institute (on Aging) devoted—at least initially—to its cause). Labeling senile dementia as a specific disease category reversed the notion of cognitive decline as an inevitable part of aging and brought both aging and memory loss more squarely under the purview of medicine.

Since this redefinition significantly increased the numbers of individuals reported to have AD, back in the 1980s Alzheimer's became the fourth or fifth leading cause of death in America—[5] seemingly overnight. The U.S. Alzheimer's Association currently purports that 5.4 million Americans have a diagnosis of AD and their annual report claims, "Over the coming decades, the aging of the baby boom generation is projected to result in an additional 10 million people with AD. Today, someone in America develops AD every 68 seconds. By 2050, there is expected to be one new case of AD every 33 seconds, or nearly a million new cases per year, and AD prevalence is projected to be 11 million to 16 million."[6] Global projections suggest that the estimated 46.8 million people living with dementia in 2015 will nearly double every twenty years to 74.7 million in 2030 and 131.5 million cases by 2050.[7] The problem with these estimates, it should be noted, is that they are taken directly from AD societies, and critical scholars suggest, "It is evident that these figures are designed to incite political action and increase funding for AD research."[8] Furthermore, "While projections are useful in highlighting the scale of the problem were risk factors to remain stable over time, this is clearly an untenable assumption."[9] AD incidence and prevalence rates cited in medical journals and by governments are nonetheless drawn from sources with such potential conflicts of interest. In fact, there is reason to believe that dementia prevalence has remained stable or even *declined* in the past twenty years.[10]

Since age is the only known risk factor for Alzheimer's, prevalence and incidence rates have been predicted to double roughly every five years after the age of 60 and claims at the turn of the century stated that 50 percent of people over 85 were affected.[11] A more recent framing by the Alzheimer's Association reports that 32 percent of Americans over 85 currently have AD.[12] If one out of every three of us in that age group has it, can it be based solely in biology? Despite what anthropologist Margaret Lock refers to as "Entanglements of Dementia and Aging," Alzheimer's has been effectively presented as a global public health issue. Perhaps as a result, even minimally efficacious medications have been championed despite the current lack of a cure or even moderate symptom reversal. A major effect of this biomedical shift, however, has been the steadfast effort to detect Alzheimer's as early as possible, ideally in its presumed preclinical period. The medical impetus to diagnose people with memory loss as soon in the disease trajectory as conceivable generates enthusiasm for classifying preclinical AD, or what is called mild cognitive impairment. As a classic case of "diagnostic expansion,"[13] this emphasis on early diagnosis designates AD as a "spectrum disorder." Drawing on seminal medical sociology, in this book Alzheimer's is shown to be a social artifact and an extension of the medical gaze that relies heavily on the technologies of self[14] commonly accompanying the rise of surveillance medicine.[15]

Significant dissent regarding the conceptual basis, the diagnostic algorithms, and the relationship between MCI and similar terms has existed since Alzheimer's was coined over a century ago, and current practitioners vary widely in their disclosure of MCI to so-called patients. Notwithstanding disputes over terminology, however, a phase of observable cognitive impairment is believed to exist prior to a person exhibiting signs meeting clinical criteria for dementia. Importantly, this potential precursory period is seen as the best time to target pharmacological interventions. This also means, of course, that clinical trials and illness narratives alike can commence much earlier in the course of cognitive decline than ever before, offering both hope and hype of delaying if not preventing Alzheimer's and understanding the earliest points of transition in first-person experiences of the illness.

Despite this scientific uncertainty and dispute involved in diagnosing the potential precursor to Alzheimer's in theory, in practice MCI is routinely diagnosed in American specialty clinics. This has resulted in the identification of individuals who have minor memory loss and thus are quite cognizant of and able to articulate their experiences. In the case of Alzheimer's, and any condition thought to have preclinical stages, individuals who seek medical attention for memory loss—even in an effort to get what is referred to as a baseline, as the prologue demonstrates—are immediately suspect.[16] In practice, most seniors seeking cognitive evaluation at specialty clinics are in fact diagnosed with AD, and the older one is, the greater one's potential for becoming an Alzheimer's patient.

Disparities between so-called lay and expert knowledges have long been of interest to the social sciences. Medical sociologists have historically conceived of the interface between doctors and patients as what Monica Casper and Michael Berg referred to as a molding process through which a person and his/her situation are constructed or reconstructed to render them manageable.[17] Such processes engage larger debates about expert and lay knowledges, and the boundaries delineating and defining them. The data I present in this book highlight the mechanisms through which such molding transpires. Molding is even at times perceived by patients as advantageous in the medical evaluation and subsequent encounters surrounding AD. Yet various points of patient resistance were also discovered.

The U.S.-based Alzheimer's Association estimates that half of those with AD are in the early stage.[18] Through the quest for earlier diagnoses, biomedicine generates patients who can and do advance different views and experiences of medical encounters and everyday life with Alzheimer's. In this way, patient subjectivity has the potential to shape clinical practice and social discourse (and vice versa). To examine this dynamic, I gathered expert testimonials from both the clinical and advocacy realms. The primary goal of this book is to investigate the diagnosis of memory loss and subsequent receipt, that is, the *managing* of memory, as an emergent sociocultural phenomenon with economic, medical, political, and historical rationalities operating. My research uncovers the social processes through which forgetful older members of society are transformed into Alzheimer's patients. That is, how seniors are socialized by medical structures and the mass media into seeing their forgetfulness as symptoms of a disease, and the costs as well as benefits of this process for those most deeply affected.

Within the long tradition of illness narratives, illnesses are seen to influence biographies and identities to instill meaning and give voice to suffering. Anthropologist Arthur Kleinman is often said to have been a seminal advocate for exploring narrative structures of illness. Kleinman and others have examined folk illness beliefs and behaviors, or explanatory models of meaning-making. Sociologists Anselm Strauss and Barney Glaser pioneered the use of grounded theory to understand the meaning and experience of chronic illnesses from the perspectives of both diagnosed individuals and their family members. These methods and an emphasis on the relationship *between* illness and identity *within* context inform the analysis presented in this book. The findings revealed here further sociological theorizing on identity and biography by arguing that illness may be both chronic and terminal, demonstrating that illness can be experienced as disruptive to and reinforcing of identities, insisting that identity be seen as fluctuating rather than a fixed, linear process, and revealing that even individuals with conditions that theoretically compromise their storytelling capacity can narrate their illness experiences. Since recovery identities are unattainable for those with AD, constructing Alzheimer's as the quintessential postmodern threat to self risks assailing both personal and social worth, which sociologists have long claimed threatens a *social death* for affected individuals.

The Study

As evident from the prologue, the future painted in medical encounters for memory loss is often one of a demented individual whose complete incapacitation is imminent. The clinical delivery of the information to Mr. and Mrs. R was not qualitatively different from the roughly fifty textbook cases of late onset (or typical) early-stage Alzheimer's disease[19] I observed at the two specialty clinics during my eighteen-month study. When I looked up the official diagnosis at the memory clinic, Mr. R's chart read: "Cognitive Impairment not meeting criteria for dementia; mild neurocognitive disorder with undetermined etiology. Causal factors: somewhat likely AD." Officially, this gentleman had *no diagnosis*. Yet when I read the information I found myself uncertain about what, exactly, was going on. If it wasn't dementia, how could it be that Alzheimer's was "somewhat likely" to be causing it? How certain could the doctors be about knowing this? And, perhaps most pointedly, how helpful was it for Mr. and Mrs. R to have this information?

Mr. R's story highlights some important issues that will be taken up in this book. The medical efforts to diagnose Alzheimer's as early in the assumed trajectory as possible—in an attempt to intervene and stop decline—generate unintentional consequences that are germane to medical sociology and have very real potential costs to individuals who are so labeled. Most centrally, the medical or scientific consensus on the etiology, the protocol for treatment options, or the ethics of diagnosing MCI[20] remains lacking. Claims made by at least one leading neurologist about "The Myth of Alzheimer's" demonstrate that contestation over Alzheimer's itself is noteworthy. Accordingly, Lock argues, "the assumed 'factness' of Alzheimer's as a disease that inevitably causes people to become demented is being questioned by a growing minority of experts."[21] Although the concept of mild cognitive impairment is relatively easy to grasp, the development of precise diagnostic criteria has been slow to emerge despite neurologist Ronald Petersen's coining the term in the mid-1990s. In part, this is related to the dispute within the scientific community regarding the exact nature of the state and whether or not it constitutes pathology. Since the transition between normal aging and dementia is largely thought to occur insidiously over many years, scientists have recently begun purporting that this period of slow cognitive decline preceding the diagnosis of Alzheimer's can be identified and quantified via clinical guidelines. In 2011, after I conducted my study, new diagnostic criteria were put forth jointly by the National Institute on Aging and the U.S. Alzheimer's Association that officially identify MCI as the stage preceding AD.

While it is far too early to understand the implications of these new criteria, MCI was initially introduced in the 1990s as a diagnostic syndrome that coincided with very early Alzheimer's pathology. Despite the lack of clinical consensus on causation, many scientists claim that MCI should be considered a cognitive syndrome that implies a likely predementia neurodegenerative process. Longitudinal studies report vast differences in conversion rates from MCI to AD, and some even reveal a full return of memory functioning; thus, the legitimacy of mild cognitive impairment as a precursor to Alzheimer's remains debatable. Consequently, there are also disagreements about treatment protocol and serious ethical considerations when employing MCI as a clinical diagnosis. In fact, a major difference between the two sites I studied in this research was the fact that one (the psychiatrically based center) did not recommend medications at all for MCI and the other (the neurology based clinic) routinely did so. The lack of consensus regarding the efficacy of treatment options led clinicians to place more or less emphasis on medications even within sites. Disparities between specialty clinics and general practitioners can be assumed to be even greater. The ethical matters involved in this debate relate to the psychosocial consequences of diagnosing individuals with mild cognitive impairment in the absence of scientific or clinical consensus regarding etiology and treatment options. The magnitude of this potential threat of a preclinical diagnosis is evident in the opening story. Earlier diagnoses extend and arguably intensify both the medical gaze and the phenomenological experiences of memory loss. The potential effect of diagnosing someone with an unknown, untreatable condition has yet to be studied, and consequently social scientists, medical practitioners, and medical ethicists alike caution against too readily diagnosing the earliest stages or identifying biomarkers of memory loss.[22] Given the conflation of terms such as dementia, memory loss, mild cognitive impairment, and Alzheimer's disease portrayed in Mr. R's story, the ethical implications are evident.

Another problematic of interest to medical sociology highlighted by the opening story is that this lack of consensus provides clinicians with a good deal of discretion in diagnosing and treating mild cognitive impairment.[23] This high level of *clinical judgment* in the diagnostic process generates wide variability among practitioners as well as between specialty clinicians (neurologists, neuropsychiatrists, and psychiatrists) and general practitioners. Without knowledge of the scientific debates within which MCI exists, Mr. and Mrs. R clearly thought that Mr. R had Alzheimer's and was on the doomed trajectory of someone with a progressive, degenerative illness. The fact that Mrs. R's mother had lived with Alzheimer's for fifteen years led them to have a very specific perception of what their future would look like. After his general practitioner assured him that his current memory loss was age-related, Mr. R proudly showed me the letter to that end from his physician. Mr. R's doctor held a view common among general practitioners. In one survey of general practitioners, 34 percent saw no benefit to an early diagnosis and 66 percent said they in fact foresaw negative consequences from making an early diagnosis.[24]

This leads to a related problem of concern to medical sociology. In some cases there is an inconsistency between the way memory specialists and general practitioners *define* pathological memory loss. The lack of clarity regarding the existence of MCI and subsequent ethical considerations significantly confounds the experiences of people seeking medical care; particularly when, never having heard of mild cognitive impairment, individuals seeking medical care for their memory (and perhaps even clinicians, if inadvertently) conflate it with Alzheimer's, a condition saturating the public media and lay discourse. Alzheimer's disease, for better or worse, is a household term with a very specific connotation. Like Mr. R initially did, the vast majority of individuals that I observed being diagnosed with MCI fully believed that they either had or would soon have Alzheimer's. Largely, this is due to the fact that Alzheimer's was mentioned during every MCI diagnosis observed in this study. Clinicians were repeatedly heard saying, "It might be caused by early Alzheimer's disease," or "It could end up being Alzheimer's, so we'll track it carefully." There is considerable dispute regarding the disparities between identifying and treating memory in specialty and general practice.[25] And although they play a major role in the "success" of earlier diagnoses and clinical trials,[26] memory clinics have long been accused of being short-sighted in their dealings with patients,[27] especially regarding the psychosocial aspects of the illness.

The lack of medical consensus, practical latitude in diagnosing, and subsequent differences between the way specialty medicine and general practice define MCI are directly related to the social aspects of health and illness so fundamental to medical sociology. These factors necessitate that the operationalization of memory loss in particular, be explicitly addressed in this study. Conceptually, Alzheimer's disease and mild cognitive impairment are used interchangeably in this research. Despite the fact that MCI is technically, and *debatably*, considered a precursor to AD, as the prologue shows, the findings from this study will demonstrate that in daily life diagnosed individuals interpreted MCI as AD, since it was the only known entity to which they could relate their symptoms. I am thus arguing that phenomenologically the participants in this study interpreted their experiences within a framework saturated by AD. That is, lay interpretations of MCI diagnoses both reflect and reinforce contemporary clinical constructions of AD. Alzheimer's and the subsequent social perceptions of it have become a common cultural trope within American society over the past few decades. Therefore, the clinical employment of a term at once foreign to respondents as a diagnostic category and yet common as everyday words (mild cognitive impairment) can in everyday life lead those diagnosed to conflate MCI and AD. For this reason, they experienced an MCI diagnosis in a manner remarkably similar to those in the study who were told they had AD.

Although the biomedical world clearly differentiates Alzheimer's disease from mild cognitive impairment for various reasons, including having distinct study samples, the diagnosis of MCI is understood by patients as a distinctly Alzheimer's-oriented condition. In the quest to understand the disease processes in clinical practice and research, the boundaries between early Alzheimer's and mild cognitive impairment become indecipherable. Thus, the loose biomedical concepts have critical implications for the everyday lives of the individuals diagnosed and for society broadly.

When individuals are diagnosed with mild cognitive impairment the primary organization established to assist those with memory loss suggests the world they are entering; the Alzheimer's Association[28] bears the name of the very disease that they fear might afflict them. Established in 1980, shortly after the founding of the National Institute on Aging (NIA), by researchers and family members of those with AD, the Association is entrenched in the biomedical knowledges and practices to which newly diagnosed individuals have recently been introduced in the specialty clinics where they were evaluated. For individuals diagnosed with AD and MCI alike, the Association supports a distinctly, if not surprisingly, disease-oriented approach. Within the Association mild cognitive impairment, to the degree it is addressed at all, becomes Alzheimer's disease in an effort to fit the condition into the organization's existing culture (including, of course, well-intended efforts to provide services to constituents in need). Here too MCI is embedded in an Alzheimer's discourse.[29]

The remainder of this book describes in rich ethnographic detail[30] what this Alzheimer's discourse is, how it reflects and reinforces contemporary cultural values and assumptions about aging and memory loss, and the everyday effect of such rhetoric on individuals currently being diagnosed with either Alzheimer's or mild cognitive impairment in America.

In chapter 2, "History and Technoscience," I challenge readers to interrogate where our understanding of Alzheimer's comes from, how definitions have changed over time, the influence of scientific quests for earlier diagnosis on affected individuals as well as society, and whether or not efficacious treatments actually exist. Despite these factors and the fact that the condition cannot be definitely diagnosed except upon autopsy, in excess of 2.6 billion National Institutes of Health dollars were dedicated to AD between 2010 and 2015 alone.[31]

The chapter examines the historical background of memory loss, including the German psychiatrist whose 1906 patient became the first case of Alzheimer's disease. I outline the new guidelines for diagnosing Alzheimer's proposed in 2011, and delineate their potential bioethical implications. Tracing the nascent memory sciences and the technological innovations that now enable earlier diagnosis of the condition demonstrates the virtual monopoly biomedicine has over AD. Sociologically speaking, diagnosing Alzheimer's as early in the trajectory as possible generates a group of patients who are both able to discuss their experiences and to practice technologies of the self, thus providing a lens for investigating the effect of this trend on illness narratives. This history allows for an examination of how AD is handled in biomedicine and the way the Alzheimer's Association has used the knowledges and practices based on this epistemology, which are taken up in subsequent chapters.

Chapter 3, "Constructing Facts in Clinical Practice," draws on eighteen months of observation in specialty clinics and interview data with practitioners to delineate the information doctors consider relevant to making a diagnosis, how those data are gathered and interpreted in clinical practice, what happens when clinicians disagree, how those seeking evaluation are told of their results, how the answers to these questions differ according to whether evaluations are conducted by a neurologist or a psychiatrist, and whether or not anything is really being done to help patients after they are diagnosed.

By investigating the daily work practices of clinicians performing cognitive evaluations and diagnosing Alzheimer's in two specialty clinics,[32] I engage the tropes of trust and uncertainty that clinicians use to understand how cultural dynamics such as organizational ethos and work practices influence the social fabric of cognitive evaluations. By way of comparison between neurology and psychiatry, I trace the distinct institutional and organizational protocol employed to accomplish these tasks at each site. Despite the seemingly obvious disciplinary differences, the data reveal codified routines that support a common goal, that of moving individuals from the category of what I refer to as "potential patients" to that of patients, and ultimately research subjects, by establishing trust and highlighting uncertainty. Work practices support the routine collection of information, standardized symptom classification techniques, and assumptions of patient incompetence while discouraging qualitative, narrative data. Understanding these clinical work practices allows me to examine why practitioners do what they do and analyze any interesting differences between what they say they do when being interviewed by me and what I observed them actually doing in practice. Most importantly, these data allow me to understand the effect of clinical practice on the subjective experiences of cognitive evaluation and diagnosis in the following chapters.

In chapters 4 and 5, "Being Cognitively Evaluated" and "Hearing 'the A Word,'" I utilize observation and narrative data to provide an intimate portrayal of patient perspectives at the two specialty clinics. You are told to count backwards from 100 in increments of 7. The clock starts ticking. You go blank. Is it Alzheimer's or general test anxiety? Do you have dementia or are you distracted? After hours of testing, you hear the words Alzheimer's disease. How does it feel? What are your first thoughts?

Chapter 4 depicts the subjective experience of being cognitively evaluated for and diagnosed with Alzheimer's at these specialty clinics, which I argue amounts to a degradation ceremony. Drawing on medical sociology's long history of research on the effect and socially contingent nature of various medical conditions, technologies, and the sciences more broadly, I demonstrate the myriad factors influencing the interactions between science and its technologies on the one hand, and people seeking medical care on the other. The common experience of cognitive evaluation is one of feeling exposed, confused, and overwhelmed. Everyday personal struggles to manage awkward and foreign symptoms are mirrored by the environment in which patients find themselves evaluated and the highly standardized battery of tests and clinical interactions they experience. Individuals being evaluated thus utilize various strategies to minimize social awkwardness and normalize clinical interactions. Accounts of diagnosis in chapter 5 suggest that while potentially removing personal blame and/or responsibility, designating a brain demented also threatens the individualism and autonomy of those diagnosed. Accepting what American sociologist Everett Hughes (1958) called the master status of Alzheimer patient is a clear threat to one's social status, thus ultimately designating the patient an outsider, as Howard Becker (1963) noted. Building on seminal social theorist Erving Goffman's work on impression management and stigma avoidance, I depict a proactive side of people with Alzheimer's disease (PWAD) that is all too often assumed to be lacking. Indeed, individuals work to present themselves favorably by employing deliberate strategies to manage their identities during cognitive evaluation and the diagnostic disclosure. Given the diagnostic advantages and disadvantages revealed, an AD diagnosis serves both a social function and a personal one, neither of which is without detriment.

In chapter 6, "Everyday Life with Diagnosis," I explore how diagnosed individuals resist seeing their lives as being over in the face of society telling them otherwise and how the diagnosis changes people, who might live with the condition for another twenty years or more. I present postdiagnosis interviews conducted with seniors to learn how it feels to live with Alzheimer's, whether one can still act strategically in social interactions, if the diagnosis provides any advantages, and if and why people with AD might choose to try and pass for normal.

This chapter explores the experiences of those who joined support groups and research studies as a result of their interactions with the specialty clinics and the Alzheimer's Association. Investigating how individuals make sense of their everyday experiences after being diagnosed, I reveal that—in contrast to unilateral fatalistic public perceptions—persons with AD strategically employ the diagnostic label (or not) as they see fit. Study respondents with AD/MCI are not passive recipients of the disease label; rather they deliberately, if hesitantly, embark upon the path of becoming Alzheimer's patients. The diagnosis causes increased tension over the management of self *and* others, which in turn prompts interactional problems and requires further management, producing *a spiral of dilemmas*. Participants heed the advice of clinicians and utilize Alzheimer's Association services largely in an effort to manage the uncertainty of their everyday lives. Since the questions that are asked both in science and in practice influence the possible answers that can be found, diagnosed individuals undergo considerable socialization into medicalized interpretations of their experiences. Most of the forgetful respondents in this study ultimately help accomplish the goal of modern medicine—as an exemplary technology of self—by being active participants in their care, as support groups and research studies model how to monitor and control both themselves and each other through a biomedical lens. Yet involvement with support groups and research also allows respondents to feel proactive and do something in the face of memory impairment. Although the support groups are based on middle-class ideals and the subjects in research studies are often affluent Caucasians, participation in these arenas can provide a sense of collectivity reported by other disease-based social movements. This positive spin allows respondents to normalize their often erratic behaviors and experiences, which is a crucial step in solidifying Alzheimer's identities. By placing hope in finding a cure and by participating in research, patients support and potentially shape biomedicine.

Chapter 7, "Advocating Alzheimer's," based on participant observation at dozens of Association-sponsored conferences and interviews with staff at the U.S.-based Alzheimer's Association, is an organizational analysis examining the inherent tensions of serving both patient and caregiver populations, the dilemma of garnering adequate sympathy to encourage philanthropy without exploiting constituents, and the one-sided portrayal of those with the condition that Association staff perceived to be necessary.

I explore the role of the leading national advocacy agency dedicated to serving people affected by Alzheimer's, focusing primarily on the effect of organizational dynamics and what Goffman (1974) called framing contests on the approach to the diagnosed individuals themselves. I draw on seminal social movement literature to demonstrate how its founding by bench scientists and caregivers places the Association in a tenuous position for incorporating the relatively new constituency of persons with early-stage Alzheimer's, who can and will advocate on their own behalf, into an organization based on biomedical principles too often assuming their incompetence. By tracing the steps leading to the 2008 appointment of the Association's first board member with dementia and the 2014 establishment of Dementia Alliance International, including the perhaps unobvious role of the contentious on-line forum called DASNI (Dementia Advocacy and Support Network International), I elucidate the challenge of trying to serve competing interests and the unique role of activism played by persons with young-onset AD and scholars within the academy itself.

In chapter 8, "Forget Me Not," I reiterate how my respondents maintain a sense subjectively of who they have always been and work to incorporate Alzheimer's experiences into their prediagnosis identities. After delineating the experiences of evaluation cum degradation ceremony, I map the identity changes that commence with diagnosis and the many turning points before Alzheimer's identities are accomplished, the various phases in this transformation from a forgetful person to an AD patient who has synthesized his or her interactions with specialty medicine and the Alzheimer's Association, including both interactional tensions and opportunities afforded. In understanding the processes through which illness realities are socially constructed, it becomes evident that there is nothing intrinsic to the feelings expressed by these respondents that necessarily and inevitably lead to a definition of forgetfulness as a disease. Instead, these identities must be reinforced by biomedical classifications and activities based on them. Diagnosing Alzheimer's as early in the trajectory as possible generates a group of patients who are able to discuss their experiences, thus providing a lens for investigating the effect of this trend on illness narratives.

I then bring the book to a close by asking readers to critically evaluate whether or not Alzheimer's is really a disease or whether we would all get Alzheimer's if we lived long enough, and who stands to lose depending on the answers; how our views on this have changed over the years; and what the answers to these questions mean for diagnosed individuals and their family members alike. Given the central place of memory in the lives of (many) Americans in modern times, I question whether or not memory loss being seen primarily (or exclusively) as a medical problem is good for seniors (with or without reports of memory loss), is good for any of us as we ourselves are aging, and is good for society at large.

Based in the theoretical frameworks of symbolic interaction and social construction, in this final chapter I reexamine the book's two overarching themes: the biomedicalization of memory loss and the sociology of illness narratives. Given the stronghold memory has over our personal lives and social worth in contemporary American society, I contemplate how our current preoccupation with memory loss and its construction as a medical problem shape phenomenological experiences of Alzheimer's, the values of society members not directly affected by the condition, and our overarching cultural views on aging. Contributing to conversations that are currently taking place in academia and popular culture alike, I interrogate what contemporary constructions of memory and so-called memory problems tell us about the role of allopathic medicine in aging processes in contemporary U.S. society.

This book aims, first and foremost, to lay out alternative and diverse frameworks for understanding the experiences of people currently being diagnosed with AD; second, to delineate how the medicalization of senility and the dramatically changed sociohistorical context of the disease influence psychosocial experiences; and third, to map out the potential consequences of diagnosing and thus socializing forgetful people into exclusively medicalized interpretations of their experiences. As the story of Mr. and Mrs. R shows, I answer these questions through empirical data from interviews with doctors, Alzheimer's Association staff, family members, and most importantly, seniors living with memory loss. I will depict an entirely different perspective on what it currently means to be living with Alzheimer's in U.S. society—one that not only debunks notions of lives devoid of all meaning and selves lost but also offers an alternative model of perseverance in the face of the adversity such social assumptions engender. My attempt to counteract contemporary misconceptions of Alzheimer's revolves around three basic claims. First, a medical/scientific consensus on causation, viable treatment alternatives, or the ethics of diagnosing mild cognitive impairment (and in some cases even AD) does not exist. Second, since this disagreement leaves practitioners without standardized protocol to follow, there is heavy reliance on *clinical judgment* regarding whether, when, and how to diagnose MCI (and to a lesser extent, AD). Last, there is significant dispute within specialty medicine and especially between specialty and general practitioners on what constitutes pathological memory loss.

I engage with recent critique of the dominant dementia framework as a lens through which to consider the advantages and pitfalls of conceptualizing Alzheimer's as we do in contemporary times and how our cultural values both reflect and reinforce the biomedical paradigm. By showing how experiences of dementia are larger than what humanities scholar Anne Basting refers to as "tales of tragedy" suggest, the paradoxical narratives of both resistance and reinforcement portrayed in this book expose the *social nature of memory* and how *self is relational*. In this way, I use AD as an exemplar of more general and processual social phenomena common to many modern Western societies: ageism and biomedicalization. Drawing on these critiques as well as recent contributions to the sociology of aging, I map out how and why contemporary social constructions of Alzheimer's are based on the dominance of cognitive hierarchies across the lifespan, fueled by the youth-based and memory-obsessed media, and American anxiety about decline and aging in our hypercognitive society. To that end, this book contributes the first empirical illness narrative, or counternarrative as I see it, of dementia to the burgeoning accounts that exist of the myriad ways of aging. By challenging our societal fear of Alzheimer's and of aging more broadly, I hope to make unique contributions to some of the most salient and enduring public, existential, and sociological debates of our times.

2

History and Technoscience

From Senility to Alzheimer's

The history of Alzheimer's disease is a long and interesting one. Based on an extensive literature review and both collection and presentation of data at numerous domestic and international scientific conferences devoted to Alzheimer's, this chapter delineates the developments and technoscientific innovations that inform contemporary biomedical knowledges and practices concerning memory loss. I will present the first two cases of what became known as Alzheimer's disease and introduce the terms senility, Alzheimer's, and mild cognitive impairment, including how they are currently conceptualized and approached. I will address how President George Bush's Decade of the Brain (1990s) affected the brain and memory sciences, including the generation of three central areas of technoscience: diagnostics, imaging, and therapeutics. Contextual factors such as historical developments, the technoscientific innovations during the Decade of the Brain, and the new diagnostic criteria proposed jointly by the NIA-Alzheimer's Association in 2011 together shape contemporary conceptions of AD in America. Persistent—often heated—debates ensued.

The Cases of Auguste D. and Johann F.

In 1910, the eponym *Alzheimer's disease* was first used by Emil Kraepelin, a German psychiatrist who was compiling the eighth edition of his *Handbook of Psychiatry*, a precursor to the *Diagnostic and Statistical Manual* (DSM). In 1906, German psychiatrist Alois Alzheimer described the first case of the condition that came to carry his name. Auguste D., a 51-year-old German housewife, presented at an asylum in Frankfurt with jealousy, paranoia, difficulty remembering, and nervous pacing.[1] She died after four years of progressive decline. Upon autopsy, her brain was found to have innumerable concentrations of tiny clusters and dead neurons in the cerebral cortex (these are called amyloid, or neuritic, plaques and neurofibrillary tangles, respectively). Discovery of the brain tissue from Frau D. at the turn of the twenty-first century confirmed that she was in fact the first documented case of AD. Dr. Alzheimer's second case, Johann F., a 56-year-old man who was forgetful, could not find his way, and was unable to perform simple tasks,[2] was observed from 1907 to 1910. He died within three years of presenting symptoms and many amyloid plaques were found in his cerebral cortex upon autopsy. Unlike Frau D., however, neurofibrillary tangles were not detected. Since dementia was at the time considered a psychosis or mind disorder, as opposed to an anatomical state, these cases were seminal in establishing a biological basis for so-called insanity, given their similarities. When Kraepelin made the assignment of AD based only on the four cases that had been documented by 1910,[3] it was despite the different neuropathology of those cases and the noted skepticism of Dr. Alzheimer himself.[4] This ambiguity regarding the "discovery" of AD has resulted in a complicated and contested trajectory.

Although the specific proteins, the plaque (beta-amyloid) and the tangle (tau), observed with AD have been identified, scientists differ on whether plaques, or beta-amyloid, hold the cure, or whether they support tangles as central to the pathogenesis of dementia. Accordingly, the problem is either the accumulation of protein or too much phosphate attaching to the tau, respectively. The amyloid and tau hypotheses, which remain predominant schools of thought, refer to themselves as the Baptists[5] and the Tauists, although there are a small number of agnostics as well. The overwhelming majority of AD research to date has been informed by the Amyloid Cascade Hypothesis aiming to identify drug treatments.

Despite the fragmented nature of scientific knowledge concerning Alzheimer's, the predominant conception of the disease process can be outlined as follows:

The current model of AD pathogenesis begins with the deposition of beta-amyloid plaques in the brain. ApoE4, a risk factor for AD, may promote this formation or interfere with its clearance. Tau, a stabilizing protein, may be threatened by the plaque deposition . . . [and] oxidative stress may further promote the aggregation of tau into neurofibrillary tangles. . . . The loss of key neurotransmitters (e.g., acetylcholine) and the breakdown in neuronal connectivity result in the clinical hallmarks of dementia such as cognitive impairment and abnormal behavior.[6]

Neuropathologically, the Amyloid Cascade Hypothesis suggests that beta-amyloid plaques deposit in the brain, causing neurofibrillary tangles that result in cell death. Atrophy occurs as a result of both neuronal and synaptic losses. This localization theory assumes that disease located in certain regions of the brain leads to behavioral changes.

The Conceptual Background

While the link between AD neuropathology and dementia is strong for people under 65, as in the initial cases, the vast majority of people currently diagnosed with AD are well over 65, where the combination of aging and comorbidities makes an explicit connection to pathology elusive.[7] Nonetheless, the aging of our population has fueled ever greater clinical efforts to differentiate between normal aging and dementia. Increased life expectancy resulting from improvements in diet, housing, public sanitation, personal hygiene, and the advent of antibiotics as well as reductions in death rates from chronic diseases has exponentially increased the number of older people with cognitive impairment. Since the National Institute on Aging and U.S. Alzheimer's Association's decision in the 1980s to redefine senility (until then a state presumed to accompany old age) as Alzheimer's rendered the condition largely unique to later life, it is not surprising that prevalence rates have risen with the aging of the baby boomers. Nonetheless, the quest to identify cognitive impairment as soon in the disease process as possible is arguably the most prominent concern at the current time, though another common fear since this redefinition is that "the precise demarcation of, particularly, early dementia from the cognitive, neurologic, anatomic, and neurochemical changes seen in normal aging is difficult to define."[8] Based on this, the less fashionable "entanglement theory" suggests that AD is processual and emergent.

Beginning at least as far back as the nineteenth century, the medical community was unclear whether senility was physiological or pathological. Throughout the twentieth century there was a great deal of uncertainty among researchers regarding whether senile dementia was a disease or a normal accompaniment of aging.[9] Late nineteenth- and early twentieth-century beliefs purported a view of disease as an inevitable part of old age[10] and "senescence" (or senility) was deemed an organic consequence of aging at that time.[11]

Social scientists view diseases as socially constructed biomedical phenomena.[12] Historians, in particular, have long argued that the over-emphasis on science and medicine results in health conditions being viewed through too narrow a lens[13] and a lack of acknowledgment of the fluidity of clinical concepts and practices. Alzheimer's is no exception. If the definitive discovery of AD as a disease category is impossible, given an inability to differentiate dementing illness from normal aging, then attempts to do so are arguably a mechanism for creating order in the complex world of memory loss, revealing what sociologist Jaber Gubrium referred to as the social organization of senility.[14]

With the advent of medical dominance in the twentieth century, however, the question of whether or not old age, and thus senility, could be cured became a subject of intense debate. Therefore, when in 1906 Alois Alzheimer described a case of dementia in a 51-year-old woman, it was done amidst an existing controversy about the relationship between aging and senility. Specifically, the notion that these neuropathological observations were found in a presenile brain was of great significance. Clinically and pathologically, senile dementia and what became known as Alzheimer's disease were strikingly similar and Dr. Alzheimer himself believed that the presentation of symptoms in Auguste D. was an accelerated version of the well-known condition of senile dementia rather than the discovery of a novel disease state.[15]

Emil Kraepelin, a founder of modern psychiatry, however, was persuasive in his claim of the legitimacy of AD as independent from the senile dementia of the time and entered it into his textbook of psychiatry as a distinct entity named after its alleged founder. Historians have suggested that Kraepelin may have rushed the definition of AD as a separate disease category unrelated to age to promote his own interests by demonstrating physical lesions upon autopsy.[16] Since the ability to distinguish between normal and pathological brains was an important component in the establishment of AD,[17] Kraepelin's endorsement was a vital factor leading to the acceptance of these plaques and tangles as a distinct disease state. The term *Alzheimer's disease*, then, originally referred to dementia in patients with presenile onset of symptoms, while *senile dementia* was used when symptoms began after 65 years of age, and was not considered a disease per se.

As early as 1933, however, German neurologists reported that the neurofibrillary tangles associated with AD were discovered in a majority of normal senile brains.[18] Allegedly, many older individuals experienced a degree of memory loss, which was observable but did not necessarily interfere with their daily living; that is, losses of memory function were considered part of normal aging.[19] A longitudinal study of older individuals depicted the following subgroups: those with preserved memory function, or normal aging; mild memory problems, or *benign* forgetfulness; and more severe memory difficulties, or *malignant* forgetfulness.[20] Experiences of benign forgetfulness, of course, were considered typical in older adults.

By the mid-twentieth century, however, senescence and senility were a unified construct and an interpretation of senile dementia as pathological quickly overshadowed previous meanings.[21] In 1968, a study reported that the same lesions observed in the brain of Auguste D. and Johann F. were found in 62 percent of all autopsies,[22] which was interpreted as suggesting that Alzheimer's was a far more prevalent phenomenon than previously believed (rather than a sign that the aging process had been wrongfully medicalized). Throughout the 1970s and early 1980s, most scientists agreed that it was pointless and arbitrary to maintain a distinction based on age of onset alone.[23] In fact, reports showing that the pathologies of presenile and senile dementia were not qualitatively different had existed for many decades.[24] With the continued discovery of pathological similarities between AD and senile dementia, debate over terminology again ensued.

Over the next decade, leading researchers, including neurologists Robert Katzman and Robert Terry, struggled to dispel the notion that AD was a rare condition (based on the projections of unifying presenile and senile dementias). In concert with the National Institutes of Health (NIH), these researchers and a number of families afflicted by dementia banned together in search of accurate diagnoses, treatments options, resources for so-called caregivers, and ideally a long-term cure. The late-stage diagnoses customary at the time justified an approach devoted exclusively to cause and cure. In 1980, the Alzheimer's Disease and Related Disorders Association (ADRDA) was formed to address these concerns. In October of that same year, a letter to Dear Abby sought advice on caring for a husband with probable Alzheimer's and was referred to the ADRDA, which made the association visible to the public. The following year, the beloved Hollywood actress, Rita Hayworth, was reported to have the disease. Together, these factors brought the scientific studies highlighting the prevalence of Alzheimer's to the attention of media and lay audiences alike. Consequently, AD emerged as an illness category and policy issue in the 1980s, more than seventy years after the first case had been documented by Dr. Alzheimer.

In contrast to the strong link between AD neuropathology and dementia observed in people under 65 years of age, the vast majority of people currently diagnosed with AD are over 65, where establishing a clear link becomes decidedly more difficult. Therefore, the definition of dementia remains a site of considerable dispute,[25] the issue being whether senility is a pathological state (localized) or an acceleration of essentially normal aging (entangled). Etiological questions of AD remain unanswered even today as there is significant evidence both for and against aging as the cause of AD. The focus on rising prevalence rates and population aging, however, prioritizes the influence of age. In fact, age remains the only proven risk factor for Alzheimer's. In contrast, in the same way that neurochemical changes in an AD brain differ from those of a non-AD brain, younger cases of AD have far more severe lesions than older ones.[26] As noted earlier, the first classification of dementia by Kraepelin in 1910 was based on presenile cases and only this (extremely rare) premature senility was originally designated as a disease.[27] Thus in clinical practice, efforts to categorize disease and implement a model of staged, progressive illness helped to combat the lack of normativity with dementia.[28] Since the 1960s, however, these two disorders began to be framed as a homogeneous entity. Given recent predictions that roughly 65 percent of people over 80 would be diagnosed with AD or predisease based on imaging,[29] the persistent questioning of the scientific basis for unifying these two terms has met with strong resistance underscored by their different rates of decline, neuropathologic changes, and actual symptoms.[30] As far back as the late 1980s, critics have claimed that the motivation to merge these two terms was a political one to increase medical legitimacy and, thus, federal funding.[31] It remains unclear whether early- and late-onset AD are the same entity, entirely separate diseases, or exist on a continuum of the aging process.[32]

Dementia's paradigm has two main implications for patients and practice: first, the narrow definition of cognition generated a need to minimize or ignore any noncognitive symptoms, and second, dementia needed to be considered irreversible to meet clinical criteria for neuropathology.[33] This view of dementia as essentially a disorder of cognition involves clinical, conceptual, and social factors, with unforeseen consequences, including giving preferential attention to intellectual deficits, thus potentially generating both over- and misdiagnosis, assumptions that those diagnosed will be depressed, leading to massive increases in psychotropic treatments, and encouraging the proclivity to loathe the forgetful that "is especially attractive in a hypercognitive culture."[34] The history of pathology and subsequent association between senility and dementia added to theories of degeneration to create a view of a dementia as a problem.

From a medical perspective, constructing old age as a period of progressive decline rendered dementia an inevitable and normal stage of life.[35] If AD wasn't seen to be pathological, the quest for a cure would prove futile, therefore frustrating the ability to manage the condition through biomedical efforts. Thus, a new disease category that was "unencumbered by debates about normalcy and pathology in old age, met a number of needs."[36] Conceptions of normal and abnormal health are intrinsically tied to cultural and political constructions of moral order.[37] As such, aging and AD can be used as a way to investigate how morality gets articulated through a picture of decline and impairment. The immediate goal of medicine was less the treatment than the discovery of the cause of AD. Proving a disease-state ostensibly renders aging more manageable and fits within the existing worldview despite the glaring descriptive tension[38] when trying to distinguish AD from normal aging, since all the symptoms of Alzheimer's disease appear, to some degree, in every brain.

Despite such disputes, the social construction of AD as a major threat to health in—and treatable part of—old age unwaveringly achieved the goal of expanding diagnostic categories of disease. It is important to situate designations of health, illness, and aging within the normative narratives or moral order surrounding these phenomena. To understand the history of the concept of AD, an examination of the larger milieu is required.

State of the Science

Contemporary clinical distinctions between cases of Alzheimer's are made according to the age of onset (prior to 65 years of age is early-onset AD and 65 or older is late onset, or "typical" AD).[39] Although the occurrence of Alzheimer's in individuals less than 65 years old is extremely rare,[40] these familial (autosomalt dominant) forms of AD typically follow a drastically accelerated version of the path found in the more common onset of Alzheimer's in the seventh or eighth decade of life and are passed to roughly 50 percent of offspring.[41] Individuals with late-onset AD can survive over 20 years with the condition whereas those with early onset live an average of only 3–5 years with their diagnosis,[42] as we saw with Frau D. and Johann F. According to the Alzheimer's Association, the average person can expect to live 8–10 years with Alzheimer's.[43] Overall, individuals diagnosed with late-onset AD can expect to live an average of 5 to 6 years less than their nonimpaired counterparts and an individual with early, or presenile, onset will have a life expectancy reduced by 15 years more than their contemporaries.[44] While the vast majority of those diagnosed with AD will succumb to the same major causes of death as the rest of us (e.g., heart disease, cancer, or stroke), those who do not will ultimately asphyxiate, aspirate, or die from infection- or pneumonia-related complications.

A multitude of hypotheses regarding AD etiology and pathogenesis remain, including genetic factors or biomarkers (APP mutations, Presenilin, APOE-4) and biochemical variables (inflammation, free radicals, estrogen deficits, excitotoxins). Additional risk factors such as increased age, positive family history, female gender, low educational level, head trauma, diabetes, midlife hypertension, midlife obesity, smoking, depression, and physical inactivity have also been noted.[45] A focus on genetic, biochemical, and other risk factors has been part of the impetus to diagnose AD as soon in the process as possible, and particularly in the preclinical stages of mild cognitive impairment. Understanding the genetics of AD is said to possibly yield valuable clues for the development of new diagnostic tools for MCI[46] and interventions to eradicate onset of familial (early onset) Alzheimer's. Recently, a new protein in the brain that may play a role in the development or prevention of AD has been discovered. The role of cerebral tans-activation response DNA protein 43 (TDP-43) in the region of brain degeneration characteristic of Alzheimer's has begun to receive attention in the hope of understanding the pathological significance of TDP-43 abnormalities in dementias. While the mechanism causing the changes associated with TDP-43 are unclear, this proteinopathy is thought to have great promise for developing disease-modifying therapies and differential diagnosis.[47] The most recent work in this area suggests that TDP-43 correlates with severe neuronal loss [48] in an entirely different way than through the "gold standard" amyloid and tau mechanisms that have long been the targets of study in late-onset dementia—thus potentially redirecting the field.[49] Some researchers, however, are cautioning that clinical presentation in AD is driven by pathological subtype, not by TDP-43,[50] and we must better understand how this protein accumulates in normal brain aging before we go too far down the path of assuming a Kuhnian "paradigm shift."[51]

Mild Cognitive Impairment: A Self-Fulfilling Prophecy?

Since the mid-1990s onward, molecular approaches to AD began to focus on prevention, namely, the identification of preclinical, even presymptomatic, phases of dementia. Claims that a preclinical stage of Alzheimer's can be observed as much as ten years in advance of decline and can be quantified have been taken at face value since the turn of the century by all but a few noteworthy players.[52] Accordingly, Kral's 1962 identification of benign senescent forgetfulness was not so innocuous after all. A quarter century after that term was introduced, the concept began undergoing numerous refinements, including age-associated memory impairment (AAMI), age-consistent memory impairment (ACMI), late-life forgetfulness (LLF), and more recently, aging-associated cognitive decline (AACD) and age-related cognitive decline (ARCD).[53] In 1993, the International Classification of Diseases (ICD–10) listed "mild cognitive disorder," and a year later the Diagnostic and Statistical Manual (DSM–IV) cited "mild neurocognitive decline." In 1997, both "cognitive impairment no dementia" (as seen with Mr. R in the prologue) and "mild cognitive impairment" entered the discourse in psychiatry and neurology.[54] Shortly after neurologist Ronald Petersen and his colleagues at the Mayo Clinic coined the term MCI and suggested diagnostic criteria, the nascent domain of mild cognitive impairment took off, theoretically replacing the concept "possible AD" or "possible early Alzheimer's" that was being used in specialty clinics at the time. MCI was "generally considered as the clinical syndrome corresponding to the earliest stages of neurodegenerative pathology," or "a transitional zone between normal cognitive function and clinically probable AD."[55] Thus the term identified a population believed to be at elevated risk of developing Alzheimer's.

MCI quickly developed a life of its own and in 2003 the International Working Group (IWG) on Mild Cognitive Impairment was held in Stockholm, Sweden, to integrate clinical and epidemiological perspectives in the area. The resultant IWG recommendations for MCI criteria included: 1) the person is neither normal nor demented; 2) there is evidence of cognitive deterioration shown by either objectively measured decline over time and/or subjective report of decline by self and/or informant in conjunction with cognitive deficits; and 3) activities of daily living are preserved and complex instrumental functions are either intact or minimally impaired.[56] MCI was envisioned in one of two ways: based on a pathological model of cognitive change for seniors or early-stage dementia. Medical initiatives to standardize diagnostic protocol led to the development of research guidelines for cognitive evaluation, resulting in the implementation of two commonly used rating systems for the global staging of cognitive impairment, the Global Deterioration Scale (GDS) and the Clinical Dementia Rating (CDR) scale. The mini mental state examination (MMSE) and mental status questionnaire (MSQ) are also used in some cases as a proxy for the global rating systems. Thus, a diagnosis is made first with the clinical determination of dementia and second, an assessment of etiology. MCI itself also has subtypes: amnestic MCI (aMCI), which is memory impairment not meeting clinical criteria for dementia, nonamnestic MCI (nmMCI), which involves decline not related to memory (e.g., language, attention, visuospatial skills), and multidomain MCI (mMCI), which never really caught on. Criticism that these subtypes were not rigorously tested led to further controversy over defining and employing MCI in practice, especially outside specialty clinics.[57]

Despite the quest for standardization, the consensus on whether, when, and how to diagnose MCI has not been achieved either across practices (specialty versus primary care) nor between disciplines (neurologists and neuropsychologists, for example, or geriatricians and general practitioners). Given the alleged difficulties in demarcating the proverbial line of pathology, significant dissent regarding the conceptual basis, the diagnostic algorithms, and the relationship between MCI and similar concepts persists.[58] Yet an enormous amount of scientific attention has been directed to *discovering* this prodromal state of Alzheimer's disease. Despite scientific controversy regarding the implementation of such diagnostic classifications,[59] in practice this has meant further expansion of what counts as pathology.

While the clinical features of individuals with dementia are "unmistakable, the ability of these preclinical features to predict future disease is less clear."[60] Yet screening for "predementia" is becoming commonplace in clinical practice. Consequently claims about conversion rates from MCI to AD vary wildly, and unpredictably so, according to evaluation site (community versus research setting or clinical- versus population-based studies), criteria used (Mayo Clinic, IWG, neuropsychological definition), and subtype. Early studies reported annual conversion rates (ACR) as small as 9.6 percent over 22 years and as large as 100 percent in 4.5 years.[61] Whereas one review reports rates of AD conversion ranging from 1 to 25 percent per year, another using pooled longitudinal data found an overall annual rate of 14.7 percent.[62] Looking back almost a quarter of a century, an even wider range, from 0.4 to 36 percent conversion per year, has been reported.[63] Early studies also found that the same numbers of MCI cases converted back to "normal" as they did to AD and a general instability across time, with as much as 40 percent of those with MCI reverting to normal.[64]

Furthermore, up to another 61 percent remained the same over 3 years.[65] Recent research shows drastically smaller conversion rates, ranging from 0 to 3 percent in 12 months to 5 to 10 percent over 10 years.[66] One study found that larger proportions of study participants improved or reverted back to normal than progressed to dementia (6–

53 percent) or remained stable (29–88 percent).[67] A meta-analysis of 41 robust cohort studies between 3–10 years in duration reports a 5–10 percent annual conversion rate, which is not only far smaller than those previously reported by Petersen and his colleagues (at 10–15 percent) but they also note that "most people with MCI [*more than 60 percent*] will not progress to dementia even after 10 years of follow-up."[68]

Beyond the seemingly compelling lack of evidence regarding the rate of conversion, extensive disparities exist in terms of methodology (longitudinal, prospective, or retrospective), sampling (numbers of study participants), age groups (i.e., whether or not individuals with EOAD were included), sample size (including whether or not the sample is comprised of individuals solely with MCI or includes unimpaired persons as well), scales administered (GDS, CDR, MMSE, or other), follow-up intervals (months or years), subtypes (whether they are analyzed separately or even reported), and recruitment strategies (where, such as research center versus general practice, and how, including media advertisements versus general or specialty visits), making comparisons virtually impossible and scientifically unsound. This is supported by arguments that "[r]isk of progress is influenced by the definition and subtype of MCI and the setting."[69]

This wide variation demonstrates the lack of consensus on conversion rates from MCI to AD and clearly calls into question the utility of diagnosing MCI. While it is noteworthy that the trend reveals decreasing claims of conversion rates in newer studies, what the data overwhelmingly suggested as late as 2009 was that "MCI can no longer be assumed to always be a simple transitional state between normal aging and dementia."[70] The lack of anything even approaching standardization in the design and implementation of these studies is mind-numbing. The very language used to discuss MCI has been fragmented and consensus between specialists and general practitioners over whether to use the term at all has not been reached. This lack of cohesion has implications not only for science and practitioners aiming to identify and treat memory loss, but for older individuals who may or may not be experiencing forgetfulness that is pathological.

Notwithstanding such epidemiological disputes, however, in practice the notion that a phase of observable cognitive impairment exists prior to a person exhibiting signs meeting full criteria for AD prevails. In fact, the NINCDS-ADRDA criteria are purported to have an 80 to 90 percent accuracy rate in diagnosing AD.[71] Yet these figures come from specialized academic research centers and are largely based on patients diagnosed later in the disease process so they cannot necessarily be applied to MCI. Nonetheless, Petersen claims that mild cognitive impairment is "a clinical entity that represents a transitional state between the cognitive changes of normal aging and the earliest presentations of clinically probable AD."[72] Thus, older individuals presenting with "subclinical" cognitive deficit are approached as if they have quantitative anatomical and structural changes distinct from either normal aging or Alzheimer's. The magnitude of these changes, however, is difficult to calculate due to the variable selection criteria employed and nonrepresentative samples. Consequently, ten years before the new guidelines were introduced, researchers warned, "MCI has been defined by the tests used to measure it, and the results of these measures have then been used as validation of its definition: a nosological tautology and self-fulfilling prophecy."[73]

Accordingly, initial conceptualizations included: MCI covers cognitive change that is possibly pathological but unrelated to underlying systemic disease, MCI is assessed in terms of memory and not other cognitive domains, and neuropsychological testing procedures for MCI are the same as those used for diagnosing AD. In addition to the lack of standard diagnostic criteria, however, at least two conceptual issues remain contested: 1) whether MCI should refer exclusively to impairment of memory or not, and 2) whether MCI is a prodome of AD or a clinically diverse group of individuals at increased risk of developing any dementia.[74] Although MCI as a separate nosological entity allegedly allows "active rather than palliative care," the demarcation between normal aging and disease remains vague and the legal implications of conceptualizing memory loss as abnormal is equally Byzantine. Due to these factors, many vociferously argued that consensus on the criteria of diagnosing MCI needed to include not only clinicians and researchers in the field, but individuals studying bioethics, legal specialists, and those concerned with classification systems.

Unfortunately, these pleas were not heeded when the proposal for changing the diagnostic criteria for AD lengthened the disease process even further. In contrast to the original criteria developed over a quarter century ago, the revised diagnostic and research standards posit a continuum of AD that extends the medical gaze to include two new phases prior to Alzheimer's: prodromal subjective cognitive impairment (SCI) and MCI.[75] In April 2011 the National Institute of Aging (NIA) and the U.S. Alzheimer's Association jointly released new diagnostic guidelines for AD that now officially identifies MCI, defined as a cognitive complaint with objective cognitive decline but intact functional ability, as the stage preceding AD. An even earlier so-called presymptomatic phase is proposed, as indicated by biomarkers, that defines the period of disease before noticeable changes in cognition occur (SCI). While this later phase is theoretical and not part of the diagnostic tools currently used, some posit that SCI may be an indication of preclinical AD that occurs before MCI.[76] SCI is defined as a subjective cognitive complaint without the measurable change in cognition required for a diagnosis of MCI. Despite possible associations between SCI and MCI, of course not all cases will progress to AD. In fact, a substantial percentage will actually revert to normal, as we would expect the numbers to be even fuzzier than those for MCI to AD conversions.

Due to the slow onset of AD, seniors already report difficulty distinguishing between age-associated memory loss and dementia. It currently takes 2 to 5 years, on average, before a diagnosis of AD is established.[77] The expanded criteria and inconclusive conversion rates potentially complicate the ability to identify pathological memory loss, lengthen the time before most people seek medical attention, and expand the duration of the disease process. The revised diagnostic and research standards posit a continuum of AD that extends what medical sociologists and bioethicists refer to as the medical gaze to include two new categories *prior to formal diagnosis*. Lock argues that this represents a strategy of "subdividing and fragmenting what is subject to scrutiny to make it manageable."[78]

From the mid-1990s MCI was considered merely a potential precursor and while diagnosed individuals scored below average for their age and education on neuropsychological tests, they did not have any functional impairment in daily living and were not necessarily expected to convert to AD. This was the case at the time I conducted my research. The new criteria inflate the already soaring numbers of seniors experiencing memory problems.[79] As others have noted, if you look at the list of affiliates, almost all the authors of the 2011 guidelines are associated with American universities and/or drug companies or the Alzheimer's Association.[80] Lock reveals that critics from within medicine, like neuroscientist Sarjay Pimplikar, caution against adoption of these recommendations, especially those linked to biomarkers, because the required PET scan studies expose people to radiation, the literature base has demonstrated that 1 out of 3 normal brains have plaque, and the countless trials done have consistently failed to show cognitive improvement even after plaques have been removed. Furthermore, the cerebrospinal fluid studies are uncertain, painful, too risky, and can have side effects. Likewise, neurologist Peter Whitehouse highlights the inherent, seemingly irresolvable entanglement of aging and dementia.[81] Based on her extensive ethnographic study, Lock argues that this focus on biomarkers, inextricably linked to the new guidelines, is "seductive hype" due to the persistent failure to achieve the desired laboratory results and remaining low efficacy of pharmacological treatments available rather than a Kuhnian paradigm shift as it is presented. That is, in an effort to maintain their legitimate jurisdiction over AD, the new guidelines are a symbol of their striving for radical change. Either way, these new criteria, whether adopted or not, represent the power of the Amyloid Cascade Hypothesis and how entrenched (most) bench scientists are in molecular approaches. This research project was conducted before the release of these guidelines, and it will be some time before they reach practice (if they do indeed achieve uptake outside specialty clinics), yet it is a prime example of the larger trend in U.S. medicine of targeting preclinical diagnoses and a classic example of what medical sociologists refer to as diagnostic expansion.[82] The new criteria codify MCI as a stage of Alzheimer's; making what social scientists, ethicists, and even pioneering neurologists have referred to as a "Hardening of the Categories,"[83] indeed a self-fulfilling prophecy. The changes in the fifth edition of the DSM-5, the new criteria proposed by the NIA-AA, and increases in biomarker testing "are likely to increase overdiagnosis because they permit labeling of asymptomatic people as having pre-symptomatic Alzheimer's disease or dementia."[84]

The Decade of the Brain

Perhaps no contemporary example better epitomizes the power of bio-medical efforts than when President George H. W. Bush declared the 1990s the Decade of the Brain. The enormous amount of research on Alzheimer's disease that was conducted under this initiative began on July 17, 1990 when the President proclaimed:

> The human brain, a 3-pound mass of interwoven nerve cells that controls our activity, is one of the most magnificent—and mysterious—wonders of creation. The seat of human intelligence, interpreter of senses, and con-troller of movement, this incredible organ continues to intrigue scientists and layman alike.[85]

In particular, President Bush noted powerful microscopes, advances in brain imaging devices, and neuroscientific mappings of the brain's biochemical circuitry to demonstrate how the alleged new era of discov-ery in brain research would fuel "our nation's determination to conquer brain disease."[86]

From 1990 to the end of 1999, the Library of Congress (LC) and the National Institute of Mental Health (NIMH) sponsored an initiative to advance the goals set forth by President Bush. In designating the 1990s as the Decade of the Brain, the intention was "to enhance public aware-ness of the benefits to be derived from brain research" through "ap-propriate programs, ceremonies, and activities." To achieve this public recognition, the LC/NIMH coalition sponsored a variety of activities including publications and programs aimed at introducing members of Congress, their staffs, and the general public to cutting-edge research on the brain and encouraging public dialogue on the ethical, philosophical, and humanistic implications of these emerging discoveries.[87]

Politically, clinically, and scientifically the 1990s were devoted to the brain. The resultant books, such as *Brave New Brain* (Andreasen 2004), *The Future of the Brain* (Rose 2005), and *The Adaptable Brain* (Levy-Reiner 1999), epitomized the aims of the "brain initiative" and squarely situated the brain as an object of the nascent field of neuroscience: "[It] holds the promise to cure and prevent a long list of diseases includ-ing Alzheimer's, schizophrenia, and drug addiction; to repair damaged nervous tissue; and to reverse the debility dealt by stroke and injury. [Thus] [n]euroscience will revolutionize the treatment of psychiatric and neurologic disorders."[88] Importantly, the Decade of the Brain served to solidify, in the eyes of many researchers, clinicians, politicians, and even potential patients, the connection between mental maladies and the brain. The brain has been an object of wonder throughout human history. One of the most fundamental questions of such inquiry is how humans can be so different from chimpanzees, for example, when our brains are composed of identical molecules that are arranged in similar cellular patterns, and our genes are 99 percent identical. Even after the Decade of the Brain was officially over, and despite remarkable scientific progress to such ends, disputes over the intricacies of "the most complex three pounds of matter ever encountered"[89] persisted, and new contingencies have ultimately surfaced.

Uniting mind (person) and brain (organ) situated conditions of the brain in a unique historical position where self is equated with brain. Neoliberal cultural values of individualism and autonomy engender a dichotomization between having a sick body and a sick brain. Consequently, acknowledging mental inadequacies (i.e., biological disease) without a subsequent threat to identity is difficult to achieve. Since our encounters with scientific objects shape our notions of self, health, illness, and human nature, medical practices seeking to distinguish the normal from the pathological aim to measure deviations from normality and label conditions accordingly.

The Memory Sciences: How the Brain Studies Itself

Since the Decade of the Brain launched extensive investigations into memory, the branches of brain and memory sciences and neuroscience have multiplied considerably. In particular, fundamental diagnostic expansions have transpired in the memory sciences through the development of imaging techniques and a psychoanalysis of consciousness. The use of memory in the courtroom over the past two decades has placed the scientific paradigms of human memory on trial in a previously inconceivable manner.[90] Both the laboratory and the courtroom have been intricately involved in the production of so-called scientific facts regarding memory.[91] Significant efforts have been undertaken in terms of memory states, such as repressed or false memories, various brain pathologies including depression, schizophrenia, and anxiety disorders, and dementias, namely Alzheimer's disease, vascular dementia, and frontotemporal dementia.

Unlike the alleged wars on such things as poverty, drugs, and various diseases of decades past, however, positioning the brain as an object of neuroscience has implications for people and their loved ones seeking or receiving diagnoses for brain-related pathologies, for scientific discourses and practices, and for society overall. Although living with and through scientific facts is commonplace in modern American society, British sociologist Nikolas Rose warns that the exciting breakthroughs of neuroscience also raise troubling questions about what it means to be human.[92] American anthropologist Joseph Dumit adds that the emergent imaging techniques making the visualization of the human brain as clear as that of a laboratory specimen, for example, simultaneously generate new types of citizens and bodies, including depressives and schizophrenics.[93]

The emergence of the memory sciences has both shaped and been shaped by the scientific and political foci on the brain. Subtle epistemic shifts demarcate how we see societies and the people living in them. The transformations in the memory sciences have engendered new types of people in twenty-first-century American culture. By manipulating the definition and organization of memory, medico-scientific discourses and practices *make* subjects. For example, shortly after the Decade of the Brain, Ledoux (2003) and Dumit (2004), respectively, addressed existential questions of human nature by introducing *The Synaptic Self: How Our Brains Become Who We Are* and *Picturing Personhood: Brain Scans and Biomedical Identity*. Since we live in an age when self or personhood is paramount, contemporary technosciences create distinct biomedical subjects. In the same way as imaging technologies generate a new type of human, a depressed human is also a type of brain, a depressed brain, which is unable to monitor its own depression; the medical practices and technologies of memory loss breed a demented human and brain unable to recount or *trust* its own memories. Technologies of knowing, such as visual imaging, create and substantiate the conflation of brain and person. Contemporary conceptions of brain functioning as the zenith of personhood threaten the societal worth of individuals afflicted with conditions such as mental illness and memory loss, but also affect the social and personal contexts of all brain diseases.

In contrast to traditional mind-body dualisms, which dichotomized live, active bodies and passive, medical ones,[94] however, contemporary biomedical imaging technologies, for example, reveal medicalized but active, irrational brains.[95] In fact, modern medicine generally *requires* active, rational patients[96] who will engage in medical discourse. Scientific "facts" allow groups of people sharing similar biological abnormalities to coalesce in the promotion of research into the cause and cure of their specific conditions.[97] This is simultaneously a potential tool for empowerment and a device of regulation. Arguably, in spite of the lack of scientific consensus surrounding many conditions, so-called scientific facts provide a means for social inter/action, a justification for certain research endeavors, and an argument for biological understandings of health and citizens. Since scientific efforts to *understand* and personal accounts of *living with* illnesses are not necessarily compatible, objective facts (based on science, medicine, technology, and nature) and subjective facts (including experience and culture) coerce and reinforce each other through means of self-sacrifice, encouragement, surveillance by others, and pharmaceuticals.[98]

Technoscience and Innovation

The research initiated by the Decade of the Brain and the resultant proliferation of neuroscience contributed to at least three areas salient to the technoscience of Alzheimer's: diagnostics, imaging, and therapeutics. Historically, these areas of innovation have taken place within a context that is saturated with biomedical knowledges that transform twenty-first-century American society and its members alike.

Innovation: Diagnostics

The area within AD which has the greatest implications for changing not only clinical practice but also the very identities of its subjects is the realm of diagnostics. The concerted effort to diagnose the condition in the earliest stages of the disease, and preclinically, is a distinct aim of biomedicine. Consequently, the state-of-the-science on Alzheimer's disease is based on at least two premises crucial to clinical practice: identifying the etiology of a disease is not a prerequisite for its diagnosis and/or treatment and scientific research and clinical diagnostics are emergent and divergent. For these reasons, I conceptualize diagnosis and the diagnostic process as forms of social artifacts and technologies customary under what British sociologist David Armstrong refers to as surveillance medicine.

Cognitive function is defined as "the sum of the brain's power to acquire, process, integrate, store, and retrieve information."[99] Thus, cognitive impairment is reduced capacity in any of these realms. There is considerable scientific agreement that at least four types of dementias exist: the Alzheimer dementias, vascular dementia, depressive dementias, and nondepressive dementia or what are called pseudodementias.[100] The majority of dementias, however, fall within one of two realms: degenerative (primarily Alzheimer's disease, including MCI and frontal-temporal disease) and vascular disease. Less frequently, Lewy-Body disease (LB, LBD), Progressive Supranuclear Palsy (PSP), Cruetzfeldt-Jacob disease (CJD) or Pick's disease, as well as depressive and pseudodementias, are identified.

Dementia, the most common of which is Alzheimer's disease, is considered "a complete and usually progressive loss of intellectual capacity with resulting functional impairment. It is increasingly common with aging but hardly inevitable."[101] Currently, the scientific construct of dementia is operationalized via one of the many sets of common diagnostic criteria. This has historically included guidelines for what is called "primary degenerative dementia" in the American Psychiatric Association's 1994 Diagnostic Statistical Manual of Mental Disorders (DSM-IV) and "Alzheimer's Disease" by the National Institute of Neurological and Communicative Diseases and Stroke and the Alzheimer's Disease and Related Disorders Association (NINCD-ADRDA). In 2012, the DSM-5 dropped the term "dementia of the Alzheimer's type" (DAT) and replaced it with "major cognitive disorder." The 2011 NIA-AA guidelines simply refer to it as "AD dementia."

Despite the obfuscating semantic terrain, most of the diagnostic criteria employed in clinical practice are based around five key features that comprise the dementia construct. These include both first-order aspects, including cognitive impairment, functional impairment, and neuropathology, as well as second-order facets describing the severity and disease course of the previous three factors, namely, progression and deterioration.

Dementias are differentiated, and cognitive changes observed, through a neuropsychological battery of tests involving at least five cognitive subtypes of intellectual functioning: memory, language, visuospatial, attention, and abstraction. Impairment must be global in scope and affect multiple areas in order to be diagnosed as dementia. This testing can range from brief mental status screening scales (e.g., MMSE or MSQ) to extensive batteries requiring several hours to complete. Results are considered particularly valid in the rare cases when they can be compared to previous tests (ideally prior to impairment). It is important to note, however, that the validity of these tests depends on factors such as education (very high or low levels can bias test results),[102] English fluency (having a primary language that is not English or even dyslexia can cause individuals to appear more impaired than they are), and cultural sensitivity (or an understanding of the ways different groups interpret memory loss).[103] Since as many as 90 percent of older individuals could be diagnosed with age-associated memory impairment,[104] part of the challenge in diagnosing as early in the disease trajectory as possible is to persuade individuals to come in and get a baseline long before there are any signs of decline.[105]

Functional impairment refers to difficulties in performing the tasks of everyday life (including ADLs and IADLs),[106] changes in behavior or personality, and trouble with occupational or social roles. The determination of functional impairment is frequently a matter of clinical judgment, since accurate assessment requires longitudinal knowledge of the person in question. Although some types of functional impairment might be evident throughout the medical encounter (affect, level of engagement, and physical appearance), ideally clinical judgment is corroborated by so-called informant (or proxy) reports in addition to the complaints expressed by potential patients.

The neuropathology of all dementias includes physical abnormalities in the central nervous system (CNS), which depend on the density and location of neuritic plaques and neurofibrillary tangles. The plaques and tangles reported by Dr. Alzheimer in 1906, although observed to varying degrees in the brains of nondemented older individuals, are most common in the temporoparietal regions of the brain in the case of Alzheimer's. The neuroanatomy of aging and dementia suggests that the demented brain experiences observable atrophy, or decreased brain weight, as a result of region-specific cell loss. A healthy brain weighs an average of 1,300 to 1,400 grams, whereas one affected by Alzheimer's weighs approximately 1,000 grams.[107] The postmortem pathologic changes of those with AD are qualitatively similar to those of apparently normal aging, however, as there is considerable overlap between the neuropathology of Alzheimer's and that evident in normal aging as well as other conditions. For example, senile plaques are found in 70 percent of individuals over 65 years old and neurofibrillary tangles are observed with many other conditions.[108] Thus, the difference is in the quantity and location of plaques and tangles,[109] which can threaten validity especially when comorbidities are present.

Additionally, monitoring neurologic function helps to distinguish between normal aging and dementia through an examination of the cranial nerves, oculomotor function, neuromuscular tone, and regressive reflexes.[110] Of course, this is not standard practice as not all clinicians have neurological training. Combined with a family medical history and ideally corroborated by a third party, the techniques of neuropsychiatric testing, a history and physical examination, and the said patient and informant reports are the contemporary staples involved in diagnosing Alzheimer's in specialty practice.

To combat the heterogeneity of the category of MCI and account for "within-person performance variability,"[111] many argue that demographics, social and life style factors, genetic factors, and health-related factors must be considered when making a diagnosis of AD or distinguishing between AD and MCI. Thus, for AD/MCI, predictors from the social, behavioral, and biological domains are essential to accurate disease classifications given the fact that postmortem results remain the primary tool for definitive diagnosis. Since AD remains a diagnosis of exclusion, or what is left after all other known dementias and conditions are eliminated, it is perhaps not surprising that there would be diagnostic inefficiencies. Since the late 1990s it has been understood that some older people who present no cognitive impairment on neuropsychological tests while alive show high degrees of AD pathology upon autopsy (and vice versa).[112]

Innovation: Imaging and Biomarkers

In the perennial drive to standardize diagnostic practices, neuroimaging technologies have become a major focus of research pursuing preclinical AD, signaling a sea change around 2005 tied to the presumed existence of a long preclinical period of decline prior to the onset of symptoms. Efforts at diagnostic uniformity encourage clinical practice to draw on technologies of knowing in the form of visual depictions or images of the brain in making their diagnosis. In this way, clinical findings are mediated and (potentially) produced through a third discipline: radiology.

Developments in brain imaging techniques include neurochemical imaging (e.g., of neurotransmitters, enzymes, or receptors) and the pathological accumulation of amyloid and/or tau, and may provide important supplemental diagnostic information on cognitive decline.[113] The hippocampus and neighboring regions of the brain control the encoding, storage, and retrieval of episodic information.[114] Histopathology, structural imaging, and functional imaging are used to reveal hippocampal change assumed to be implicated long before an AD diagnosis.[115] Modern neuroimaging can be subdivided into structural and functional techniques. Both structural and functional techniques can reveal abnormalities in AD as well as an arguably intermediary level between individuals with Alzheimer's and no dementia. The former provide information about the size and other morphological characteristics of brain structures, while the latter detect regional changes.

Structural techniques utilize magnetic resonance imaging (MRI)-based volumetric measurements to monitor brain atrophy within specified regions and such quantitative imaging is used as a marker of disease progression. With MCI and AD, imaging has focused on volume reductions affecting medial temporal lobe structures like the hippocampus and entorhinal cortex.[116] In fact, it is atrophy within specific regions that signals MCI.[117] It remains unclear whether or not this atrophy is a specific marker for AD pathology since volume loss is still believed to occur in up to one-third of nonimpaired older adults.[118]

In contrast, functional technologies employ single photon emission computed tomography (SPECT) or positron emission tomography (PET) measurements to predict progression. Computed tomography (CT) studies demonstrate atrophy in the left medial temporal lobe[119] and lower lobe volumes,[120] low parietal-temporal perfusion and left/ right parietal-temporal asymmetry in MCI[121] registering between that found in normal aging and AD. This, bench scientists argue, suggests that MCI and AD have similar anatomical foci, with MCI being differentiated mainly by degree of impairment and functional, rather than structural, change.[122] Since SPECT can allegedly predict MCI accurately approximately 50 percent of the time, the delineation of MCI and AD can in theory be made.[123]

Since at least the early 1990s, researchers have also been comparing the cerebrospinal fluid (CSF) of patients with AD to cognitively unimpaired individuals to identify biomarkers indicative of AD pathology.[124] Results suggest that in the early stages of AD, CSF levels of tau protein and beta-amyloid peptide may be similar to cognitively unimpaired individuals and thus the diagnostic utility of these assays in MCI may be minimal. Further research on how such measures compare with other predictive markers such as those based on neuroimaging and psychometric criteria is being undertaken, and the recommendation that standardization of methodology and establishment of larger cohorts and more heterogeneous populations be pursued [125] no doubt contributed to the new diagnostic criteria in 2011.

With the mapping of the Human Genome, many of the genetic markers of Alzheimer's have recently become detectable.[126] Only in a very small fraction of cases (between 2 to 5 percent according to the American Alzheimer's Association) are genetic factors believed to be the sole determinant of the disease.[127] For individuals with MCI or AD who do not have a family history of early-onset Alzheimer's (pre-65 years old), however, the presence of these genetic factors is extremely unlikely.[128] Since any person carrying the allele e4 isoform of apoE is believed to be at increased risk of developing late-onset AD or will experience a more rapid progression to dementia,[129] the identification of the genes involved in the etiology of both AD and MCI is believed to provide opportunities for improvements in diagnoses and prediction of progression.[130] While studies suggest that genes involved in lipid metabolism, hypertension, homeostasis, and homocysteine may prove fruitful,[131] it is important to clarify between genetic risk factors and hereditary genetics. There is a hereditary component for the less than 5 percent of people with early-onset AD. For late-onset, the roughly 95 to 98 percent of typical cases, the existence of some genes may increase risk but there is no conclusive evidence on how or why only some individuals with these genes ever develop Alzheimer's. This makes it worth repeating that these are susceptibility genes, not predictive per se. Again, the only known risk factor for the vast majority of cases is increased age and even that isn't linear.[132]

Innovation: Therapeutics

Most therapeutic efforts to treat Alzheimer's to date have been directed at the "downstream" phases of the pathological process, that is, management of symptoms. In the mid-1970s, the Cholinergic hypothesis suggested that a deficiency in the neurotransmitter acetylcholine was a major factor in Alzheimer's pathology.[133] Fifteen years later, the first cholinesterase inhibitors (CIs) were developed to combat the cholinergic deficit found in the AD brain, and they remain the only FDA-approved medications for treating the condition's symptomology. In 1993, Tacrine, the first treatment available, was approved for use in the early stages. Subsequently, Donepezil (1996; for all stages) and Rivastigmine (2000; for mild to moderate stages) became available, with minor improvements in efficacy and only in some cases. Galantamine, the fourth CI, was FDA approved in 2001 for mild to moderate stage Alzheimer's. All three of the more recent developments in CIs require less frequent doses and are believed to have fewer side effects. The CIs were originally intended to stabilize or plateau symptoms for up to one year. Although more recent studies have suggested that the benefits of CIs can be observed for over a year and that there might be some additional advantages that even slow the progression of decline,[134] unfortunately "[t]here is no evidence of long-term efficacy of currently approved pharmacological treatments in MCI, and only modest evidence for symptomatic treatment efficacy in AD."[135] The last FDA-approved treatment, Memantine, an NMDA[136] receptor antagonist, which targets the latest stages of the disease, came onto the scene in 2003. According to the American Alzheimer's Association, these five Alzheimer's drugs are only effective for about 6 to 12 months for about half the individuals who take them and do not treat the underlying causes of dementia.[137] No new classifications or pharmaceutical advancements have been reported since Memantine was approved in 2003 and adverse effects of CIs are now widely documented.

As a result of repeated failed efforts that threaten the legitimacy of the Amyloid Cascade Hypothesis, energy devoted to therapeutics for treating Alzheimer's has been refocused since the turn of the century. The past focus on drug trials directed at symptomatic treatment alone (CIs) has been redirected at prevention and slowing disease progression itself. This turn both reflects and reinforces the impetus to identify AD cases as early as possible in the trajectory of decline, which critical scholars of medicine suggest increases medical jurisdiction or expands the medical gaze through techniques of surveillance medicine.

Of the noncholinergic agents believed to have some link to potentially treating or preventing AD, antioxidant strategies have received the most attention. For example, vitamin E, selegiline, zinc, and ginkgo biloba may have benefits for people with AD and possibly MCI, both individually and in combination.[138] The American Alzheimer's Association website now lists vitamin E under Medications for Memory Loss despite it being the only one listed that is not FDA approved.[139] Both clinics where I observed routinely recommended 800–1000 IUs of vitamin E and a few clinicians even admitted to taking it themselves. A number of clinical trials have also explored the possibilities of nonsteroidal anti-inflammatory drugs (NSAIDs) in suppressing inflammation thought to promote decline. Ibuprofen has been reported to reduce plaque formation in transgenic mice with familial AD.[140] Alas, most clinical trials in these areas have also proven ineffective.

Neuroprotective, neurotrophic, and neuroregenerative agents showing promise in slowing progression or recovering function have been a focus of inquiry since the turn of the century.[141] For example, estrogen and testosterone might be protective if started before symptoms appear.[142] Recent evidence suggests that cholesterol functionality (namely, high-density lipoprotein or HDL) is impaired in AD and that this alteration might be caused by AD-associated oxidative stress and inflammation,[143] so cholesterol lowering agents, statins, and beta-blockers are being studied as well.[144] As the copious list of possible causal agents reveals, the cure that is seemingly always just around the corner is in fact, according to some, elusive precisely because the entanglement of dementia and aging make Alzheimer's a "stubborn conundrum."[145]

Many scientists believe that the most promising research involves treatments directed at preventing the formation of beta-amyloid or accelerating its clearance and that recent mappings of the beta- and gamma-secretease properties provide encouragement in discovering the inhibitors of these enzymes. Although a human anti-amyloid strategy, the beta-amyloid vaccine, under clinical investigation in the early twenty-first century purportedly offered great hope, a 5 percent incidence of encephalitis in participants brought the study to a screeching halt. Further studies aiming to modify the disease process itself, including targets such as beta-amyloid, tau protein, inflammation and insulin resistance, as well as better understanding of healthy brain function and aging, remain at the forefront.[146]

Against this backdrop of political and biomedical attention to the brain and its associated disorders, President Ronald Reagan's 1994 speech entitled "Alzheimer's Letter," which divulged that he himself had been diagnosed with Alzheimer's, had the potential to be pivotal. President and Nancy Reagan showed great strength of character in their decision to disclose this information at a time when the condition was highly stigmatized and questions about Reagan's mental acuity during his presidency had been circulating. While the speech expressed optimism that "[i]n opening our hearts, we hope this might promote greater awareness of this condition. Perhaps it will encourage a clear understanding of the individuals and families who are affected by it," the remainder of this book reveals a reticence to recognize that potential and the various sociocultural obstacles that continue to impede their lofty goal.

The Future Is Wide Open: Getting outside the Black Box

What becomes overwhelmingly obvious after tracing the history of diagnosing and treating AD is that we continue to have more questions than answers. Critique, even from within, abounds. Lock argues that three interrelated tensions remain unresolved: the relationship between mind and body, whether AD is on a continuum with normal aging or pathological, and a revitalized version of the nature/nurture debate brought on by the focus on genetics. In addition, Peter Whitehouse, a founder of the so-called cholinergic center in the cerebral cortex that has since been the target of all existing drugs, questions this now thirty-five-year focus: "[A]nti-amyloid compounds have largely failed, casting doubt on whether drugs that target amyloid are a viable therapeutic strategy."[147]

Neurologist John Hardy also voices increased skepticism about the utility of the Amyloid Cascade Hypothesis that he himself coined. There appears to be path dependency within the molecular approach to AD:

> Despite inherent problems with standardization of both clinical and neuropathological AD diagnoses, and explicit doubts expressed by certain researchers about the very concept of AD, the basic science paradigm that has held sway for over 20 years in the Alzheimer's research world continues to be dominant—it is a model in which amyloid deposition in the form of plaques is for all intents and purposes regarded as the master key.[148]

Furthermore, with the discovery of genes associated with early-onset AD, neurologist Bradley Hyman and colleagues began to question whether early- and late-onset AD are the same process at differing speeds or distinct processes that share some common traits.[149] Neurologist Marsel Mesulam suggests that early-onset is a matter of excess production whereas typical AD is due to accumulation, that is, the brain's inability to get rid of normally occurring plaques. John Hardy and others question whether AD is one entity or has subtypes.[150] Based on decades of autopsy studies, epigeneticists and others suggest that all brains would develop AD if they lived long enough. Still others argue that aging is a continuum that cannot be divorced from its context and recent data suggest that amyloid beta (A4) precursor protein (the APP gene) could even be protective against AD in some places, both of which lend support to the notion of entanglement theory. Neurologists, epigeneticists, and social scientists alike argue that localization theory ignores everything extraneous to the body, and thus will never be able to adequately address dementia. Accordingly, "by reducing causal explanations for AD to molecular changes alone, medicalization sidelines socioeconomic, political, and public health arguments in connection with risk for AD."[151] This controlled chaos is the underpinning on which memory loss is currently being diagnosed, treated, and experienced.

The potential effects of encouraging more and earlier diagnosis are daunting. One meta-analysis of clinical tools used in general practice found that at 6 percent prevalence, for every 100 patients screened, two-thirds would be correctly identified while an additional one-quarter would be wrongly diagnosed.[152] The multibillion dollar research industry dedicated to Alzheimer's is steadfast nonetheless. In the past five years, the NIH reports allocating 2.6 billion to Alzheimer's research alone, with generous annual increases and projections for 2016 at $638 million, and the U.S. Alzheimer's Association has contributed at least an additional $335 million since 1982.[153] When Alzheimer's is searched within project titles among the additional $12.7 billion NIH devoted to aging research writ large between 2010 and 2015, another roughly 2 million can be identified. The recent trend in "healthy aging" studies that fall increasingly under the jurisdiction of AD research since the 2011 reclassification, render the monies invested in the cause of epic proportion. Yet definitive diagnosis remains possible only upon autopsy and postmortem studies reveal as many false positives as negatives. The overwhelming majority of the projects funded by these agencies nonetheless focus on clinical studies of cause and cure, including diagnostic techniques and pharmaceutical treatments aimed at reducing the behavioral and psychosocial problems presumed to accompany the condition. Noticeably absent are exploratory qualitative studies, namely, of the subjective experience of AD. This has led political economists of aging and critical gerontologists and social scientists alike, such as Carroll Estes and Margaret Lock, to claim that the "Alzheimer's Industrial Complex" both reflects and reinforces the conundrum that is Alzheimer's. Despite the persistent lack of scientific consensus and warnings to proceed with caution, "The desire of politicians, dementia organizations, and academics and clinicians in the field to raise the profile of dementia is understandable, but we risk being conscripted into an unwanted 'war against dementia.'"[154] The following chapters will demonstrate how real in its consequences the metaphorical war against dementia is for those who are diagnosed and their loved ones.

3

Constructing Facts in Clinical Practice

Interpreting, Diagnosing, and Treating Memory Loss

Despite its discovery well over a century ago, diagnostic consensus on the disease classification of Alzheimer's remains lacking in the scientific community.[1] Debate, sometimes heated, persists about when and how to test for it, what to call it, whether to diagnose the condition, and which—if any—treatment regimen to follow. Yet, "despite the paucity of evidence, biomarkers and amyloid scans are entering everyday practice, especially in memory clinics."[2] Disputes are taking place both among specialties, such as neurology or neuropsychiatry, and between specialists and general practitioners. Among specialty clinics, though, it appears there is an imperative to identify memory loss as early as possible in the disease trajectory, and ideally in the preclinical (or even presymptomatic) phase. It is important to understand that memory clinics were first introduced in the 1980s with a primary goal of recruiting patients into clinical trials of cholinesterase inhibitors—who were then used to market the said drugs.[3] No evidence exists to suggest that memory clinics are beneficial yet attention has not been paid to the potential stressors, increased use of biomarker testing and neuroimaging, and the associated consequences of specialty clinics.[4]

I was interested in examining the concrete, routine work practices[5] that specialty clinics used to manage these diagnostic uncertainties and disciplinary divergences. To investigate these matters, I spent eighteen months doing participant observation of cognitive evaluations, including intake testing, clinical team meetings, and diagnostic disclosures with twenty-two clinicians and then compared my observations with what I learned from the eight in-depth follow-up interviews I conducted with various clinicians at the two sites.

Based on my efforts to understand the differences between what clinicians said they did and what I observed in the specialty clinics, the conceptual goal of this chapter is to map the contemporary diagnostic practice surrounding memory loss in American specialty medicine. Describing the daily practices of cognitive evaluation within two specialty centers, one largely neurological and the other psychiatric, reveals a shared process through which older adults become Alzheimer's patients despite seemingly evident disciplinary discord. While these clinics indeed have historical, contextual, and cultural differences, they ultimately produce strikingly similar effects in terms of the *structure of the diagnostic process* itself. That is, the fundamental tenets of specialty practice result in tangible outcomes common across the realms of neurology and psychiatry.

The biomedical knowledges and practices that convert *ideas* about human memory into scientific *facts* about human memory transform individuals seeking medical attention into what I term potential patients by socially constructing the definition and organization of memory[6] in a particular light. Contemporary clinical assumptions within the memory sciences guide the medical encounter in an attempt to produce the appearance of order[7] around a condition that is the *dis*order du jour by implementing increasingly more complicated and foreign technologies and by deliberately exploiting uncertainty. Since routine practices must be achieved in these settings, "scientific practice [still] entails the confrontation and negotiation of utter confusion."[8] That is, clinicians' and researchers' "deployment of uncertainty is reflexively implicated in bio-clinical collectives' search for rules and conventions, and that the collective production of uncertainty is in fact central to the 'knowledge machinery' of regulatory objectivity."[9] Trust was also employed; trust in their expertise and team approach. In practice, forgetful individuals become patients through mechanisms of technoscience, or medical guidelines and technologies, which quantify deficit and establish parameters of normalcy. This chapter will trace the clinical process of making what is perceived institutionally as biographical nonsense into biomedical sense and the strategic employment of trust and uncertainty in that quest.

How clinicians conceptualize illness has important ramifications for both the delivery of medical care and its experience by so-called patients.[10] Perceptions about AD, and how it is subsequently reacted to, managed, and both objectified/subjectified are highlighted to demonstrate how medicine is caught up in and driven by its own developments. Following historian of science Peter Keating and sociologist Alberto Cambrioso, who characterized contemporary biomedicine as a bioclinical hybrid intricately linking basic science and clinical care (i.e., bench and bedside),[11] this chapter shows how people seeking evaluation become hybrid patients/research subjects upon entering these memory centers. Uncovering the mechanisms through which the legitimacy and authority of medical knowledge and practice regarding memory are organized and substantiated in practice despite numerous points of potential resistance demonstrates the work that must be done to achieve this end.

Neurology and Psychiatry: Never the Twain Shall Meet?

The state-of-the-science on Alzheimer's disease is defined at the intersection of the fields of neurology and psychiatry. The neuropathology of AD results in an inability to definitively diagnose premortem. Instead, examination of brain tissue upon autopsy locates and quantifies the characteristic plaques and tangles containing amyloid and tau proteins. Although brain biopsies were performed in the 1960s, the efficacy of these procedures was low and they have since almost completely ceased. Lumbar punctures are performed in rare cases, but the potential for error prevents the procedure from gaining much popularity with the general public. In practice, clinical distinctions were historically made between probable AD and the somewhat more tentative possible AD; to date there remains no definitive diagnosis except upon autopsy. The struggles to manage such clinical ambivalence have implications not only for the disciplines involved in diagnosing memory loss and a pharmaceutical industry eager to find treatment options but also, and more concretely, for all people diagnosed now or in the near future. The resultant implications for potential patients are ultimately remarkably similar in both the neurologic and psychiatric models observed in this study. Disciplinary ways of knowing, diagnosing, and treating dementia require the employment of various techniques and technologies in evaluating potential patients.

The Brain Clinic and the Health Center

Although the data presented in this and the following chapters will reveal significant similarities in clinical practice and patient experiences of the diagnostic process of memory loss, there are at least three important differences between what I am referring to as *the Brain Clinic* and *the Health Center*: the history, including the disciplinary background and center affiliations; the context, including the physical settings and the geographic regions; and the culture, including the perception of patients and types of interactions. Specifically, the Brain Clinic exudes a lively, almost frenetic, feel that contrasts sharply with the leisurely ambiance at the Health Center. It is noisy and people are rushing around, whereas few are present at the Health Center at any given time and its nearly abandoned halls are silent. There is also a sense of high-tech and cutting-edge science at the Brain Clinic whereas the Health Center has more of a feeling of empathy and interpersonal relationships and does not suggest the fervor of science-in-action. The Brain Clinic staff appeared more stereotypically professional and the environment was more sterile than the laidback and personalized setting of the Health Center.

To medical sociology, factors such as history, context, and culture matter insofar as they constitute what could be conceived of as the philosophy of a given site. My use of culture intends to acknowledge that there are, in addition to daily practices, standard ways of doing things within organizations (i.e., formal protocol and informal belief systems are often shared in common). In particular, in this study these factors affected how the diagnosis was delivered, the treatment options offered, and the ways in which the prognosis and the future were presented.

As a result of the historical, contextual, and cultural dynamics within the two centers,[12] one painted a picture of a progressive, terminal illness, an emerging science, and a need for continual medical supervision, while the other addressed how to continue living—even with increasing decline—despite the newly acquired condition.

As the Brain Clinic saw most patients exclusively for diagnosis, talk of the therapeutic future was glaringly missing (except to consult their primary care physician). The exchange typically ended upon diagnosis, as would be expected of any specialty referral, despite the gravity of the news being delivered. The Health Center, in contrast, began a relationship with patients *upon* diagnosis by encouraging them to continue coming to them for follow-up appointments and to partake in support groups recommended by the center. Importantly, this also involved recruitment into research studies, including individuals diagnosed with no cognitive impairment who would be given information for or enrolled into normal aging studies or as control groups in memory studies.

In conclusion, rather than aiming to compare neurology and psychiatry to decide which discipline was better in certain areas, I will demonstrate the ways in which social structures, or institutional dynamics, affect clinical evaluation within a given context. Factors such as history, context, and culture matter in the clinical practice of diagnosing memory loss in that they have tangible consequences for the people seeking their services. Although these sites vary considerably in these areas, the remainder of this chapter will depict how the resultant experiences of the process are in reality remarkably similar for potential patients.[13] For this reason, the disciplines of neurology and psychiatry are conceptualized from here on as creating similar conditions for people seeking cognitive evaluation for their memory at specialty centers.

Shared Biomedical Principles

The disciplinary perspectives theoretically vary according to the respective approaches taken on dementia—neurology offers the hope for a cure to ameliorate the devastation brought by Alzheimer's, whereas psychiatry largely purports to enhance the resources to help people *live with* the condition. Despite such different approaches, my data reveal these are relatively inconsequential in the overall process of diagnosis at both locations. Whether the unit of analysis is the disease process or the person with a chronic illness does depend upon disciplinary practice, however. The view of memory loss as a disease or a chronic illness, a focus on the brain or the person, affects the clinical treatment options distinct from the diagnostic process itself. Tracing the larger conceptualization of normal memory and aging and subsequent practices of diagnosing pathology *within* these disciplines fosters an analysis of the conditions in which diagnoses of Alzheimer's disease or mild cognitive impairment are constructed and rendered.

Ultimately, the processes through which people become dementia patients at both centers can be characterized by three common components, including compiling evidence, constructing a diagnosis, and rendering a diagnosis. This is largely the result of three underlying assumptions shared by both centers regarding the clinical objectives in dementia care, including the need for standardized protocol, the questionable competence of patients, and the importance of patient management. In general, the processes whereby individuals seeking examination of their memory are transformed from potential patients to patients commences with some common fundamental assumptions.

Cultural and disciplinary presumptions are routinely, if unwittingly, integrated into the diagnostic process at both sites.[14] These hidden biases affect the identification, delivery, and treatment of people with memory loss. The assumptions upon which clinical objectives and practices for diagnosing memory loss are based presuppose that standardized protocol and interactions are essential, and that patients are incompetent and thus require clinical management. These convictions underlie each of the three components involved in the diagnostic process and significantly inform clinical impressions at both centers.

First, since at least the early 1990s evidence-based medicine (EBM), or the reliance on current scientific knowledge bases to make decisions, has been embraced as an attempt to standardize clinical care.[15] While in theory EBM provides clinicians with the ability to follow standard protocol, in reality it generates multiple interpretations and new contingencies for practitioners. Accordingly, clinical uncertainty must be systematically managed during the medical socialization process. Clinicians are driven by a need for precise information with which to make a diagnosis, since the diligent procurement of information relevant to making an accurate diagnosis is the hallmark of clinical practice. For both theoretical and practical purposes, such information is thought to be best attained via standardized procedures for collecting and quantifying the data.[16] Maya Holmes and Seth Ponte, while pursing joint MD/PhDs in medical anthropology, found that the systematic processes of standardization, namely the so-called problem-oriented medical record, were essential tools for managing uncertainty in the process of constructing a clinical diagnosis.[17] For example, following uniform protocol both expedites the process of fact gathering and allows for a linear comparison of all patients. In this way, employing standardized practices and clinical judgment to determine the relevance of the data presented prevents potential patients from straying too far off topic while also providing space for generalized assessment across patients who may otherwise be very different. Sociologist Nancy Davenport's ethnographic study of a family practice team on an in-patient ward echoes many of Holmes and Ponte's findings by showing that residents are taught the act of narrative storytelling, whereby "narrative templates" are used "in a process that is routine, habitual, and iterative," with the ultimate goal of "building a patient story."[18] Sociologist Carol Heimer has talked about this process as the difference between the clinical need for generalizable "cases" and individual expressions of subjective "biographies."[19]

The primary clinical objective of accurately diagnosing memory loss is also based on a second assumption regarding the perceived status of the person seeking a diagnosis. There is a presumption that patients are incompetent since they are seeking medical evaluation for memory loss. The standard patient presentation, which some argue operates as a disciplinary technology to manage uncertainty in clinical decision making,[20] is especially suspect when patients are recognized as cognitively impaired. By definition, then, clinical impression reveals cognitive biases[21] that assume that potential patients are unable to participate in an acceptable manner due to cognitive deficits. This is clearly demonstrated in the value ascribed to "informant" reports at both sites:

> I am [in the informant interview] trying to get some information from the family about their observation and changes, and trying to get some information about who this person [the patient] was pre-morbidly. A nice baseline. What their kind of personality was and their cognitive strengths and such, and then trying to see how they've changed. If there has been a significant change in . . . their condition, if there is an undetected condition going on. (Clinical Nurse Specialist)

Particular weight was given to whether or not the potential patient was capable of accurately recounting events; that is, whether their stories could be trusted. For example, "Her [the patients] story really wasn't corroborated by her husband. He recognized far more impairment"

(Registered Nurse), and "He [the patient] doesn't really sound like a good historian, what did the informant report?" (Neuropsychiatrist). Thus, due to the assumption of patient incompetence, informant reports are used to corroborate the stories told (of the existence, duration, and severity of symptoms) by patients themselves and establish a view of individuals seeking a cognitive workup whereby personhood is suspect a priori. As we see, in the event of any discrepancy or if the potential patient is not deemed reliable, informants' renditions reign supreme.

Presumed patient incompetence necessitates patient management, the third assumption. The strategies used to accomplish this task are at the core of the diagnostic process; managing patients serves a multitude of purposes. Clinicians need to maintain order and perform the tasks necessary to the diagnostic process as proficiently and expediently as possible. The most efficacious means to ensure high quality, standard practice is allegedly through strict patient management. Since patients whose competence is questioned are believed to require additional supervision, potential patients must be coerced by clinicians into following the stated objectives of the clinic. By establishing the rules for participating in the medical encounter, managing patients is at the core of making a diagnosis. These institutional conditions produce potential patients and begin the process of patientization for those seeking medical attention for their memory.

Each of these three assumptions situates clinicians in a position of expert authority over potential patients and their families. As such, clinicians become the arbiters of truth. The standardized routine of the medical encounter dictates a prescribed set of regulations that are unlike everyday interactions, thus ensuring that (only relevant) information is garnered as efficiently as possible. The clinicians are the conductors of this ritual and determine the speed and tone of the interaction. The assumptions of incompetence have obvious ramifications for the status of those with memory loss. Such stereotypes infantilize potential patients and engender assumptions of their alleged neediness. The perceived need to manage patients is fueled by both of the previous assumptions. If patients must be managed, then clinicians are positioned to perform this role with help from the structural dynamics of medical encounters, primarily the problem-oriented medical record.[22]

The data presented below will demonstrate how the clinical aims of these two sites are also quite similar. In particular, a shared logic infuses the basic processes of compiling evidence, constructing a diagnosis, and rendering a diagnosis at the centers.

Compiling the Evidence

At both sites, the primary objective of the clinical interaction with people seeking medical attention for memory loss and their loved ones was to elicit from potential patients and their families all the information deemed clinically relevant to determining a diagnosis. In general, the intake information at both centers includes (to a greater or lesser extent) a family and medical history from the potential patient, a physical/neurological examination, neuropsychological testing, and an informant interview with any family member(s) present. These data are taken as the evidence upon which a diagnosis can be constructed.

Potential patients' initial contact at the neurology clinic was with a male medical resident, typically in his late-20s to mid-30s, doing his neurology rotation. The process of the history and physical (H&P) takes approximately an hour and includes first noted symptom(s), past medical history, familial medical history, medication history, and various neurological inquiries to detect (or preclude) other disorders. A general physical exam measures health status, reflexes, coordination, and flexibility. After this, a neuropsychologist administers an hour-long battery of tests on verbal, visual-spatial, semantic, and global memory functioning. This process was so uniform that I observed few divergences from the script in the almost fifty cases I attended despite different clinicians and patients (i.e., the battery of tests is linear in presentation). Simultaneously, the nurse met with any family or friends who accompanied the patient to discern onset, first symptom(s), and rate of decline. This typically lasted an hour and included proxy reports of the patient's cognitive functioning, mood, and activities of daily living (ADLs).

At the psychiatry clinic, the initial contact was with a female clinical research coordinator in her twenties. Demographic data were collected, study consent obtained, and information regarding where the results were to be sent was gathered in the first thirty minutes. Then the clinician (an RN, a psychiatrist, or a clinical psychologist, all females in their 30s to 50s) brought the informant into her office while the potential patient was getting a CT scan and lab work done. The clinician talked with the informant to elicit what was going on with the potential patient and why they had come into the clinic. This interview lasted approximately thirty minutes and established what was referred to as a clinical impression using the family member/friend as a proxy. Then the clinician conducted the same interview, often lasting thirty-five to forty-five minutes, with the potential patient. On occasion, this procedure involved *some* components of a physical and/or neurological examination but this was not standard practice (and was rarely observed except with the neuropsychiatrist). The potential patient typically went back to see the research assistant to take the majority of the neuropsych tests. In some cases, the clinician conducted the neuropsych battery herself but the nuts and bolts were commonly collected by the research assistant.

Since AD remains a diagnosis of exclusion, both sites focused largely on eliminating other potentially treatable/ nonprogressive conditions that could be causing the memory loss, specifically psychiatric syndromes, Parkinsonisms, vitamin deficiencies, overmedication, strokes, and age-related memory loss. In formulating the exact type of dementia, clinicians were aiming to rule out vascular, depressive, and pseudodementias. For example, the following quotes were typical at the neurology clinic: "A lot of what we [clinicians] do is eliminating other things it [memory loss] could be" (Resident Neurologist); "We look at all the other possibilities, other dementias, strokes, depression, medication interactions, metabolic deficiencies et cetera to make sure there are not other causes" (Neurologist); "There's nothing to help us think this isn't AD-like" (Neurologist); and "With the non-AD dementias, you can tell a lot by looking for Parkinsonisms and ruling them out" (Resident Neurologist).

Likewise, clinicians at the psychiatric site expressed similar sentiments: "Any system that goes awry can cause memory trouble" (Clinical Nurse Specialist); and "It's [sleeping medication dosage] a lot and it's definitely going to affect a person's memory, probably more likely if you are older. This is not the dose you would give if you just wanted to help somebody get to sleep" (Psychiatrist).

Yet certain information more clearly signaled a diagnosis of memory disease. Increased age and a family history of dementia, the best-established risk factors, were seen as particular indicators that a person likely had abnormal, or non–age related, memory loss: "He's very young [55 years old] and things causing memory loss, like AD, are unlikely. It's not impossible, but it's so rare" (Neurologist); "She's 80, it's not MCI [it's AD]" (Neurologist); "If you guess AD in a 75–80 year old person you're probably right without knowing anything else" (Neurologist); and "There is a very strong family history of AD. What a consolation. Next patient!" (Neurologist).

Lingering symptoms, a slow rate of progression, decreases in daily functioning, complaints of predominantly short-term memory loss, and change in weight/appetite were the signposts clinicians expected to see with typical AD: "Dementia is an impairment of daily function" (Psychiatrist); "From a cognitive perspective, AD is slow progressing" (Neurologist); "We often hear people forget that they ate. Forgetting is part of the problem. We do hear this with AD . . . some people lose their appetite for unknown reasons" (Neurologist); "Things are really falling apart around her. This is not subtle, from what I'm hearing, it affects her well-being" (Neurologist), and "Whatever's going on, he's not failing. He is just noticing problems. He is not at a stage of dementia yet" (Neurologist).

Specific examples of memory loss, such as repetitive questioning, inability to remember common words, missed appointments, or difficulty learning new things, were also seen as indicative of an imminent AD/MCI diagnosis. The telltale signal was a change from prior functioning: "The triggers are if they can't do something that they could in the past" (Neurologist); and "Explain any changes, with examples, in your brother and why you are at the clinic [today]" (Psychiatrist).

The level of functional ability or impairment was another important variable in the diagnostic equation. In particular, changes in ability to perform day-to-day tasks such as cooking, doing finances, or keeping appointments were key indicators obtained from potential patients and their families. Probes such as "Does your memory interfere with your daily living?" or "Is there anything you can no longer do?" were standard at both sites.

On the neuropsych testing, people with AD were expected to do poorly on certain tasks, including naming animals, listing D words, performing calculations, drawing intersecting pentagons, the memory questions on the mini–mental state examination, and abstract reasoning. During the team meetings to determine diagnosis, the following statements were common across sites:

This is characteristic ADish distortion [holds up drawing of clock]. (Neuropsychiatrist)

This is an early AD drawing [holds up picture of shapes that are slanted, smaller]. (Neurologist)

It's garden variety AD. He's totally disoriented. It was hard to get him to concentrate. (Clinical Psychologist)

This is a memory-dominant picture. (Neurologist)

Cues won't help with AD. The word was lost in the process of storing information. (Neuropsychiatrist)

Related to eliciting information, another clinical objective was to measure decline, achieved by examining the information collected from potential patients and their family member(s) and comparing them with other clinical and empirical data (e.g., averages for age or education). Symptoms were ranked to establish that they surpassed the threshold beyond which was deemed normal. The clinical intention was to demonstrate pathology; a diagnosis could not be made without such evidence. The following excerpts were typical:

Basically you come here for two things: to find out "Is there a problem?" to get an objective observation of what is going on with your mom. If there is, we try to find out how severe it is and in what areas. Then we try to figure out what the cause is. (Psychiatrist)

Whether it's serious or not, the most important thing [for making a diagnosis] is what injuries—where we know the name and what it looks like—that can be traced, are visible, when we evaluate. (Neurologist)

The process of collecting data focused primarily on eliciting relevant evidence in a systematic fashion and quantifying deficit in an effort to demarcate any departure from normalcy and justify the medical management of so-called cognitively impaired individuals by assigning a diagnosis.

Constructing a Diagnosis

Both centers purported a multidisciplinary or team approach to constructing a diagnosis. If the employment of the notion of consensus is arguably a management strategy—the proverbial "them" as expert versus "us" as patients scenario—then it is no surprise that both centers boasted a team orientation to enlist trust. The following framings were common: "We think people get the best care by having this team approach" (Neurologist); "We really go for a team approach here and we aim to get a whole bunch of minds together on this and not just have one perspective" (Neurologist); and "We really bring everyone together to talk about what is going on so not just one person is making the decision [of what diagnosis to give]" (Registered Nurse). More elaborate explanations were also observed:

> The primary purpose [of the team meetings] is teaching but there are other purposes too: 1) to be able to quickly evaluate the data, 2) having all the disciplines available at once, 3) it puts the NP [neuropsych testing] into context quickly, which heightens efficiency, and 4) it streamlines the diagnostic process. (Neurologist)

> One of the strengths of these centers like [ours] is that we have a consensus diagnosis so it is not just one person doing it but a team. We all vote on it and if we all agree we give that diagnosis and if we don't then we figure out what needs to be done to reevaluate. (Psychiatrist)

The objective at this stage of the process was to screen for relevant facts from all the information gathered and situate patient deficits into preformed clinical categories. Naming symptoms fits cases into preexisting classifications that clinicians were able to understand and treat since putting a medical label on it meant looking for certain symptoms.

Consequently, this also served to enhance the robustness of the original categories themselves and reinforce their utility.[23]

As with compiling evidence, constructing a diagnosis assumed patient incompetence and the need for patient management. This was supported by the significance clinicians assigned to the informant interviews when determining the etiology of a given set of symptoms. Potential patients embarked on their career as patients, unbeknownst to them, during the assignment of medical labels occurring at this point in the process. Patients allegedly needed management because they were perceived to require coercion in availing themselves of treatments, to be deficient by definition, and to need increasing help in the future. As the following chapter details, for those people receiving a diagnosis of AD/MCI, the first step in the process of adopting Alzheimer's as an identity coincided with the ascribed medical classification and the subsequent commencing of patienthood.

Despite the shared trope of team meetings and the extensive editing of biographical stories into medical facts performed by clinicians, there were important differences in the construction of diagnoses at the neurology and psychiatry centers, including both the formal and informal procedures involved in rendering a diagnosis at the two sites and the roles of medication, the brain, and the mini–mental state examination (MMSE) in making a decision.

First, the objective of the meetings varied between the centers. Both models were invested in presenting their diagnostic process as a collaborative effort—as the gold standard of specialty clinics—despite the fact that, in practice, there was essentially one key figure during the meetings at each site and significant variation between the centers in the proceedings themselves. Specifically, the neurological model utilized what they called their team meeting as a teaching session and, like grand rounds, it was not uncommon for literature to be cited, drawings to be put on the board, or discussions regarding classification systems and etiology to emerge. The attending neurologists (or neuropsychologists, to a lesser extent) made the following remarks:

> So if in a three-year study you measured hippocampal volume at time zero and then looked at hippocampal volume on placebo versus Aricept, then I think you might be able to say something about pathologic progression.

This recent study at Columbia by Yakoff-Stern looked at blood flow by education—MMSE-matched—and found hypoprofusion in the highly educated. They can compensate on the testing we give them.

Observational and retrospective studies show all cognitive functioning is better if you're on Statins approximately 10 years.

Christine Yaffe has shown that although ERT [estrogen replacement therapy] is a good growth factor, if you already have AD it doesn't work. It may delay onset, but it's not retrospective.

If you go long enough and your plasticity declines, everyone will have it eventually, and maybe there is some subclinical pathology that is there your whole life and kids would have Alzheimer's disease if they didn't have the brain plasticity that they do.

In fact, the entire process simulated playing a game or solving a puzzle. In concert with the ethos of teaching, the main objective of the team meeting was to formulate a differential diagnosis, including all possible conditions involved. Reminiscent of what Holmes and Ponte, as medical residents themselves, referred to as a mechanism for the "construction of a coherent narrative structure in which chaotic experiences are reorganized and reinterpreted to fit neatly into a linear plot with a predictable ending,"[24] or what Davenport refers to as diagnostic storytelling, the procedure was relatively standard for every case and relied on involvement from all the clinicians present. The following exchanges were common: "So, I think AD is still at the top of the [differential] list. She could have LB, maybe regular PD on top of LB"; and "He's got a lot of FTD flavor. I think we all sort of lean toward FTD.[25] Anyone think it's Alzheimer's with a lot of frontal? I think we need to keep it on the differential." More ostensibly teaching focused interactions were also observed:

What might cause dementia? With these caveats? What other diseases cause dementia? [Long pause] So the differential diagnosis includes AD, LBD, VaD, CBD, PSP, MSA, and maybe depression.[26] The caveats are the tremor, the rapid change, and her gait.

I'm bouncing around between PSP, vascular, and LBD. The testing goes against LBD. She has little amnestic (memory) problems. It is not PSP neuropsychologically. Maybe it is some PD and AD.

ATTENDING NEUROLOGIST: So the differential?

RESIDENT: I was wondering if it's dementia?

ATTENDING NEUROLOGIST: Yeah, but what's one other thought? Is there another dementia that you can think of that tends to present a lot of visual spatial trouble? Let's say he's kind of a little more Parkinsonian than MCI on exam today.

RESIDENT: I don't think that Lewy-body has that much visual spatial.

ATTENDING NEUROLOGIST: It does. So Lewy-body . . . He definitely wouldn't even meet possible criteria nevertheless, when you get this feel for . . . and Lewy-body, among all these disorders, I think is the least well-defined. The clinical criteria are the least useful.

RESIDENT: Is it possible that it is Alzheimer's?

ATTENDING NEUROLOGIST: I think so. I think that's what I would call it.

Formally, the patient had at least three people speaking on her/his case, presenting the so-called facts (or translating the biography into biology) to the attending neurologist who had yet to meet either the patient or the family. As the final quote shows, the attending neurologist teaches or leads residents to the desired end through "narrative templates."[27] While each team member reported his or her findings, the attending neurologist copied down all the information he deemed significant for making a diagnosis. The attending physicians presented a unified front as the cornerstone of specialty clinics:

We see patients in teams that consists of a nurse, who spends a lot of time with the family thinking about what the family has noticed about the person, whether they feel the disease has been superimposed on that person, they also get quantitative information on the personality, on the function of day to day life, and make sure that we get good information from all the sources we are hoping to get, so other physicians and other data.

The second part of our team is a resident physician—neurologist, psychiatrist, geriatrician or sometimes internists—and they go through the functional complaint with the patient and often the family as well, they think about medical issues, superimposed medical problems, superimposed psychiatric problems, they think about metabolic status, is there a deficiency in sodium, thyroid, these sorts of things. They think about whether there's some sort of reversible factor that may not be related to the memory problem as a degenerative dementia. And they do the history and also go through the medications and also do a neurologic and a general medical exam. And then there's a third part of the team which is the neuropsychology team which does neuropsychological testing and it also probes for mood, depression, things like that.

After these three groups have met with the patient we sit together and think about the problem, think about what the disease is, what we need to do to confirm that, how would we treat, whether we should or not, try to decide whether we are going to reassure people by saying we think things are okay, whether we think we need to follow them, or whether we think we need to intervene in some way.

In this manner, the construction of a diagnosis was presented as an interactive, negotiated conversation between all the clinicians present. While intended to be a multidisciplinary process of learning and mentoring, the emphasis on empirical research (evidence-based medicine) meant that the attending neurologists were ultimately the arbiters. These team meetings allocated approximately one hour for each patient and were on the same day as the evaluation.

The psychiatric clinic, in contrast, held weekly team meetings for consensus diagnosis of all patients seen that week. Attendees included the director of psychiatry,[28] three to four clinicians, the three clinical research coordinators, and three to four research staff. The potential patient and his/her family left after the administration of the tests and a "family conference" was scheduled for approximately two weeks from the screening date, to render the results. While the research coordinators typically played a central role in administering the cognitive tests, the clinician who saw the potential patient and conducted the evaluation was the only individual who spoke on the case at the team meeting. The presenting clinician read from the typed handout she had prepared and circulated to all attendees in advance. She went over the age, race, and marital status of the patient and noted the source of the information (e.g., medical chart, patient, informant, etc.). Then she reviewed the "history of presenting illness," stating onset, duration, and concrete examples of memory loss. Next, she discussed past medical history, medications, social and family histories, and any psychiatric conditions. Then she read her dictation on the neurological exam, the lab results (noting any abnormalities), and CT scan results (if available; often they were not).

Next, she presented the findings of the neuropsychological exam, again highlighting areas of deficit and comparing the potential patient to previously calculated averages for the age group and education level of the person being tested. Finally, the director of the clinic called any clinicians present to vote on the diagnosis and each of three to four clinicians stated what they saw as the primary syndrome (e.g., dementia), causal factors (e.g., AD, cardiovascular disease, PD), and primary diagnosis (e.g., "probable" or "possible" AD).

At the Health Center, the consensus diagnosis meeting was conducted more like a business meeting and was far more scripted with the one clinician who saw the patient reading—typically verbatim—a one- to two-page summary of all the data evaluated. It was far more systematic and less interactional with the clinical ethos of standardization more visible than at the neurology clinic. Frankly, it was difficult to discern how the process would have been any different had the correspondence taken place via email or the summaries left in clinicians' mailboxes simply led to voting. What was touted as a democratic process in practice more closely resembled an autocratic one whereby a single clinician interpreted and presented all the data. Each of the three to four clinicians voted on the diagnosis and I never observed any disagreement between them. The tallied results yielded a diagnosis without discussion. As a result, the psychiatric diagnosis meeting allotted approximately fifteen to twenty minutes per patient. So, while both sites touted a team approach relying on interdisciplinary expertise, in reality this amounted to little more than a trope, as both the Brain Clinic and Health Center essentially had one key player (attending neurologist and presenting clinician, respectively).

The role of medications was another important departure between the two models. The neurology center routinely recommended a pharmacological treatment (Aricept) for everyone receiving a diagnosis. The notion that people with dementia *deserve* medications and should be adequately aided in that process was central to attending neurologists' framing: "He deserves whatever treatment is available. He deserves Aricept," "She deserves Aricept. . . . It's good, overall, on the average patient, so we have to try it," and "So, she deserves Aricept and Vitamin E."

There was also an explicit sense from the attending neurologists that the actual diagnosis mattered very little in terms of treatment as many dementias are prescribed the same medications: "In the end, we'd treat it [AD or Lewy-body disease] the same way either way," "The treatment [Aricept] is appropriate either way [for AD, LBD, or mild dementia]," "All these [LBD, PD, AD, VaD] get the same treatment," and "So let's say that we decide that she definitely has early Alzheimer's disease. The course would be the thing. . . . It almost doesn't matter if we decide that she has AD today. We'd still do the same things." In this way, the neurology center's primary intervention revolved around medications. A major structural difference between the clinics was that the psychiatry site was not a primary care center and thus not allowed to prescribe medications despite the ability of some staff to do so. Since the local context of the psychiatry center prevented a focus on prescribing medications, although recommendations were made to the referring physician, medication regimens, side effects, and expectations were rarely topics of discussion. Instead, far more attention was directed at postdiagnostic care and services.

The third difference was the centrality of the brain or the mind at the sites. In concert with localization theory that permeates modern medical approaches to AD,[29] the regions of impairment were central identifying markers of diagnostic categorization at the Brain Clinic. Visual representations of the brain and links between symptoms and location within the brain, including comments such as "AD effects parietal temporal a lot," or "Injury to the frontal lobes equals memory problems" were regularly employed at the neurology center. For example, "A lot of diseases affecting the brain make you look like this. For the most part, if I had to localize it, I'd say frontal problems," "We're seeing some right parietal, some right hippocampal, not much left parietal or temporal," and "Memory doesn't have to be hippocampal for clinical memory loss. The other anatomical location is frontal."

Visually displaying scans for the team to view was the rule, not an exception; I did not observe a single meeting where an MRI image was not available. After the clinicians presented their reports and the diagnosis was decided upon, everyone would stand around while the attending neurologist and the residents pointed out atrophy, white matter, lacunae, and any signs of possible strokes, commenting: "That's not as much atrophy as I expected from the testing," "She's even less preserved than I thought she'd be," or "Look at all that white matter disease in the hippocampal region." Such emphasis on scans demonstrates how the everyday work practices of clinicians reinforce MRI technology and imaging routines, as outlined by sociologist Kelly Joyce,[30] and reflects the contemporary preoccupation with being able to "picture" or make visible that Joseph Dumit argues such technologies offer.[31]

For neurology, not surprisingly, the brain played an integral role in the diagnosing of memory loss. In fact, the cerebral cortex—and its various occipital, parietal, temporal, limbic, and frontal lobes—was the primary unit of analysis. The site of etiology is a telltale factor in diagnosing various forms of dementia. The neuroanatomy relevant to localizing and diagnosing Alzheimer's includes primarily the back of the brain (the occipital lobe), which processes visual information such as recognition, and the top right quadrant (the temporal lobe), storing the hippocampus, which has a role in memory and emotion processing. Thus, cases of AD were ostensibly "discovered" when imaging scans revealed atrophy in the hippocampus and/or the temporal domains. The scans were also used to legitimate diagnosis. As one neurologist put it, "They [MRIs] make me feel better [about making a diagnosis]." Cultural narratives in the media, popular science, and hospitals that suggest that MRI images provide unbiased knowledge and thus reveal the truth about the health of a person's body, erase how doctors use medical images in conjunction with other tests to make sense of a potential patient's situation.[32]

In practice, the neurology clinic utilized MRI and occasionally a PET/SPECT scan taken in advance, brought to the appointment, and interpreted on-site at the time of the visit; whereas the psychiatry clinic primarily employed CT scans, which involved a printout of lab-interpreted impressions (which allowed little room for clinical judgment) typically not available at the team meeting. At the psychiatric clinic, however, not only were there no discussions about the specific sites of pathology, but little was mentioned at all regarding imaging in particular, or the brain in general. Thus, as the neurologists aimed to advance the disease classification of AD and MCI, they had significant power as instillers of scientific knowledge.

The results of the copious randomized clinical trials (RCTs) conducted at the centers also directly informed both the practices adhered to and the information relayed to people seeking evaluation at the clinics. These trials had varying effects on both scientific advancement and phenomenological experiences for individuals with memory loss. The psychiatric clinic, which focused squarely on the mind, was far less involved in the taxonomy of memory loss or the certainty of the diagnosis itself. Rather it focused on studies regarding healthy aging, sleep patterns, caregiver health, and clinical assessments, as well as follow-up care and meeting the psychosocial needs of a clientele who were likely to be given a diagnosis with serious emotional, financial, and social ramifications.

Lastly, when constructing a diagnosis, both sites employed various allegedly objective tests to demarcate seemingly arbitrary points beyond which memory loss was deemed pathological. At the neurological center, the mini–mental state examination (MMSE) was framed as the gold standard of global memory functioning upon which to evaluate cognitive impairment: "The MMSE gives a nice thumbnail sketch which is widely known, easily translated to others [read, nonspecialists]. It is a way to talk about cognitive function in a broad sense." After hearing the presentation of the history and physical, the attending neurologist would typically ask each person to make a guess as to the MMSE score before hearing the result of the neuropsych tests: "Who wants to guess this guy's MMSE?" or "Does anyone want to take a stab at her MMSE score?"

The MMSE was clearly not seen as an infallible measure nor was it the deciding factor in any case. In fact, such efforts at guessing the score were often by way of testing the efficacy of the measure against clinical impression, which was deemed more reliable than neuropsych testing (by the dominant neurological paradigm of this site at least). Consequently, neurologists routinely made comments such as, "I'd just throw it out. I don't think it tells us much. I think it's a classic example of how the mini-mental can really just not be down the right road," "The results from any one trial are only as good as the one trial," or "I wouldn't put too much emphasis on any one set of tests. This may just be a baseline." The latter comments also justify the need for continued medical surveillance.

Not surprisingly, at the neurology center the history and physical/ neurological (H&P) exams were seen as far more crucial in determining etiology:

> There are no neuropsychological criteria for dementia. It's all the history because the neuropsych can't tell you how functionally impaired somebody is. They can only tell you how they do on the tests.
>
> So I think the H&P I still consider the primary tool. There are several reasons: obviously, it picks up on a lot of features that the neuropsych may or may not pick up (like behavioral abnormalities) and it also goes back much further . . . that is very valuable in helping to narrow down the diagnosis. So, I think the H&P is certainly and the (neurological) physical exam obviously is important because there are some kinds of disorders that have various kinds of problems on physical examination others which don't have any abnormalities on physical exam. (Neurologist)

This clearly alludes to the hierarchy of disciplines within the Brain Clinic, wherein neurology dominates.

At the psychiatry center, in contrast, the MMSE rarely came into play in constructing a diagnosis. It was often not mentioned at all until after the diagnosis was agreed upon and then it was requested only by the research staff trying to determine if the person would be eligible for research participation: "I guess that MMSE disqualifies him for most of our studies," "He sounds good for research, what's his MMSE?" or "Will she qualify for any studies? What's the MMSE?"

In the rare cases when a physical examination was done at the Health Center, it was an extremely abbreviated version. Instead, the focus was far more on postdiagnosis outcomes, such as "Something I see as a major part of my role [is] crisis intervention. If someone needs to talk to me, I want to be available." In some cases, they positioned themselves in contrast to the neurological model, "An AD diagnosis is a death sentence. It's terrible when people are diagnosed and then left hanging. That's why we hesitate to refer people to [a neurology clinic]."

Thus, the emphasis on measurement validity and discrepancies between clinical impression and any single test result did not carry the same sense of urgency at the Health Center as it did at the Brain Clinic. Nonetheless, clinicians at both sites collected copious amounts of data and performed exhaustive tests ostensibly to locate the cause of memory loss. Under this ethos, in the clinical process the patient is, frankly, a potential disease. The objective of specialty practice appeared to be to isolate etiology to a specific site using general medical technologies, or technoscience. That is, the goal is accomplished by using "narrative templates" to "provide the preliminary structure, the warp and weft, for building a patient story that holds together long enough to diagnose, treat, and discharge the patient."[33] Beyond concrete procedures, another primary way both sites constructed a diagnosis was through the rhetoric of a team meeting where multidisciplinary experts were said to reach consensus despite the fact that, in reality, one key informant appeared to control the outcome. The results of these technologies of knowing were then employed as legitimators of a diagnostic label in the process of relaying information to those who had been evaluated. That is, I am arguing that employing the trope of a team approach helped clinicians at both sites to establish trust and bracket the uncertainty of making a diagnosis that could only be definitely made postmortem by theoretically instilling greater confidence in the diagnosis.

Rendering a Diagnosis

After compiling all the evidence perceived to be relevant and subsequently constructing a team or consensus diagnosis, both sites followed a formula for delivering diagnoses to patients and their families that varied in only minor ways between clinicians or sites. In general, a clear distinction between normal aging and the pathological, dementing process with which the person was being diagnosed was a primary objective of this component at both centers. Consequently, the belief that patients require pharmacological treatments or psychosocial interventions to manage their symptoms and that hope for such treatment exists were the aims of the Brain Clinic and Health Center, respectively. Further, due to the downward trajectory presented, both centers encouraged participation in research. It is at this point that the full incorporation of potential patients as patients is realized by clinical standards, and what Keating and Cambrioso refer to as the hybrid patient/research subject[34] can potentially begin.

As with compiling evidence and constructing a diagnosis, delivering the diagnosis was based on assumptions of the need for standardization, patient incompetence, and patients who require management. The latter two become central when making an AD diagnosis. First, an AD diagnosis meant that the family member(s) had become caregivers for the now bona fide patient (or would in the near future). At this point, much of the discussion appeared to be aimed at enlisting family members in the management of patients. Also, due to the legitimization of the patient's incompetence via an AD diagnosis (or impending incompetence in the case of MCI), patients needed to be managed to make sure they adhered to the treatment regimes and necessary follow-up care required.

At both centers, efforts to differentiate dementing illnesses from the decline and gradual slowing accompanying the aging process were essential to the process of rendering a diagnosis. Clinicians spoke at length and with fervor about the importance of understanding the difference between aging and dementia. Due to current disagreements and previous conceptualizations of memory loss as a normal part of aging, clinicians worked to dispute this connection when giving a diagnosis, saying, "Memory trouble is abnormal," or "Alzheimer's is progressive and so the decline progresses faster than memory loss." More explicitly,

> What we are talking about it NOT normal aging. When it is severe memory loss, what we call some form of dementia . . . when it is something like that it is clearly not normal. Not everyone has these types of experiences as they get older. (Psychiatrist)

> She's really on the cusp. She's not that far from normal that PCP/ GPs [primary care providers/general practitioners]—and even some neurologists—can tell. We used to think this was normal aging, but not anymore. That's the way a lot of clinicians see things—and we're trying to change that. (Neurologist)

Since these clinicians wished to help, they presumably wanted to do something for the people they were diagnosing. Within allopathic medicine, the primary way to do this is by treating the condition with pharmacotherapy and encouraging continued surveillance. Only if such individual experiences are found to be clinically pathological can clinicians claim jurisdiction over managing patients. According to such logic, most of these patients required medical management, especially since their insight/awareness was suspect:

> It will get worse but the bigger question is when. It's a matter of years, not months, of progression for you. . . . If anything, you're older than that and doing quite well. We time it by how well you're doing when we raise the concern. The clock starts ticking now and it's hard to say how long it'll be. (Neurologist)

Both sites employed unequivocal impairment and decline as justification for the management of patients who otherwise might not abide by the appropriate rules of conduct.

As a result of the newly discovered neurodegenerative process underlying the patients' symptoms and behaviors, clinicians at both centers saw the need for treatments aimed at addressing the problems, including pharmacological interventions to stabilize decline (primarily at the Brain Clinic) and nonpharmacological regimens to decrease further decay (primarily at the Health Center), and continued medical visits to document deterioration (at both sites). Emphasis on the notion that *something* could be done as a result of the diagnosis, intended to instill hope (that help is available), was common across sites: "We always start with Aricept here. I'm optimistic, gung-ho, that we'll be treating AD within the next few years" (Neurologist); "As long as you are on *something*, that's the important thing" (Registered Nurse); "If all other things are being addressed, your memory will be protected. We have limited control over this but we are doing all we can to help" (Psychiatrist); "We are optimistic that of all the major diseases, AD might be one we can treat and even stop" (Neurologist); and "I'm sure in your mind you know one possibility is Alzheimer's disease. We can never be sure of that but it is something and we can try to do things about it if it is that" (Psychiatrist). The correlation between having a neurodegenerative condition and the need for treatment further reinforced the role of clinicians in properly managing those being diagnosed. As the experts holding the available knowledge (order) within an ambiguous realm (disorder), clinicians positioned themselves as the beacon of hope during the diagnostic disclosure.

It is clearly explained at both centers that although a cure was not a viable option for people being diagnosed with dementia, *finding a cure* and/or *living with the condition* depended on people like them participating in clinical research in order to better understand the intricacies of dementing illnesses. At the very least, they might receive medical treatments prior to their general availability: "Regarding our clinic, I really think you should call us periodically and participate in research" (Psychiatrist); "I really believe in research and I think in this area, people who participated in research as a group, if you compared them to non-research, have done much better" (Neurologist); "It's important that we follow this closely. Keep in touch with the clinic and get involved in research" (Psychiatrist); and "Our job is to educate you, get you involved in research or treatment that might help you" (Neurologist). In this way, clinicians had something to recommend and patients had something to do to fight against the irreversible process of degeneration, if not for themselves then for those who would come after them or for the good of society and/or the advancement of science. In the words of one senior neurologist, "I think having research options [e.g., drug trials] available to people gives them hope, gives them a sense that they are participating in this, not just being a passive observer."

Despite the clearly shared objectives of distinguishing dementia from normal aging, their presumed need for treatments, and the making of patients and research subjects, the difference between the centers was arguably the largest in the realm of the evaluation process. The presentation of the diagnosis, the recommendations made, and the role of the person being diagnosed varied considerably between the two sites.

The terminology used to deliver a diagnosis at each center was based on their respective approaches to constructing diagnoses. Clinicians aim to identify and eradicate medical conditions. As demonstrated in research on medically uncertain conditions, clinicians are forced to manage in different ways when a cure is not available, including by exploiting the open-endedness of science.[35] In specialty clinics, the same conscious employment of ambiguity used in the "collective production" of new clinical guidelines and standards of approaching AD more broadly[36] can be said to serve as a mechanism for softening the diagnosis, managing mixed diagnoses, and encouraging research participation. Although utilized to varying degrees, it was observed most strategically during the rendering of diagnoses and primarily at the Brain Clinic. These ranged from vague statements such as "We can't eyeball the hippocampus and diagnose," or "Our definitive diagnosis is still clinical—the only way to know for sure is to take your brain out and put it under a microscope," to very detailed explanations:

> Once we do tests at autopsy, it's possible you might have had AD. The best I can do is give you my best guess, which is not meaningless—it is based on the tests, exams, etc. Adding it all up, my best guess is that you probably do have AD, very minor, and only possible AD. There's no way I can be sure, but you're having enough trouble to start treatments.

> The way we make a diagnosis about these things is to add it all up (from the neuropsych testing, the H&P, the scan, and our interviews with your wife)—given what we know—and decide what is *probably* [emphasis in the original], say 90 percent or better, going on.

Another noteworthy difference regarding the presentation of the diagnosis was the amount of information disclosed to the patient, and in what format. The neurologists were willing, if hesitant, to withhold the so-called A word if an informant requested it for fear of "making mom terribly scared" or "freaking him/her out." Indeed, it was not uncommon for an attending neurologist to come in and render a diagnosis without ever mentioning the word Alzheimer's, whether or not this was explicitly requested by an informant. In this way, the neurologists saw their role as tailoring the diagnosis to each patient/family and utilizing the craft of "reading the patient." In particular, the extent of conversation between the clinician and the patient and use of the term Alzheimer's or medical labels more generally differed significantly. The Brain Clinic conducted the delivery interactively, with both patients and families involved. Thus, the following queries and introductions were standard practice: "What's your agenda today? What are you looking for? What should we tell you about?" "Tell me the main reason you came here? What's the biggest issue, what would you ideally like us to help you with?" "My job is to ask you a few questions to hear in your words why you're here and go over the results of the tests you took and talk about the future" or "Why are you here today? What has your memory problem changed for you? How does it affect you?" Subtle inquiries were also observed:

> CLINICIAN: Something needs to be talked about. Did [your PCP] talk about AD?
> POTENTIAL PATIENT: It would be my concern, it's always important.
> CLINICIAN: Did he mention AD?
> POTENTIAL PATIENT: No, if he had I'd probably have fainted.
> CLINICIAN: Well, it's our job to talk about it and check it out.

The Health Center, in sharp contrast, was far more prescribed and impersonal in its diagnostic format. The conversations were similarly scripted in the process but they seemed more like a business exchange, which did not vary considerably from diagnosis to diagnosis or between different conditions. In this way, they matched the professional objective stance of psychotherapy more generally. These disclosures also ranged from somewhat vague statements such as "Your [neuropsych] tests with [the Research Assistant] were really bad, particularly in memory," or "It's [test results] not terrible but you just did not do well on this," to far more direct, instructive commentary: "Definitely contact your MD if there are any changes and come back here for a follow-up and to learn how to cope with anxiety and stress," or "There is some dementia and dementia has some other causes and we've ruled out the other things and it's probably of Alzheimer's pathology." In the extreme case, they could resemble a routinized checking of boxes:

> CLINICIAN TO SON: So, based on that [results of tests showed possible AD], I have a check-list I have to cover. First and foremost, contact the Alzheimer's Association. I know your mom may not need/want all of this right now but . . . [and she goes over Family Caregiver Alliance, support groups, Durable Power of Attorney, contacting her MD, stopping driving, long-term care/day care placement, and participation in research virtually without pausing for a breath].

The second factor was the use of medical labels themselves. The issue of disclosure in dementia has long been a source of intense debate[37] and it is said to parallel past issues in cancer care, whereby an estimated 50 percent of clinicians routinely withhold a dementia diagnosis.[38] The Brain Clinic was very flexible with what and how they would diagnose. They were involved in a process of reading the potential patients to elicit what they were looking for and felt it was appropriate to never use the term Alzheimer's in some cases. To that end, the diagnosis was positioned as a skillful negotiation requiring clinical judgment, as for example: "You're not doing as well as you should be," or "You do have some memory loss and more than is normal for your age. It's not terrible. But it's clearly *an abnormality* [emphasis in the original]." More elaborate efforts included:

> [On the neuropsych testing] I'd like to see you better on your memory. There could be lots of reasons for it; I'm unsure why it's happening. Some people have normal aging, some very early AD, some small strokes. We don't know yet as much as we should regarding who's who. You don't have orange flags; your problems are very subtle. We see what you're seeing. But where you are heading is unclear. I don't think it's AD, if I had to prioritize who I'm most worried about, you'd be low on the list.

A similar tone was observed in the team meetings: "We won't be as optimistic and hopeful here. You couldn't ask for a more prototypical case of AD," and "We're not allowed to mention the word AD in front of her, but we should be forward about home modifications, etc."

The Health Center, however, required that everyone be made aware of their diagnosis and be present for it. For a discipline focused on behavior modifications and a site targeting postdiagnostic services, there were obvious reasons for their different approach to delivering a diagnosis. Being aware of the diagnosis was a necessary first step in psychosocial treatment options, for example. Much of this mimics the disciplinary patient/therapist relationship of establishing trust and confidentiality in psychiatry generally: "It is written into our protocol that all patients must be present for the diagnosis," "We tell them everything since it doesn't work to have secrets. It is important to establish trust," "If someone doesn't want the diagnosis disclosed to the patient, then we refer them elsewhere," and "We can do it [family conference] separately, but we don't feel we can't tell people. They signed a consent and at the end of the day it is *their* [emphasis in the original] medical care."

In a similar vein, the family conference was intentionally scheduled for a few weeks after the testing:

> It is a long day and people can barely retain what is said. Plus, the time gives them a chance to process what has happened, allows for the coordination of as many people as desired at the diagnosis, and makes it a separate experience from the testing. We encourage people to be available by phone for them to call because this is a family discussion that needs to happen and it encourages psychological bonding. This way they all hear the same thing and they can air any questions or concerns at that time. (Codirector and RN)

Since such open discourse was necessary to achieving the therapeutic aims of the Health Center, it is not surprising that nondisclosure was intolerable in their setting. Without such so-called awareness of diagnosis, people would be unable to participate in the endeavors the clinic hoped to accomplish. The political-moral dimension of this intention was also a central component to their disclosure practices.

Beyond disclosure, the treatment plan or recommendations made were the single largest difference between the sites. While both centers highlighted such things as diet and exercise through comments such as "Mental and physical exercise helps cognition" (Nurse), "Physical exercise would be helpful. If you're going to do one thing that's not medicine, I'd encourage you to do exercise" (Psychiatrist), and "What's good for the heart is good for the brain. I think exercise is really important. Of all the things we do here, we see our best results there" (Neurologist), the emphasis at the Brain Clinic was squarely on pharmaceutical treatments, which were framed as at least moderately efficacious in stabilizing decline even for those with MCI. Accordingly, drugs were a way of getting at neurons: "With Alzheimer's there are some medicines to help." More explicitly hopeful explanations were common:

> There is a lot of work around the causes and treatments [of AD] and we've found there are a lot of options. You're not on any of them . . . . There are

3 meds if you have memory problems and think it is AD—we can never be sure—because most people decline and the meds try to stabilize that. Your memory doesn't get all better. Maybe people are more alert, focused, or in a better mood. You'll notice changes. If not, that doesn't mean it's not working. There isn't a downside; there aren't bad side effects, so why not try it? (Neurologist)

I think because our physicians are kind of on the cutting edge and they feel that the safety risk is so minimal, and they know that in some of the animal models it's been successful, and they are quick to treat. (Clinical Nurse Specialist)

Aricept makes your thinking more efficient. It's been proven in studies to work 1–2 years and there's no reason to think it stops working then, there just aren't any studies done on that yet. We might get even more meds as you go. It doesn't completely stave it off—people will get worse over time. Overall, the meds slow it down. (Neuropsychiatrist)

As MDs used to say, it's normal aging if you're getting along okay. Some MDs with expertise say no, you're not supposed to have decline as you age. If we don't think about it as AD—we couldn't treat you. You deserve to be treated and it could help you. You're having problems—not bad ones—but ones affecting you every day. (Neurologist)

The Brain Clinic also invariably suggested the use of Vitamin E and folic acid, lowering cholesterol, and stopping driving.[39] For example,

I'm going to suggest 1 milligram of folic acid as well since it might protect the brain and certainly doesn't hurt. We also think Vitamin E may protect the brain, not a mega dose, but 800. I'd like your cholesterol to be under 200; we now think high cholesterol is bad for memory.

I'd like to see you on Vitamin E. There is one study where high doses seemed preventive of AD. It was only one, but it's probably not harmful and may be helpful.

Driving is about mapping representation. In real life, that means combined with memory loss and mapping troubles, your driving should be reevaluated. . . . I'm telling you my legal obligation, I'm not telling you I think you should stop driving.

The Health Center, in contrast, made recommendations to the referring physician but actual conversations regarding the various medications and the expectations of them (beyond a continued relationship) were rare. In fact, people seeking diagnoses and their families often had to inquire themselves about pharmacological options. Clinician responses to family questions about available treatments included: "We don't prescribe since we're not a primary care center. We'll make a referral to your doctor and it's your choice whether or not to take the medications. Everyone makes their own decision" (Nurse); "We tend to recommend Aricept. It's been around the longest and has the least side effects, but we don't prescribe here" (Psychiatrist); and "No, it's mild cognitive impairment, we don't recommend medications unless it's a diagnosis of dementia" (Psychiatrist).

At the Health Center, the recommendations made included a vast array of items not covered by the Brain Clinic, including: contacting the Alzheimer's Association (the national advocacy organization), legal/financial issues, on-site support groups, medication monitoring (by way of informant or other noncognitively impaired person), home safety, driving safety, day care/respite care, and long-term care placements. In this way, the recommendations were directed at both patients and their families and were tangible things to manage ambiguity, encourage open communication and acceptance of the situation, and otherwise cope with the condition. In these ways, the recommendations made for both patients and care partners were compatible with the psychiatric emphasis on issues related to the therapeutic aims of their site. The Family Conference Summary[40] was a checklist used to review (often verbatim) relevant items with patients and their families during the delivery.

Clearly, the list of recommendations from the Health Center was comprehensive and addressed many issues that would come up over the course of the illness trajectory, which was a significant departure from the Brain Clinic. Although clinicians typically checked only those items relevant to discuss at the present moment, the scripted list often relayed a tone of impending doom (as demonstrated vividly with Mr. R's case in the prologue), for example: By way of introduction to the checklist, "These are the things you can expect to happen," "I'm not going to report you to the DMV at this time [MCI diagnosis]," "You don't need these things *yet* [emphasis added] but you will in the future," or "Next are your medications, they need to be taken and monitored closely. And communicate any changes you might need. Regarding the medical bracelet, I'm not recommending it because it is not something you need at this point." These quotes reveal some of the obvious (potential) drawbacks to the Health Center's comprehensive list of recommendations, but most of the items were indeed focused largely on *coping with* the condition as opposed to trying to fend it off with medications.

The perceived role of the person being diagnosed, in concert with the various foci of attention during the construction of diagnoses, also varied between the centers. Whether the potential patient was seen as a disease process or a person coping with a chronic illness (likely some combination of both, of course) had concrete ramifications on the subjective experiences of those seeking medical attention for memory loss at the respective sites (as will be elaborated in the following two chapters).

Conclusions

Despite the noted differences, the general processes of diagnosis, namely, the ways of constructing and rendering the news of AD/MCI, resulted in strikingly similar approaches to potential patients. Both centers alluded to managing the uncertainty of a dementia diagnosis through the promise of various treatment regimes and participation in research. Although the Brain Center focused more squarely on pharmacotherapy and related randomized clinical trial research while the Health Center addressed psychosocial interventions and research on quality of life, normal aging, and behavioral studies, both achieved order through standardized protocols and interactions, assumptions of patient incompetence, and presumptions that patients require medical management. Furthermore, both sites fostered trust through the trope of experts coming to a consensus via team meetings and instilled hope by employing ambiguity and encouraging research participation.

Individual biographies were made into biomedical cases[41] through the processes of compiling evidence, constructing a diagnosis, and rendering a diagnosis informed by the clinical assumptions of standardization, patient incompetence, and the need for patient management.

These data demonstrate the ways in which the scientific context in general as well as within these particular disciplines justifies the management strategies employed to elicit allegedly relevant facts from patients and their families. Most centrally, an (objective, nonimpaired) informant from whom reliable data could be collected was essential to constructing a diagnosis. Without the corroboration of such informants, clinicians would be forced to rely exclusively on their clinical impression, neuropsych testing, imaging technologies, and patient accounts. The informant served as a proxy for the patient and validated the clinical management of the person with memory loss. Thus, the person seeking diagnosis was (cognitively) impaired until proven sound (in the rare cases where someone was not diagnosed). In this way, patient management played a profound role in the diagnostic procedures at both sites.

Specialty clinics address aging, memory, and disease in a manner that confounds the confusion of normal memory loss and aging.[42] Through the formal cognitive assessment of older adults, tests geared to measure mental status and cognitive impairment become facts[43] and the management of old age follows. Further, early diagnoses potentially prolong the phenomenology of AD (and aging in the case of MCI). If solutions can be seen as providing the framework for interpreting and addressing problems, then hegemonic knowledge claims about the utility of diagnosing AD as early in the disease process as possible generate a right way of relating to oneself, the family, medical practitioners, and society.[44]

Drawing on exclusively quantitative methods for formulating a hypothesis, gathering evidence, and testing the hypothesis, specialty medicine "has become a theory-bound and paradigm-dominated . . . positivist representation of reality."[45] Inevitably, not all potential patients view memory loss in a light consistent with biomedical and technoscientific knowledges. The legitimacy and authority of medical knowledge requires a particular perception and organization of memory loss.[46] Accordingly, various views of aging and memory loss shape medical practice, patient compliance and resistance, and the incorporation of an Alzheimer's identity.

Scientific protocols and rhetorical devices such as team meetings and problem-oriented medical records are tools for converting biographical stories into clinical facts, while simultaneously socializing medical residents into becoming future physicians.[47] Since "diagnostic stories are shaped by what residents think they can *do* for the patient, practically speaking, and by the habitual hospital activity,"[48] what clinicians think they can *do* and how they do it will differ according to whether patients went to the Brain Clinic or the Health Center.

These techniques for reinforcing the legitimacy and authority of medical knowledge and practice are substantiated across disciplines. As argued elsewhere, these "images and records appear to create and control both medical practice and the patient's medical experience."[49] While this chapter highlighted how routine practices of cognitive evaluation generate processes through which patients (and ideally research subjects) are made in the clinic, that is, how forgetful individuals become patients through the mechanisms of technoscience, the following two chapters will address how these processes of constructing clinical facts and the resultant interactions encourage a distinctly medicalized view of memory loss for individuals undergoing cognitive evaluation and how potential patients respond to it.

4

Being Cognitively Evaluated

Learning to Medicalize Forgetfulness

Mrs. V is a well-dressed, savvy 78-year-old Jewish woman who has been experiencing minor memory loss for a year or so and came to the clinic alone. Widowed twelve years ago after her husband died in his sleep, she has a boyfriend of ten years. During the H&P (history and physical) exam, I learn that she was unable to move into an elite retirement community (where her boyfriend intends to live) because she failed a basic cognitive screening test, and is very anxious to find out whether she has "the dreaded disease" or not. While she and I are sitting in the waiting room for the neuropsychologist to call her name, she expresses her anxiety about the test. I offer not to observe her NP testing in the event that it might make her uncomfortable, but she says it is fine for me to watch. As soon as she is asked the first question on the neuropsych exam, her nervousness is palpable. It is painful to watch as she twitches, sighs, and at one point even tears up with frustration. I find it difficult not to avert my eyes and want to reach out to her across the room. When it gets to the Boston Naming Test, the neuropsychologist begins using a timer that beeps in intervals. Each time it goes off, Mrs. V throws her hands up and says, "Oh, that thing is driving me crazy! It makes me even more jumpy." Although the neuropsychologist does acknowledge Mrs. V's discomfort, she continues to use the beeper anyway. At no point does the clinician ask Mrs. V how she is doing or whether she needs to stop to take a short break. After what seems to me like an eternity, the testing ends and Mrs. V and I leave the room. She looks at me and says, "It's bad, isn't it?" I feel terrible giving her my standard response that "I'm not a medical doctor," so I add, "I don't know that I would do too much better than you did. They are meant to be hard." Two weeks later, Mrs. V is ultimately diagnosed with AD and at that point somberly expresses her concern to me about her boyfriend having to take care of her, that this diagnosis might be the end of her relationship with him.—Field notes

The majority of older people I talk to express concern about some degree of memory loss. Some of this reflects the global impetus for earlier diagnosis of dementia despite the clear identification of risks associated with this trend,[1] but it also represents the success of the neoliberal goals of self-regulation. This chapter examines how most of the roughly 50 study participants I observed being evaluated, including the 28 with whom I conducted in-depth follow-up interviews at the Brain Clinic and Health Center, came to see their memory loss as a disease and began to define themselves as patients. That is, the first crucial step in the process of becoming an Alzheimer's patient for these seniors (average age of 73.5) was to receive the primary diagnosis. Despite the noteworthy disciplinary differences outlined in the previous chapter, phenomenological accounts of being evaluated at the two sites reveal *experiences* that are strikingly similar. Investigating the subjective experiences of neuropsychological testing and diagnosis depicts first, how the medicalization of what I term potential patients transpires and second, the social significance of being evaluated and diagnosed for the eventual incorporation of Alzheimer's identities (or not).

Medical practices and knowledges directly influence prevailing lay and professional perceptions about being in the world. Contemporary notions of personhood, or self, are shaped by notions of rugged individualism and personal responsibility for one's health,[2] the expectation of a silver bullet remedy,[3] and a perceived dualistic relationship between mind and body.[4] Existential quandaries regarding the definition of personhood for people with purportedly compromised cognition abound within both the neurological and psychiatric models: Can people with memory loss be trusted to accurately tell their own stories? How does their assumed lack of credibility affect the communication between clinicians and potential patients/their families? What does this suggest about the ability of potential patients to benefit from medical interventions or adhere to treatment regimens? Whereas the previous chapter discussed how the answers to these questions affect clinicians interacting with potential patients and their families, here I examine personal experiences of being the object of scientific scrutiny and how clinical processes shape and are in turn shaped by potential patients.

Engaging the age-old agency-structure debate, the phenomenological experiences of being tested for and ultimately diagnosed with Alzheimer's/mild cognitive impairment are influenced by institutional factors, social forces, and personal dynamics alike. The clinical procedures associated with evaluating and diagnosing memory loss of course shape subjective experiences; that is, institutional processes influence the encounter while simultaneously generating new types of Alzheimer's patients—those who act and react. Although individuals being tested and diagnosed report strikingly similar experiences of specialty practice, there is profound variation in the personal reactions to being tested and diagnosed. In the language of symbolic interaction, people select and interpret the environment within which they respond; thus meaning changes over time as actors form variable definitions of the situation. Furthermore, what is experienced personally cannot be easily reduced to neat categories and bears the stamp of the many social contingencies affecting those labeled with this diagnosis in the twenty-first century.

Not surprisingly, potential patients differed in a number of important ways, including their beliefs on aging and disease in general, their views about Alzheimer's in particular, and their trust in medical personnel. Yet people undergoing cognitive workup reported similar types of reactions to the testing process and the eventual diagnosis despite these noteworthy differences. During cognitive evaluation, perhaps as a result of the deficit-model outlined in the previous chapter, respondents worked to implement various strategies to ensure that they were taken seriously and treated in a way that preserved their prediagnosis self-concept as sentient and autonomous. The following chapter will reveal that the same range of strategies were used during diagnostic disclosure.

While experiences of evaluation and diagnosis are deeply personal and idiosyncratic, and reactions are far from universal, respondents reported common phases in the process of coming to see themselves as Alzheimer's patients, including: negotiating their forgetfulness, converting forgetfulness into symptoms, using clinical facts as status passages, and eventually embarking on a path of Alzheimer's. Rather than presuming a linear progression or uniform staging, these respondents present various routes and emphases within the common phases. In reality, individuals do not necessarily move smoothly or universally from start to finish despite what the clinical management strategies outlined in the prior chapter suggest. As study participants retrospectively narrate their stories, however, many do structure the events chronologically.

While each case tells a unique story, in aggregate my data reveal common themes in the lives of these forgetful individuals. I now turn to a detailed description of each of these phases.

Negotiating Everyday Forgetfulness (Pre-Evaluation)

Managing Impressions

Personal beliefs and medicalized approaches to memory loss in specialty clinics together shape how potential patients are conceptualized and treated as well as how the testing and diagnosis are experienced. At both the Brain Clinic and Health Center, the unique objectives and contexts of research-based memory clinics were palpable. The diagnostic settings and aims are integral to the processes by which memory loss is interpreted, portrayed, and subsequently narrated.

As a result of contemporary conceptualizations equating personhood with cognition, public perceptions presume a self annihilated by dementia.[5] Such pejorative representations flourish in the public media and scientific literature concerning Alzheimer's despite vehement and now abundant opposition from people with AD themselves.[6] These phenomena penetrate all aspects of our lives and serve as powerful ideological forces regardless of whether or not we have AD (or know someone who does). The less commonly acknowledged ways in which people with AD infiltrate medical and social practices that are the focus of this book, however, are of equal importance.

There has been extensive research on the effect and socially contingent nature of various medical conditions,[7] technologies,[8] and science more broadly.[9] These studies delineate the myriad factors constituting the social worlds of science and technology on the one hand, with people seeking medical care on the other. Disparate philosophies between those providing and seeking help in terms of the identification, meaning, and management of memory loss are crucial to the phenomenology of cognitive evaluation and subsequent diagnosis.

Although the decision to seek medical attention is often a negotiated process within families, in clinical practice persons with memory loss are often not granted much agency. Nonetheless, prior to coming to the Brain Clinic or Health Center, the individuals in this study were frequently involved in a lengthy process of coming to terms with what was commonly perceived as a gradual slowing of their minds. For most seniors, the recognition of memory loss was initially an internal dialogue, and for many it eventually progressed into a frank discussion with loved ones. While memory loss was a scary situation that led some to seek evaluation sooner than they might have done otherwise, for the majority of others it was an expected stage of the life course, leading them to the Brain Clinic or Health Center simply to ease their minds or to appease their families. Regardless of the reason for seeking evaluation, all study participants had experienced changes in their memory that they and/or their loved ones deemed significant.

Study narratives demonstrate a variety of reactions to and impressions of the battery of tests administered and the medical environment itself, especially the proverbial sterile and foreign atmospheres of clinical practice that structurally minimizes patient variation. Efforts at what Erving Goffman long ago coined "impression management" required the utilization of important strategies to ensure interactions that were familiar to them and to avoid being labeled incompetent. They were, in effect, actively engaged in Goffmanian presentations of self[10] despite the significant institutional and interactional obstacles ostensibly involved in conveying a self which was experiencing cognitive difficulties.

Reactions to diagnosis also cover a wide spectrum from shock to sadness, fear, and relief. The experience of being diagnosed, however, is intimately linked to the tone used, the information given, and the hope for the future depicted by the specific clinician rendering the diagnosis. Many study participants were as adept at navigating the interactions surrounding diagnosis as they were during the neuropsych testing process itself and undertook calculated efforts to ensure a perhaps more fundamental *preservation* of self[11] to combat the perceived threats the medical encounter presented for them.

Distinguishing So-Called Symptoms from Everyday Forgetfulness

People with memory difficulties described consistent complaints in managing their daily lives. Broadly, they noted trouble in the now well-documented areas: misplacing objects, repeating questions, missing appointments, or multitasking. In particular, finding words, remembering names, and recalling recent events were more challenging than they had been in the past. More extreme and less typical examples included taking thirty minutes to prepare a sandwich, not knowing how to turn the shower on, storing ice cream in the cupboard rather than the freezer, spooning pancake batter onto the stove top instead of into a pan, or using a knife in place of a fork. Potential patients reported changes in their everyday functioning and/or the effort involved in managing their interactions. An academic, salesman, doctor, and housewife—all in their 70s—noted the following significant changes, respectively: "I was an avid writer in the past but now words just don't come to me. I get trapped in my thinking. When I'm writing [the idea] just wilts away" (female, AD); "I am clumsier than I used to be. I can't find the words anymore and I am not as articulate" (male, AD); "I just feel like I'm constantly checking back on myself to see, did I do something or not? It makes me feel bad that my memory isn't so good, and it's frustrating because I can't do what I want to do" (female, AD); "The biggest changes are that I only cook simple meals, I am less social, and I have stopped driving" (female, MCI).

Countless other examples signaled noteworthy changes to study participants that ultimately led to their decision to seek cognitive evaluation: "I have all this information and I can't sort it out. I just have blank spaces" (male, AD); and "I've been a long-time bird-watcher and now I can't tell them apart" (male, MCI). These narratives reveal a keen subjective awareness of decline largely deemed absent in biomedical and media representations of the condition.

Despite the fact that they all eventually sought medical evaluation for their experiences, potential patients interpreted the presumed cause of these changes in various ways. A 72-year-old recently retired doctor told me, "I came to the clinic to find out if there were physical causes to my cognitive problems. And I'm concerned about Alzheimer's disease" (male, MCI). Another 68-year-old woman with an extensive family history of early-onset Alzheimer's candidly stated her reason for seeking evaluation as: "My memory is going away for no reason. It's getting a little scary here" (female, AD). In contrast, one gentleman stated simply: "I came here today because my wife wanted me to. I doubt there's anything really wrong" (AD).

The medicalization of memory loss risks conflating age-related and atypical memory loss. Everyone experiences at least occasional forgetfulness. Seniors who had watched their aging ancestors grow forgetful were particularly confused about where to draw the line between normal and abnormal memory loss. Ageism further conflates advanced age and memory loss.[12] Thus, unless there was a family history of Alzheimer's,[13] most people either delayed their medical visit or went seeking a stamp of approval that their forgetfulness was simply that which accompanies normal aging. A smartly dressed, professional-looking 77-year-old man succinctly summed up this sentiment: "One day I thought, 'Man, I'm forgetting a lot of stuff, and recent stuff.' I remember stuff from long ago. And then I heard about this program [at the specialty clinic]. . . . I came down here to get tested, wanting to be declared normal. That was my whole deal" (he was diagnosed with MCI). A 65-year-old social worker echoed this opinion: "I felt worried but I wasn't sure how much of a problem it [her memory loss] was." When I asked what made her come to the clinic, she said, "Well, I wanted to see if I could get better" (no formal diagnosis was given). Similarly, a health-seeking bachelor said he sought diagnosis "to learn how to prevent memory loss" (Mr. B, MCI). Mrs. V, a widowed retired academic who was planning for a future move into a wealthy assisted living facility said, "If I hadn't been going for an application to live at [name] and needed to do the cognitive testing, I never would've felt that what I was experiencing wasn't normal forgetfulness" (she was diagnosed with AD). Another retired professional ultimately diagnosed with MCI expressed his confusion: "I kind of blame myself a little bit, like, 'You should've known that!' or 'Why didn't you check your book?' I think it's hard to separate. I don't know whether to blame it on myself or just on the aging process." It is noteworthy that the last respondent never even mentions disease as a possible cause of his memory loss.

For many, interactions with their primary care physician exacerbated their confusion since their memory loss had often been classified as normal aging by them. Thus, the beliefs of their general practitioners often obfuscated, and routinely delayed, their seeking medical attention. This led many respondents to be skeptical of the validity of their cognitive workup or AD/MCI diagnosis. A savvy, personable yet serious 68-year-old man who did not recognize his future son-in-law at a large social gathering expressed a common opinion: "As far as I'm concerned, it's age. My doctor and my therapist both say it's just aging" (MCI). Others, like this divorced retiree, expressed their confusion over what constitutes pathological memory loss:

> I would talk to my doctors about it and they'd sort of smile, you know, "You walk down the hall and you forget why you went down there," that sort of thing. So I never took it too seriously until I began to realize it was perhaps affecting certain things that I do such as, I'm retired but I do all the book-keeping, paying the bills, and this and that, and appointments that I missed or something. It started to bother me that these things were happening because it was a new experience for me. (male, MCI)

Despite the reasons for seeking medical evaluation and any barriers thereto, the vast majority of seniors in the study held strong convictions about what it would mean to have a condition as devastating as "the A word." The fear they openly expressed included statements such as: "The biggest issue is I'm frightened to death of getting Alzheimer's." Ms. S, the single 80-year-old woman who made that statement, was one of the few people I observed who was not diagnosed with cognitive impairment. Regardless of whether they had personal experiences with someone who had AD, the concerns that reigned supreme for many mirrored the representations of the condition in biomedical science and the mass media. The stories of unmitigated tragedy are familiar to us all: complete dependence, loss of control, and annihilation of one's previous self. When asked what Alzheimer's meant to them, respondents echoed these sentiments of catastrophe: "I think of people with AD as handicapped" (female, MCI); "I'm really afraid of Alzheimer's, that I won't even recognize myself anymore" (male, AD); or "My aunt was very kind before she got Alzheimer's and the complete personality change was so hard to watch. She went from being really nice to something else and was no longer herself" (female, AD). More vivid descriptions were also common, like those from an 82-year-old widow and 70-year-old retired architect:

> It means devastation. Well, if it progresses more and I can't do what I need to do. I mean, all the things that I do normally, I mean so far, I want

to be able to do those [things]. And I've thought about, you know, the fact that I'm getting older and I will die one day. But I don't want to be an invalid for a long time before that. (female, AD).

[Alzheimer's] is a hell of a way to go. . . . There was a man who was in a book club with me, a couple's book club and he was a professor at Berkeley. A wonderful, charming man, lovely man. So he'd come to the meetings with his wife and he started not to make sense. And he developed into Alzheimer's. And he got terribly violent, it was so uncharacteristic of who he'd been. He would've been shocked to know. It was really terrible. (male, MCI)

Since pejorative societal perceptions of Alzheimer's prevail, many of the people seeking cognitive workup did so out of fear—to establish a baseline from which to compare any future decline. Indeed, many of my participants would be referred to as the worried well by social gerontologists. Clearly, these individuals were proactive in their health care and were savvy about such matters, which may not be reflective of a general population with less education, less affluence, and less access. Sociological research suggests, for example, that people for whom English is not their first language, who are from disadvantaged backgrounds, who have less formal education, who are ethnic minorities, and for whom medicine is not an organizing framework generally seek evaluation when their problems are much further advanced than their wealthier, more educated Caucasian counterparts.[14]

Importantly, respondents also had a certain faith in traditional medicine that resembled the quick fix mentality of many twenty-first-century Americans. Largely, these were people who either had a family history of dementia and/or wanted an expert both to verify that their experiences were real and to determine if they were abnormal. If their forgetfulness was deemed pathological, most of these health seekers were eager to find treatments that might help them and to enroll in research studies. A small but critical minority of respondents sought care at the request of their family and/or outright rejected biomedical interpretations of their forgetfulness. Ultimately, every study participant went to the clinic searching for an answer to the questions we all have about how much and what type of forgetting is normal.

Converting Forgetfulness into Alleged Symptoms

Cognitive evaluation is a process of transforming subjective experiences into standardized medical facts.[15] This redefinition also transfers the status of the forgetful person into a potential patient with Alzheimer's. As an important status passage,[16] being diagnosed with AD or MCI ascribes an identity of patient, which ultimately engenders the ability to implement the status as deemed necessary or desirable. In reality, however, even these promedicine health seekers felt compelled to perform significant interactional work to avoid assuming the role of patient—especially the deeply discredited Alzheimer's patient—as what symbolic interactionists call a master status. In so doing, people seeking evaluation played a role in shaping medical encounters and thought structures surrounding memory loss and diagnostics, which has consequences for biomedicine itself that will be discussed later.

Based on the clinical assumptions outlined in the previous chapter, the phenomenology of neuropsychological tests and diagnosis within the Brain Clinic and Health Center were similar. Narratives reveal experiences of the specialty clinics that are far outside the typical symbolic universe of respondents. The settings and interactions felt foreign, deficit-focused, and impersonal; some clinicians used harsh tones, scripted and convoluted terminology, and conveyed little hope; and potential patients worked to manage these dynamics during both the testing process and the delivery of a diagnosis (the latter of which will be discussed in the following chapter).

Facing Neuropsychological Tests

The environment within which the neuropsychological battery of tests was administered felt foreign to the overwhelming majority of respondents, and the sterile and uniform context created interactions that were awkward since typical norms of engagement did not apply. Following the characteristic standardization and routinization in clinical settings, questions were asked in a systematic manner with little, if any, room for anecdotal information, as my field notes portray:

Mrs. S, originally from the east coast, moved to the Bay Area 25 years ago and has since been widowed. She has no family nearby as both of her sons remained in Connecticut. She has been experiencing forgetfulness and is very [visibly] worried that it is Alzheimer's. Her Aunt had Alzheimer's and she has vivid memories of the toll it took. Mrs. S began telling [the neurologist] about her experiences with depression. This 80-year-old woman was talking about how she always wanted a daughter [her 2 daughters-in-law are not very involved in her life] and said that when she thinks about the miscarriage 45 years ago she gets particularly upset because maybe that would have been a girl [who would've helped her with her present troubles]. Mrs. S began to cry quietly. At almost the exact moment, the doctor's pager went off. He immediately grabbed the pager, looked at it, and picked up the phone without excusing himself or even making eye contact with Mrs. S. By the time he finished his call, she had fought back her tears and didn't bring up her depression again (nor did the doctor).

The inflexible, alien atmosphere of clinical testing generated various contingencies for those being evaluated. The remarks of Mrs. C, a slight, soft-spoken 76-year-old recent widow are illustrative: "Well, you've got me all off. I have no idea what's going on. I've never been through anything like this so I have no idea" (female, AD). In follow-up interviews with individuals diagnosed at the specialty clinics, this awkwardness was often reported to me: "[The testing process] was really hard. They were unlike other tests" (female, AD); "I never even knew there was such a thing as a 'cognitive test' before I went in there" (female, AD); and "It was awkward. I just felt uptight the whole time" (male, MCI).

Further, since this format does not permit the reciprocal dialogue typical of most conversations, people felt particularly bewildered. The cognitive evaluation was unlike any other encounter most participants had experienced in their lives. There was nothing to relate it to, as it was neither a standard medical visit nor a therapeutic one.

Respondents felt that the highly structured routine of clinical practice masked their individual variation (or even personhood), leaving them feeling like Marx's proverbial cogs in a wheel during a most vulnerable time. In this severely sterile environment, it was nearly impossible to discern the new interactional norms. What was clear (and in some cases even welcome) was the assumption of medical authority. As a result, my observations revealed that the evaluation process often felt impersonal, confusing, humiliating, and atypical, and the experience was exhausting and overwhelming for many. Interactions like the following were typical: "*Now we're going to play with some blocks here. Some are all red, some are all white, and some are half and half. I'll make a design and you watch me and then make the same one*" (Clinical Research Coordinator; field notes); and "*Now let's go back one step. What are the words you repeated after me? Patient: I'm too tired to even think. Clinician: You don't remember?*" (Neuropsychologist; field notes).

When I conducted follow-up interviews with Mr. R (from the prologue), a 69-year-old housewife, and a 70-year-old recently retired businesswoman, they corroborated my observational data.

> I think she needs to improve some of her practice and I think she could get a better feeling for the person she's talking to, as a psychiatrist. I didn't feel at all that I was talking to a psychiatrist. It was all medical, just straight medical. (male, MCI)

> I don't think she's that busy to be that uptight and so hard and fast because I didn't see that much activity there [at the clinic]. (female, MCI)

> I complained to [the tester] about having to draw these lines and everything, which I never could have done in the beginning. Unless I could have a ruler so that I could measure and, you know, do it that way. Just free hand, there's no way I could ever have done it. And she just said, "Well, some of us don't have gifts in certain areas." (female, AD)

These quotes illustrate a reliance on heavily rehearsed scripts that left many potential patients feeling the clinicians were robotic and they themselves were "like a number" rather than a person.

When doctors did things like answering phone calls or pagers while talking with potential patients or using digital timers that would beep when the time allotted for a task had elapsed, study participants felt exceedingly uncomfortable. On occasion, clinicians were observed not responding to questions asked or salutations offered, as shown in the exchanges below with a soft-spoken, eager-to-please woman and an earnest retired professor of finance, both in their mid-70s:

CLINICIAN: Write a sentence, anything.
POTENTIAL PATIENT [writes]: "Have a great day!"
CLINICIAN [Without even acknowledging the sentence]: Okay, now take this paper, fold it in half, and place it on the table.

CLINICIAN: Do you think you're depressed? Do you feel sad?
POTENTIAL PATIENT: I don't know the definition of depression.
CLINICIAN [without hesitating or looking up, clinician reads monotonously from her form]: Do you feel down for no reason, are you crying, do you feel life is not worth living, do you feel hopeless or helpless?

Clearly, such strange interactions were disorienting for many people and arguably exacerbated the level of anxiety and discomfort during evaluation for at least some.

A related concern was that the prescribed nature of the interaction did not allow for acknowledgment of personal variation regarding things such as education, native language, and prior difficulties with test taking in general or with specific areas being targeted. Some respondents, for example, noted that they had always had trouble with names or calculations and did not feel this was taken into consideration on the tests, which would inevitably deem such shortcomings as symptomatic and "marks against me." Despite the fact that clinicians adjust (statistically) for age and education when quantifying the test results in practice, the impersonal testing environment at the Brain Clinic and Health Center led people taking the tests to feel there was little done to account for idiosyncratic differences regarding these matters.

Whether or not respondents were subsequently diagnosed with AD/MCI, almost without exception they felt they had done poorly on the tests. Arguably, the awkward and for some dehumanizing encounter in which they were tested shaped these views. For participants, this exchange initiated the process of thinking of themselves as potential patients. Mrs. R, from the prologue, was a 67-year-old recently retired kindergarten teacher who was subsequently not diagnosed with any cognitive impairment. Nonetheless, the following quote reflects a common interpretation of the testing process and supports prior claims that "the diagnostic process can be distressing, alarming, and stigmatizing":[17]

> It was daunting to take those tests. You know, you feel like you're not do-ing well but you don't know. On the one where there were the stories and you had to recall, when I was into the next story I was back still wonder-ing about stuff from the previous story. I couldn't let it go. And there was one of the tri-tests (that's what I call it because we had a kindergarten thing that was similar to that, matching the pattern) and I couldn't get that one at all.

Others who were ultimately less fortunate in terms of the eventual test results corroborated this sentiment, reflecting an incipient perception of patienthood. A health-seeking lifetime bachelor living alone, an austere museum docent with a substantially younger second wife, and a retired carpenter all reported an awareness that they were not performing well: "I knew I wasn't doing well. Maybe the trouble I was having, maybe some of it was my brain changing with age, but I think some of it was like stage fright" (male, MCI); "[The clinicians] gave me a list, like a number of names and words and how many of them can you remem-ber, and I didn't remember as many as I thought I should. I thought I should have remembered more" (male, MCI); and "I thought I'd have the brains enough to do it in seconds. It's not hard for anybody else, I know. They're all so easy and I can't do it" (male, dementia of unknown etiology).

Some felt that this realization added further pressure and angst to the already unnerving experience of being cognitively evaluated. In the words of a widowed homemaker, a visual artist, a public speaker, and a retired physician, "stage fright" was exacerbated by the situation: "[Be-cause I knew I wasn't doing well] I probably concentrated harder on the test, trying extra hard to do it" (female, MCI); "Especially when you feel that the people who are giving the test are being negative, [it] makes it almost impossible [to do well]" (male, AD); "I thought [the clinician] was kind of hard and cold. I didn't warm up to her very much. I think maybe that was some of the trouble when I went to see her. I kind of clammed up" (male, MCI); and "I was really nervous. I was anxious to know how I was doing" (female, AD).

An additional factor discussed by respondents was the experience of having something medically wrong with your brain as opposed to other body parts. While many people seeking medical evaluation for their memory feared a possible AD diagnosis, others cherished their physical health. In large part, this may be connected to a person's views on age-related memory loss, public perceptions of Alzheimer's, and the independence associated with being ambulatory. Suggesting a Cartesian dualism, concerns of losing competency were evident in statements such as "Every one of your areas is important to you, but if you have trouble with your brain the others aren't going to work" (male, MCI); and "Having your *brain* tested is deeply personal. If there's something wrong with my brain, there's something wrong with *me*" (female, AD; emphasis in the original). The primacy of one's brain over other body parts was also commonly voiced, as it is by Mrs. V from this chapter's opening field notes:

> Despite being really healthy physically, I am lacking mentally and that is really hard for me. I don't want to be known for my intellectual shortcomings. (female, AD)

Likewise, Mr. N, a 76-year-old museum docent with a wife 22 years his junior:

> MR. N: If it's my knee to me that's mechanical and today you can put a new knee in there.
>
> RB: How is that different with your brain?
>
> MR. N: Well, first of all, the thought of their even going in there [brain] and looking at it is inconceivable. But if the knee doesn't work I still have my brain, I can still think and talk and communicate but with a problem in my brain nothing else will work. Nothing else can work. I don't know, some is mechanical and some is more personal.
>
> RB: Are you saying that compared to the rest of your body there is something about your mind that is different than any other part of your body?
>
> MR. N: Absolutely, as I say, I could function with, I mean, Christopher Reeves gets around but if he didn't have his brain . . . (male, MCI)

On the other hand, trepidation over pain or losses due to physical impairment was also expressed in statements such as "Fortunately, everything physically works. It's just my mind. I guess if I was a writer it would be a problem, but I'm physically dexterous and I'm certainly . . . very comfortable" (Mrs. B, AD); and "I'm just glad it's only my mind. I have no pain" (male, AD). A staunchly independent 77-year-old woman who was widowed early in her marriage and raised two children on her own discussed the problem in great detail:

> I want to be able to drive. I want to be able to go to my exercise class. I want to be able to do pottery. I want to be able to do my own shopping and cooking. I am very fortunate and I am content. . . . I'm physically well; I don't have any ailments. I can still do my exercises and whatever I want to do. (female, AD)

For others, the location of their problems exacerbated their circumstances since being physically healthy made their troubles invisible, and therefore it was more difficult to get support when needed. Mr. S, a 72-year-old bachelor, offers an interesting perspective:

> I think those handicapped people are lucky. They *look* like it so they get help but I look healthy but I'm not and people don't understand me. When I say I have memory problems, people don't know what that means; they don't help me. (male, other cognitive impairment)

These quotes suggest a dichotomy between the supremacy of mind or body for individuals diagnosed with pathological memory loss; that is, based on social values and individual beliefs, brain disorders appear to be the ultimate assault or the lesser of two evils. For most, of course, it is somewhere in between or perhaps even vacillates back and forth according to context (e.g., in social settings versus at home, with intimates versus strangers).

Employing Strategies to Preserve the Self

As a result of the negative experiences outlined above, many of my respondents resisted assuming the relegated status of Alzheimer's patient by making deliberate efforts to try and combat the awkwardness and prevent themselves from feeling degraded. Phrases such as: "Right off I'm sunk," "There's just nothing up there," and "That's just a wild guess" were common responses when an individual did not know the answer to a given test question. Subtle strategies such as statements like "I was not listening, I don't know," "That's a good question," and "The details I wouldn't remember," as well as asking the clinician to repeat questions were also observed regularly. In addition to these rhetorical tactics, field notes also reveal more concrete strategies such as using humor, noting deficits openly, and making references to past achievements during the testing process: *"The short term memory just . . . isn't there. That's why I'm here (laughing)—didn't they tell ya?"* (male, AD); *"I'm not very good on my animals either. I'm supposed to know that. I really don't know my animals"* (female, AD); *"[Memory] is my worst thing in the world. I think I'm getting all nervous"* (female, AD); *"It's discouraging when your mind can't remember things that used to be so easy. I used to be able to memo-rize long poems"* (female, AD); *"I've forgotten how to do it. And I used to be a math whiz in school"* (male, AD); and *"I used to be considered real bright. I used to be a petroleum engineer but now I've lost it!"* (female, AD). Mr. H, a 77-year-old retired manual laborer and one of the few working-class participants in the study, was not at all subtle in express-ing his dismay:

> MR. H: I really graduated and everything but it's been a long time ago. Nobody can't do that [calculations]. This is stupid! Don't let nobody see this. I flunked. Does everyone do this bad?
> CLINICIAN: Everyone does their best and there's a range.
> MR. H: This is really making me feel bad. I didn't give you much. (male, dementia of unknown etiology)

As Goffman argued long ago, in everyday interactions if one party pauses too long, perseverates, or cannot recall something, then the per-son's interlocutor will typically fill in the holes in an effort to remove the social awkwardness and/or to restart a stunted conversation. This back-and-forth symbolizes the joint interaction and reciprocity of daily encounters. In clinical practice, however, cognitive evaluations do not follow such norms. As a result, while potential patients employed the standard strategies we all use when gaffes are made, interactional tensions arise when clinicians fail to assist in easing the awkwardness caused by forgetfulness.

Consequently, many people came to feel less than, if not outright inept, in the process of having their memory loss evaluated. For people who were nervous test takers or generally worried, the environment often intensified their anxiety and they felt deeply exposed. In response, all individuals undergoing evaluation at these specialty clinics—whether ultimately diagnosed or not—struggled to manage their interactions to circumvent taking on the identity of being demented or incompetent, an objective they achieved with varying degrees of success.

Internalizing the Test Results

Participants also had various reactions to the testing process. Many were frustrated and afraid of their own failings, while others expressed feeling weak or vulnerable at the hands of the clinicians who were unimpaired, "looking for flaws," and "eager to check boxes." Potential patients responded with shame, embarrassment, and anger at the inability to perform at previous levels. During the neuropsych testing, a wide range of emotions were observed. For example, Mr. H berated himself, Mr. A was deeply ashamed, and Mrs. V was incredulous, respectively:

> I don't know what happened to my brains. God, I hate this stuff. That's catching me. Until I came into this room, I was happy. Now it's very stupid! (male, dementia of unknown etiology)

> Never in my life did I think something like this would stop me. This is my worst thing ever. (male, AD)

> Boy, I feel like an idiot. I don't know why I can't do it. . . . cherries, I got cherries again, pliers, god, this is tough—maybe that's why I'm here. I can only get so many words and then I just blank. . . . drill, peaches, I thought it was gonna be ball but didn't. I lose it, once you go to the next thing— cherries, pliers, god I can't get any farther. It's not there. I can't believe I can't list 4–5 words at a time, or 12–15. (female, AD)

Follow-up interviews echoed these sentiments. Mr. C, for example, was clearly still disturbed by the tests when I interviewed him almost three weeks later, and remnants of Mrs. B's feelings of shame are evident over a month after the testing occurred.

> [Doing poorly on the calculations on the test] bothered me because I worked in retail all my life and I could do figures up and down and back and forwards, and I would get upset with some of these kids, that they couldn't count out even change, I would get upset about that [and yet I couldn't do it]. (male, MCI)

> I don't want to waste time. I don't want to repeat myself. It's embarrassing. (female, AD)

For many people, testing was an arduous process, which upon completion seemed to demonstrate blatant problems (even to those who were ultimately not diagnosed). Given the intention of uncovering a deficit, potential patients felt surveilled and judged on tasks they knew to be their greatest weakness. Mr. C and Mrs. B went on to reveal the sense of fatalism many respondents expressed, "It's awful . . . because the clinician will put it down as a step towards Alzheimer's and you're just saying you can't remember. And then some I remembered later, but it was too late" (male, MCI); and "They [the clinicians] seemed as though they were just there to make it hard for me" (female, AD). More detailed descriptions of this Sisyphean process were also elaborated, including by these two women with commendable support networks (coming with a husband and daughter, in the first case, and four daughters and one son, in the second):

> The tests pointed out my weakest place. They went to my worst area. They focused on my shortcomings and I like to excel and it's hard [for me] not to. I'm healthy physically, I don't have physical problems and it's mentally that I have trouble and that's what the tests focused on, so they were really hard for me. (female, AD)

> MRS. M: We went up to the big hospital and I had to go in for an overall, for all day. And they were trying to pick out all sorts of things like

> memory loss and other things like that. At that time I found it very
> unpleasant in the way they put it and the way they were asking. They
> were trying to prove that I did not have the possibility to have the
> memory that I knew I had.
>
> RB: Are you saying you think they were focusing on your mistakes?
>
> MRS. M: Yeah, yeah.
>
> RB: How did that feel?
>
> MRS. M: Frustrating is probably a mild way to put it. (female, AD)

In this way, potential patients vehemently contested such deficiency perspectives[18] equating them with their shortcomings on the tests. They recognized some degree of impairment; that is why *they had sought evaluation* in the first place. Nonetheless, study participants felt the tests were overwhelmingly focused on finding or highlighting their deficits rather than their strengths and nowhere was there room to account for personal characteristics (such as a lifelong inability to recall names, compute math, or general test anxiety) or environmental constraints (like the awkward, anxiety-provoking test setting).

Despite personal variability between clinicians at the centers, respondents had strikingly similar experiences of the neuropsychological tests relied upon to determine their level of cognitive functioning. In particular, the standardized testing environment engendered feelings of awkwardness, confusion, nervousness, and a sense of being degraded. Perhaps most significantly, this was true *whether or not they were ultimately diagnosed*. There was a perceived emphasis on deficit, a sense of fatalism, and general indifference that failed to account for individual variation. To combat these experiences, people seeking medical care for their memory actively and deliberately employed strategies to manage their interactions *well in advance of receiving the test results* to avoid taking on the master status of the demented person or Alzheimer's patient. Such stigma avoidance strategies included using humor, showing awareness of their deficits, and making references to their past achievements. These strategies proved to be an instrumental mechanism for their perceived preservation of self in the face of the assumed incompetence they confronted during clinical evaluation.

People who seek medical evaluation for their memory loss undergo a lengthy battery of neuropsychological tests to determine the cause and severity of their forgetfulness. Being cognitively evaluated was a significant status passage for seniors in this study. As the first step to seeing oneself as an Alzheimer's patient (even potentially), the testing process was of paramount social and personal significance. These findings delineate the initial establishment of a long process of identity transformation that starts the moment someone opens the door at the memory clinic.

The clinical assumptions of standardization, patient incompetence, and patient management outlined in the previous chapter are evident during the evaluation process. After completing what amounts to a degradation ceremony, most respondents—even those not subsequently diagnosed—do envision their forgetfulness as a problem or disease, and consider themselves a patient of neurology/psychiatry; that is, medicalization works by (re)shaping not only the knowledge about AD/MCI (as the previous chapter outlines) but the knowledge of self and aging as well.

The experiences of these tests were based on clinical, social, and personal factors. Respondents resoundingly reported that both the atmosphere and clinicians were sterile, foreign, and impersonal during the testing process, as is well documented in bioethics and the medical social sciences. Since respondents had various levels of confidence in the ability of the clinicians to quantify and evaluate their forgetfulness, they experienced the evaluation process differently depending on the views they held about memory loss, aging, and disease, and their relationships with the doctors in general and the clinicians at the specialty clinic in particular. Most respondents resisted some of the negative associations during the tests by deliberately making efforts to manage their identities in a way they found more consistent with how they defined themselves and that was less threatening socially. In particular, using humor, acknowledging deficits, and referencing past achievements were tactics respondents implemented during the testing process. Such strategic efforts at impression management are noteworthy, considering the prevalence of assumptions that cognitively impaired persons are incapable both of such volition and the means by which to demonstrate it.

5

Hearing "the A Word"

The Road to Becoming an Alzheimer's Patient

With few exceptions, the individuals who participated in my study came into the clinic hoping to have concerns about their minor memory difficulties put to rest—chalked up to age, ideally. For most of them, sadly, that hope was shattered with just two words.

In stark contrast to the restlessness I feel when watching someone struggle to come up with answers on the neuropsych exam, after hearing someone get the news that they have Alzheimer's 41 times, the experience still immobilizes me. I have grown accustomed to the moment that my mouth dries out, even though I enter the room knowing in advance what they will be told. And, of course, the painfully long silence and blank stares that I have, without exception, observed following the utterance of the words "Alzheimer's disease."— Field notes

Over a decade after observing my first respondent being diagnosed with Alzheimer's, I can vividly recall the physical reactions and stifling silence that felt like hours each and every time I watched it. I often felt that the person being diagnosed heard not a single word after those two dreaded ones.

Using So-Called Medical Facts as a Status Passage

Assuming Abnormality

Despite the trend of earlier diagnosis, very little research has been done to understand what it is like to be diagnosed. Not surprisingly, the nearly fifty individuals I observed undergoing a cognitive workup and/or with whom I conducted qualitative in-depth interviews after diagnosis, depicted the event of being given the news of their condition as momentous. Obviously, going through the testing is an important status passage, or turning point,[1] for persons who will eventually take on an Alzheimer's identity. American sociologist Howard Becker argued, in his seminal study of criminal deviance, that the process of being caught and labeled deviant by a person in a position of authority was the most crucial step on the road to accepting the master status of a deviant, or outsider.[2] Likewise, being evaluated and diagnosed by a medical professional is critical to assuming the status of Alzheimer's patient. Medicalization works by informing not merely the knowledge of practitioners (as outlined in chapter 3) but also the self-knowledge of potential patients. Status passages are fundamental to social processes, structures, organizations, and interactions. Since meanings materialize from all parties participating in the diagnostic process, the degree to which experiences were medicalized by potential patients fell along a continuum.

Due to the prescribed clinical processes of evaluating memory loss and the various personal reactions, the experience of receiving a diagnosis served as a second status passage, which could be desirable or undesirable, voluntary or involuntary, individual or collective, and self- or other-initiated.[3] There are varying but limited amounts of control for the individual being evaluated and the potential passage was legitimized by a medical label. In the tradition of status passages, the centrality of the label differs significantly for potential patients. The idiosyncratic, interpretive role of status passages, then, allows for the intentional orchestration of assorted strategies for managing the information being received and the interactions based on them in a manner similar to that used during the testing process itself.

During the rite of passage amounting to a degradation ceremony[4] that people found themselves involved in, potential patients were transformed into ill people. This ascribed role was given meaning by the clinician rendering a medical label. The clinician's tone, the information given, and the prognosis conveyed shaped the experience of diagnosis for potential patients and families alike. Since the subjective experiences of being told the diagnosis were significantly influenced by all these factors, the overall variation between respondents diagnosed with AD/MCI was profound. For many, however, the strategies used to avoid taking on the master status of diseased person or Alzheimer's patient were particularly pervasive in this context. The clinical assumptions of standardization, patient incompetence, and patient management outlined in chapter 3 were palpable at this stage of the process and both potential patients and their families expressed their dissatisfaction with this (as we saw with Mr. and Mrs. R in the prologue).

Although far more visible at the Health Center, both specialty clinics utilized a formulaic set of procedures for delivering a diagnosis of AD/MCI. With varying degrees of emphasis, clinicians explained the test results, distinguished them from normal aging, labeled a medical condition, if applicable, and made treatment recommendations. The belief that deficits could be quantified was standard at both centers and perhaps best demonstrated in the rhetorical devices clinicians employed to justify the diagnostic label of Alzheimer's, as these common strategies from my field notes reveal: *"Many of the things you're experiencing fit the pattern, fit certain deficits. Memory certainly is a problem,"* or *"Your results were not as good as they should've been."*

For mild cognitive impairment, the discourse tended to be slightly less medicalized yet was still reflected as an observable, standardized pattern of deficit (that is, as a discernable medical fact). As my fieldnotes depict: *"When we evaluate tests, we see if there are patterns. How we relate that is that the disease causes impairment here and not there, etcetera. You do not have a pattern for Alzheimer's, Picks, or other diseases"* (71-year-old male, other cognitive impairment); *"You're not fitting a clear picture of Alzheimer's"* (87-year-old female, MCI); and *"We did find on the neuropsych testing that there were some problems on memory. . . . It's not quite as good as we'd expect for someone of your age and education"* (76-year-old man, AD).

The clinical notion that there is a typical and observable *pattern* of memory loss simultaneously normalized and medicalized the symptoms a person was experiencing as part of the biomedical lexicon. Although this may have served to manage the uncertainty of (or provide "order" to) an otherwise overwhelming circumstance for some people, being compartmentalized was very troubling for countless others, especially those who felt that memory loss was a normal accompaniment to aging. Such claims to expert knowledge led some to feel surveilled and potentially suspect of medical intentions.

Becoming a Partial Person

Unfortunately, when an individual is given a diagnosis of AD/MCI, he or she also embarks on a career or trajectory[5] of incompetent or at least soon-to-be incompetent person or "patient." Often both the delivery of the information and the recommendations made were unfortunately aimed more at the family members present than the older individual him/herself. In the clinical efforts at patient management, the details of the diagnosis were too often directed at family members or informants, who were systematically recruited to help handle and monitor the behavior of the patient postdiagnosis. The experience of Mr. and Mrs. R in the prologue illustrates this aptly. During their follow-up interview, they spontaneously brought this up with me:

> MR. R: [When I got the diagnosis] I was shocked and I was really annoyed that [the clinician] was not talking to me, rather than to [my wife]. She wasn't even looking at me the entire time until I said something; it was like I wasn't there. I had to tell her, "Look at me."

When I directed my eyes at Mrs. R, without skipping a beat she said,

> MRS. R: It's true. I felt the same way. [The clinician] was making [the diagnosis] to me, like I was a caregiver of his, which I'm definitely not. I may be some day, or he may be a caregiver of me, but . . . not yet.

In contrast, my field notes also revealed doctors explaining to family members how certain behaviors were symptomatic of the disease and thus the diagnosed individuals were not to blame. Mr. T, for example, came to the clinic with complaints of memory loss and a strained relationship with his wife. Shortly after retiring a few years prior, Mr. T seemingly lost interest in all the plans they had for travel and adventure during their retirement.

> *Clinician [to wife]: As far as his lack of motivation, it's not that he doesn't want to (and the same with his irritability too)—it's just part of it. It's not him; it is part of the disease.*

> Clinician [to Mr. T and daughter]: Apathy or low motivation are actually symptoms. These are injured in the process of memory problems [that's why he is not motivated].

During the delivery of a diagnosis in research-based specialty practice, the assumptions of standardization and patient incompetence proved to be essential instruments in the process of patient management. Once patient management was assured, the preliminary step to the making of research subjects was solidified. Whether or not the status passage resulted in the acceptance of the role of patient—what Howard Becker referred to as a master status—or not, without a diagnosis the legitimacy of partaking in drug trials, for example, would not exist.

Embarking on the Path of Alzheimer's

Receiving a medical diagnosis for one's atypical experiences has been found to serve a number of important functions, both personally and socially.[6] The reported advantages of a dementia diagnosis include "developing a better understanding of the situation, an end to uncertainty, the ability to plan, access to practical and emotional support, and the chance to develop positive coping strategies."[7] For some individuals, being diagnosed removes the blame and responsibility associated with abnormal or otherwise inexplicable behaviors. Consequently, previously suspect actions are legitimized; for example, they are not going crazy or being recalcitrant, they have a disease. The social function of a medical diagnosis is to allow access to the resources and compassion they are entitled to by definition of their disease. Talcott Parsons's historic "sick role" status,[8] and the accompanying temporary release from social responsibilities, is deemed appropriate for those found deficient via bona fide medical evaluation and not for those with emergent, contested, or undiagnosed ailments.[9] Unfortunately, an inherent tension exists in that what is routine for doctors (searching for deficit and giving bad news) is deeply personal and often cataclysmic for individual patients and their families. In this way, clinical routinization constructs an irreconcilable difference between cases and biographies[10] that leaves many respondents trying to resist being seen as a generic object of medicine or feeling stigmatized and/or lacking in autonomy and control.

Variables related to both the specific clinician rendering the diagnosis and the individual receiving it, however, significantly influenced subjective experiences of the diagnosis, of course. Given the clinician variation discussed in chapter 3, numerous factors potentially affected reactions to the diagnosis, including the tone used, the information relayed, the prognosis given, and the setting of the evaluation.

Reacting to the Tone

The general tone used by the clinician was easily detected and significantly affected most people's experience of receiving the diagnosis. Ultimately, many respondents perceived an impending doom. Such derogatory insinuations led to strong reactions such as, "[The diagnosis] was like she was reading a death notice to me"; "It felt like it was an execution"; and "It sounded imminent to me. I felt like, 'Well I hope I make it through the year.'" Not incidentally, all three of these quotes are from persons diagnosed with MCI, and were corroborated by family members, especially spouses such as Mrs. R from the prologue: "I was ready to have [my husband] get all of our affairs in order. . . . In case he wasn't able to think in six months or something. You know, I just didn't know." Reactions to the pejorative framing of now bona fide patients and the search for deficit were also problematic. The perceived sterile and exclusively deficit-based reporting disturbed Mr. D especially, "[The tone of the diagnosis] was quite negative . . . this kind of looking at you negatively and finding the bad rather than the good" (male, AD). Likewise, both Mr. C and Mrs. B struggled with the grim atmosphere and being reduced to their presumed shortcomings, "I was down after [the diagnosis] because of the [negative] way she reported it" (male, MCI); and "When I had my MRI at Kaiser the doctor said that there were some minor things and all, but not to worry right now at all. That they were minor. And I think that's what [the clinician] saw, and she made it major" (female, MCI). Interestingly, as these quotes suggest, many of the respondents who had negative reactions to the tone used by clinicians were not even diagnosed with Alzheimer's, but with MCI.

There were also a number of strong reactions to the impersonal nature of the delivery of the diagnosis itself. For some, this added to their feelings of discomfort while others simply saw it as unfortunate. The following detached scenarios, while outliers statistically speaking, are illustrative. My observations of Dr. P, who was nearing the end of his neurology residency, suggested a brusque, impersonal tone:

> *Clinician: Overall, your neuropsych testing is most consistent with what we'd see with early Alzheimer's . . . an MRI would be nice—to differentiate between AD and vascular dementia [note: this is the first time he had mentioned either term]. Overall you are doing well. You are doing the right things.*
>
> *[He stands up, abruptly shakes her hand, and leaves the room. The entire exchange takes less than five minutes.]*

This was the thirty-second time I had watched someone get such news yet I found myself sitting there feeling the same way Ms. K, the potential patient, presumably did: immobilized by shock and battered by the whirlwind storm that had just descended. This pleasant 72-year-old woman had come to the Brain Clinic alone. Of all the diagnoses I had observed, this one hit me the hardest. It felt like an eternity passed before I gathered my senses enough to look blankly at Ms. K. The silence was stifling yet neither of us seemed able to think of anything to say. I did not know this woman. Eventually I stood up, walked over to her, touched her arm, and asked her if there was anything I could do to help, although I already knew the answer. She shook her head no, looked at her feet. I said goodbye and left her alone in the office. I do not know how long she stayed in that room.—Field notes

A follow-up interview with Mr. and Mrs. K after he was diagnosed with AD at the Health Center depicted a similarly blasé approach to rendering what for many is probably the worse news they can imagine.

> Mrs. K: We went to the doctor and they tested him and everything else was fine except short-term memory, which was nonexistent. And so he had a mild dementia but we just kept on doing things. And then finally we went back to his doctor, and I asked his doctor, "What are we dealing with here?" And his doctor walked . . . to the desk [looked at something] and he turned and looked over his shoulder and said, "I think it is Alzheimer's"—just like that. (female, husband diagnosed with AD)

The response to such impersonal interactions was palpable, again evidenced in the case of Mr. and Mrs. R from the prologue. The following exchange took place during my second follow-up interview with them over two months later:

RB: Have you given much thought to your visit to the [Health Center] now that you've seen your PCP and he says it's just normal memory loss?

MR. R: I thought she was just reporting. I didn't get any feeling of personal contact from her.

MRS. R: Empathy.

MR. R: Empathy. That's a good word.

MRS. R: [There was] no empathy.

RB: How did you feel when she was discussing your test results?

MR. R: I was angered! I wanted to know what was happening and all, but I didn't like the way she was telling it. I wanted her to *talk to me* [emphasis in the original].

MRS. R: She [the clinician] doesn't come through. She really didn't seem to be working with patients. She was just analyzing and giving, what do you call it? A diagnosis. But it was all clinical.

Perhaps most interesting, these reactions were reported by potential patients whether they were ultimately diagnosed with anything or not. Importantly, this was also true for family members, such as Mrs. R: "I wondered, 'What in the world is going on here? [The clinician's] acting like he's not a person.'" The environment in which the diagnosis was rendered affected individuals strongly and in a variety of ways. Many respondents detected a fatalistic and impersonal tone, which shaped their phenomenological experiences of the diagnosis.

Absorbing the Details

The amount and/or type of information an individual wanted to know about his or her condition, and occasionally even the diagnosis itself, differed between potential patients. While some people wanted all the details they could garner, others preferred learning a bit at a time to prevent being overwhelmed. As an observer, I found that an individual's stance could usually be discerned by the number of questions they asked after receiving the diagnosis. Whereas some people had numerous questions, most thanked the clinician and left abruptly after receiving the diagnosis. A few respondents acknowledged the tension over knowing how much information to share, such as one 88-year-old retired businessman:

> I think that's always a problem with doctors, to know how much of it to tell. We have a friend who's just been told that he probably has one to five years to live. And he says, "You know, I wish they hadn't told me." And somehow, I guess, that doctor must have thought that this person wanted to hear. And I think it's a tough call. (male, MCI)

In particular, whether or not the word Alzheimer's was used varied between clinicians. On occasion, this led to confusion when study participants were trying to make sense of it postdiagnosis. Ms. M, a calm, diminutive 82-year-old woman with long white hair in braids, said: "I'm not sure that they ever came right out and said Alzheimer's. They seemed to do a lot of skittering around. But I think it's sort of taken for granted that that's what it is" (female, AD). Likewise, Mr. Z, a tall, smartly dressed 69-year-old gay man matter-of-factly stated:

> I'm not sure if they actually used the word Alzheimer's or not, but there was a period there of maybe three or four months in which I really didn't know what I was doing. And the one thing I remembered the doctor saying was that they've tried everything else so you must have Alzheimer's. (male, AD)

For some individuals, the details about the test results were actually more important than the diagnosis being given. Mrs. R, from the prologue, had this to say:

> Because of my educational background [as a kindergarten teacher], I would have liked to see the [test] results. You know, "This is what you scored on this and this is what it means on this test." But you don't [get that]. You just get told you did well or you did poorly. That's pretty amor-

phous. [Also] I do think that I could have had a little better understanding of what some of the tests were that they were giving me. I think that would be one little bit of feedback . . . that would really help me. Let us know a little bit more specifically what those tests were. (female, no cognitive impairment)

As Mr. and Mrs. R's case highlights, many respondents wished they had more time to process what had been said to them that day. Over two months after receiving the MCI diagnosis at the Health Center, the emotion was still palpable despite recently being informed by his PCP that it was not AD.

> MR. R: It was clinical and she just poured it out and that was it. "Here it
>   is! Take it or leave it!"
> RB: And then she said goodbye?
> MR. R: Well, she did say, "How do you feel about this? Do you have
>   questions?" . . . I think she did ask if we had questions, but I was kind
>   of in shock or something. I didn't know what to say to her.
> MRS. R: I guess [one recommendation] would be to block out a little
>   longer time for that final interview, so that we could have time for
>   what she said to soak in. [Give us] long enough to get back to her. I
>   think that would help a little bit. . . . It takes a little processing to hear
>   what she had to say. And I don't think we had time to really process. I
>   would have liked an extra five minutes or something to think about it
>   [to decide if I had any questions].

Often, feelings of being rushed or general confusion resulted from the use of scientific and/or vague rhetoric, as the following field note excerpts from resident neurologists suggest:

> *Memory is in the hippocampus, we like to think about where things reside in the brain. Visual spatial is the right parietal. And tasks, changing track are in the frontal region. Memory and visual spatial are typical of AD. Frontal is not so typical of AD, but not unheard of. You fit #1, #2, and #3 diagnosis of AD yet you are better in some places not expected. It's a little bit of a mixed bag, but we agree overall with the AD diagnosis.*

The PET tells if there is low metabolism or low energy weight within the brain but doesn't tell if there is actual atrophy [decrease in size] or shrinking.

This demonstrates how the unfamiliar jargon drawn from discourse based in medical vernacular was confusing and impersonal to many people who underwent evaluation.

Consequently, the use of diagnostic ambiguity in the clinics, of it being "a mixed bag," for example, satisfied some potential patients while disconcerting others. Whereas a few respondents were either suspicious of such tactics or used them to justify the seemingly arbitrary nature of the diagnosis, far more interpreted such elusiveness as indicative of the promising nature of emergent science (the latter of which will prove important to assuming Alzheimer's identities in the following chapter). Phrases like the following from my field notes were particularly common during diagnoses by neurologists at the Brain Clinic:

To be honest, we don't know enough about what these things look like. There are over 200 causes of dementia. Of dementia today, 50 percent are AD, 30 percent are multi-farct [or small mini-strokes], and the remainder is something else.

We see that something is going on but we have no reason to think it's even predementia. Some people with MCI go on to develop dementia and some don't. It's a new term and we don't know who is going to go on to dementia and who is not.

And truthfully, it's not possible to diagnosis 100 percent—we can just see how well it fits for typical cases. In the majority of cases, if we can't pin it down, it's a good thing. If it's a tumor, bleeding, stroke, AD—we are familiar with that and can treat it.

As with the amount of information given, the employment of ambiguity as a strategy to manage the medical uncertainty of associated behaviors subsequently led many individuals in my study to have unanswered questions even months after the diagnosis was made. Such misunderstandings remained after they left the clinician's office and new ones also surfaced. Although some questions were very specific, there were fundamental misconceptions regarding the actual diagnosis given and subsequent prognosis. While general diagnostic confusion surrounded Alzheimer's diagnoses, my field notes and follow-up interviews demonstrate that MCI was particularly fraught:

Clinician: Do you have any questions?

Mrs. A: The thing that bothers me the most is the Alzheimer's disease. I don't fully understand if I have it or not. It sounds like you're saying it's coming.

Clinician: It's either in the brain or not. I would bet that you do. If there were a test, I'd do it but there isn't.

Mrs. A: What does that mean?

Clinician: I'm trying to be honest with you but admit that we don't know everything. If new meds came out to treat AD, I'd want you to have them. (female, MCI)

RB: What were you told about your memory [at the clinic]?

MR. C: They gave me the closest thing to a failing grade as they could. In other words, they call it . . . [long pause] do you know the term that they use?

RB: Was it Mild Cognitive Impairment?

MR. C: Yes.

RB: Did it seem to you that it would be a precursor for anything else?

MR. C: Well, that was the biggest question. Yes, I didn't know whether it would or would not.

RB: And you left there not knowing that?

MR. C: Yeah, yeah, because they didn't dwell on the subject. The word came up a couple of times but not much. (male, MCI)

MR. R: [The clinician] didn't mention how long she thought this process of hers was going to take. (male, MCI)

MS. Z: One thing she did that she could have explained a little more. I can't remember the initials now, but . . .

RB: MCI?

Ms. Z: Yeah, what that meant and what it didn't mean. I think that would have been really handy if she had even had a handout or something about it that we could have brought home with us. Because sometimes when you first hear something, you don't necessarily zero in on what the person had said to you. So I think she either needed to spend more time explaining it, or have some, ask if we would like to look at this later or something.

RB: Because you had never heard those terms before?

Ms. Z: No. Right. I'm fairly well read, but I had not heard those terms. (female, MCI)

Mr. O: Our friends who were the first ones who had gone to [the Health Center] for this and then told us about it, when I mentioned to her that MCI was new and that it wasn't conclusive and all of that. She said, "We are so relieved to hear that because we felt . . ." So she had come away, even though they hadn't expressed it, they had come away with the same fearfulness from it [she too had been diagnosed with MCI]. So I know it's not just us. (male, MCI)

Questions about the difference between dementia and normal aging were especially salient both for people seeking evaluation *and for* their families, as shown in their routine queries during diagnosis: "So wait, does my mom have dementia or Alzheimer's? What's the difference between normal aging and Alzheimer's?" (female, mother with AD); "Is Alzheimer's something different from just aging memory loss?" (male, wife with AD). This confusion was revealed in my follow-up interviews with them as well. Mr. C asked me: "What's the difference between MCI and the early stages of Alzheimer's?" (male, MCI); and Mrs. B wondered: "How sure are they that this isn't just about age? And how sure can they be, really?"

The amount and type of information given, the feeling of being rushed or put on the spot, and clinicians who employed ambiguity added elements of uncertainty for respondents. Whether they had too much or too little information or were simply feeling inundated with obscure details, the amount and type of detail clinicians relayed to study participants significantly affected their subjective experiences of being diagnosed.

Imagining a Future with Alzheimer's

Another crucial factor regarding the delivery of the diagnosis was the picture of the future portrayed by clinicians. A few exceptional doctors were particularly adept at focusing on what remained and were able to achieve the perfect balance between cautious optimism and clarity of detail. Two of the most seasoned neurologists at the Brain Clinic, the director and the other senior neurologist attending, and the RN at the Health Center, were particularly impressive. For example:

CLINICIAN: Tell me about your memory?
POTENTIAL PATIENT: They're gone but there's a lot left. I used to be very bright.
CLINICIAN [without missing a beat, and reaching over to touch the patient's arm]: You're still very bright.

CLINICIAN [coming close to and crouching down to look the patient in the eyes]: Let me put it this way, no one your age [78] with these problems dies from it. This is not about your longevity. Something else is going to get you first.
BOTH: [laughing].

CLINICIAN: I wouldn't be pushing you if I didn't think you were going to get better. I think it'll [medication] help you—but not if you don't get the right doses. We say we'll see you in one month because in a month you might be doing quite better.

CLINICIAN: We're really going to need to be aggressive here. There's your walking, your independence, and your memory. Nothing is severe—they are all really minor.
HUSBAND: Well, it sounds hopeful.
CLINICIAN: I'm not pessimistic.
POTENTIAL PATIENT: Well, I'll take a crack at it. As you can tell, I'm not a true believer.
CLINICIAN: It's good to be skeptical—it's better than believing everything.

CLINICIAN: Studies are now looking into whether taking AD medi-cines will slow down progression if you have MCI. We don't know yet. In the meantime, we have to decide. With a person like you with some trouble, I'm inclined to start [Aricept]—as we go through this—because I want your memory to be as good as it can be for as long as possible.

While these practitioners were among the most skillful and compassionate I observed, or what sociologists refer to as charismatic leaders, other clinicians, in contrast, were scientific and scripted in their delivery or focused their attention more on the family members present than the individuals being diagnosed. The prologue depicted a heartbreaking scene with Mr. R straining his neck to see the picture the clinician drew for Mrs. R of his brain atrophy. My field notes depict a negative framing and, in extreme cases, a sense of impending doom: "Your tests with [the research assistant] were really bad, particularly in memory" (psychiatrist).

There were two adult children on the phone, three people [the potential patient and her two sons] sitting in the office, the clinician, and myself for the family conference. The small office was cramped with the five of us in there. The clinician was on one side of a desk, the potential patient and two sons were on the other, and I was sitting to the side between them. There was no speakerphone so the clinician spoke back and forth between the people on the phone and the people in the room.

> *Clinician: This is what we did when Mrs. [L] came in here. . . . We went over her medical history, we talked about her past and her family's history, we did the Neuropsych testing, and we did the blood work. . . . There is some dementia and dementia has some other causes and we've ruled out the other things and it's probably of Alzheimer's pathology. The potential patient opened her eyes and mouth widely and gasped. Clinician [without looking up from her forms]: Specifically she had prob-lems with [robotically goes over test results line by line].*

Fortunately, Mrs. L's friend grabbed her hand and squeezed it. I caught her eye and we were both fighting back tears, but I forced myself to maintain eye contact until she looked away—something I came to feel strongly about after observing my first few diagnoses. Although some of this relates to the tone and type of information relayed, the additional factor of prognosis clearly affected both those who were being diagnosed and their families.

Like the counternarratives of Mrs. B and Mr. C, some respondents had their own views on the future that did not allow room for pejorative portrayals or demonstrated differences of opinion within families:

> MRS. B: I didn't even think about [my memory loss as] being important until my daughter decided it was. I managed to keep appointments; even if . . . well I do write things down on my calendar. But I hadn't been aware of missing anything much. I mean, there are things that I didn't remember, but nothing that was important. Little things that didn't change my life at all.
> RB: And do you think that's still the case?
> MRS. B: I think it still is.
> RB: Are you worried about it getting worse?
> MRS. B: Well, I wonder about it. Is that possible? But I think, with the amount of time I have left, it won't make much difference. (female, AD)

In similar vein, Mr. C demonstrated strength of character and an acceptance of his symptoms, "I just feel like as long as I can get up and see the sunshine and have the love and support of my family then the memory loss is really not that important to me" (male, MCI). Such alternative narratives reveal a concerted resistance to structural constraints framing biomedical interpretations of AD as uniformly catastrophic (or even pathological).

The portrayal of the future depicted by clinicians significantly affected the experience of people being diagnosed. As would be expected, whether the scene was characterized by optimism or skepticism, whether the delivery was aimed at the individuals being diagnosed or family members, and whether the terminology used was perceived as scientific and scripted or accessible and compassionate all affected the experience of the medical encounter.

Experiencing the Environment

As seen in the testing environment, the setting of the diagnosis itself at both the Brain Clinic and the Health Center was also experienced as impersonal or awkward, even if one was not ultimately diagnosed with Alzheimer's:

> Well, with that kind of a talk [diagnosis] . . . rather than her sitting behind the desk, when you're giving that kind of information, a circle or a semicircle, or something without the desk. Somehow I didn't mind it with the early questions, but with that, somehow the desk didn't fit in for me. That day I kept thinking, I pictured we would be in a different room. (male, no cognitive impairment)

> One of the things I got out of that [the Brain Clinic] was that they were not there to tap you on the hand and say, "Don't worry." They go as far as they can go. They are doing two jobs, they are diagnosing you to the best of their ability, and they are also doing the job of adding you to their fund of knowledge. (female, MCI)

> We were sitting out there where you can see right down the hall and I saw this whole group standing in the hall and that's where I saw [the neurologist] for the first time. But they stood there for a long time and I almost assumed that they were talking about me because everyone but [the neurologist] was, was, I'd recognized them. (male, MCI)

> MR. L: I thought, for what to me was the importance of the occasion, they were cramming seven to eight people in the room. [It's] a pretty minor criticism. I know they are a teaching university.
> RB: Is that your biggest concern about that? Did it bother you?
> MR. L: Yes, a little bit because there was hardly enough room for everybody to breathe. Most of them were standing. [To get diagnosed] with all those people sitting around looking at you [was strange]. I felt like a spectacle. (male, MCI)

Importantly, these clinician- and setting-specific factors set the stage for the experience of the diagnosis regardless of the label itself. In addition to the tone used, the amount and type of information given, and the prognosis presented, environmental aspects also influenced the phenomenology of being diagnosed. That is, the clinical context itself fundamentally shaped patient experiences.

Responding to "the A Word"

As reported elsewhere, the variability regarding the tone used, the information shared, the portrayal of the future, and the testing environment, led to mixed reactions to the actual diagnosis.[11] When being informed of an AD/MCI diagnosis, many people highlighted their feelings of shock and confusion. Notions of "This can't be happening" ring through the narratives of both diagnoses. Perhaps not surprisingly, the respondents felt shocked, fearful, sad, uncertain, angry, and overwhelmed:

> I could hardly believe it. I had known a number of people who had this problem, but it simply just never came into my mind that I might have it at any time. (female, AD)

> When I was diagnosed I thought it was a mistake . . . because I had wonderful days, as clear as they could be. (male, AD)

> I had a brother and mother who had Alzheimer's and so when I first found that out I can remember what they went through, and it just blew my mind. . . . That was a real blow. (male, AD)

> When I got the results and heard the word it was *shocking* [emphasis in the original]! For a couple days I was really stuck and in shock and I didn't know what to do with the information. It was really a downer. It really was a "You've got this thing and you're never going to get better" and that there wasn't an end in sight. I spent a number of weeks trying to figure out what was going on and confused and in a daze. (female, MCI)

> They mentioned Alzheimer's, which made me blanch a little bit because I wasn't really ready for that. (male, MCI)

When you get the results back it's really a reflection on you in a deeply personal and a unique way and to have failed these tests was really sad for me. (female, AD)

During a physical exam, the nurse practitioner who I was sent to started talking about this and that and something else. And talk about stupid, I was I had no idea that there was anything like this [Alzheimer's]. And she asked me lots of questions, and she asked me to do some drawing and things. And I was just listening to her talking about the tests and all of a sudden I hit the floor [with the news of the diagnosis]. And I wasn't expecting that. And little by little over a period of time I began to accept it . . . but [at the time] I couldn't believe it. I had just stopped working maybe three to four months before. It just hit me. I just felt frozen to the spot. (female, AD)

Family members reported equally varied reactions to the news: "[The diagnosis] was like a black cloud, that's the only expression I can think of" (female, husband diagnosed with MCI); and "[My husband] went through a period of being very angry, for him, and upset. He got mad at the psychologist, and when we . . . went in with our son to an attorney because I wanted to bring stuff up to date, and he [husband] turned around, in the office, and said, 'I don't have Alzheimer's'" (female, husband diagnosed with AD).

Yet many other diagnosed individuals and their family members reported feeling relieved at the diagnosis.[12] Now that there was something to call their condition, people did not feel personally responsible (i.e., crazy or lazy) and could elicit help as needed. During follow-up interviews with one couple, the wife reported: "I was almost relieved with the diagnosis because I had known for years and I just wanted it confirmed" (husband diagnosed with AD). Other spouses elaborated further during such dyad follow-up interviews:

When we did go to a neurologist, they found Alzheimer's but her whole attitude changed after she was diagnosed. It was a like a big load [was lifted]. Now she knew why she felt like she did. (male, wife diagnosed with AD)

I think in a way [my husband] got some relief from [the diagnosis] because looking back . . . after his first diagnosis we would go to meetings with groups that we had met with before. And when he introduced himself he would say, "I have Alzheimer's." I think it explained to him some of these very confusing things that were happening to him. At least it gave him a handle, like: "It isn't all my fault. It isn't, you know, there's a reason for this. It isn't just me. You know, I'm not just doing stuff wrong. There's a reason." And I think he found some release in that. Some help. (female, husband diagnosed with AD)

Two gentlemen showed clear insight by noting that their Alzheimer's diagnoses were not distressing because it was expected, given their persistent memory difficulties, and it allowed them to elicit help/support: "This was probably coming on for longer than I realized, so [the diagnosis] was not a traumatic thing. It happened gradually; it was sort of subtle"; and "I was really relieved [to have the diagnosis] because I could publicly say, 'I have this and that's why I act a [certain] way.'" Others diagnosed with Alzheimer's displayed decidedly mixed emotions that either varied from time to time or included a whole spectrum of reactions, as these two married women with supportive husbands and adult children show: "Sometimes [the diagnosis] makes me cry to talk about it and other times I think I'm lucky, very lucky. I'm not over worrying about kids in the service, at war [or something like that]"; and "Although [getting a diagnosis] was good in that [it proved] something was going on . . . there was something to blame [for the problems], it was also shocking, and hearing the words was really hard. I didn't really know quite what to do with them."

Interestingly, there were again counternarratives from Mrs. V (from the excerpt introducing chapter 4), Mr. N (who had a much younger wife), and others who were far less concerned with what the medical label might imply than with the imminent loss of tangible valued things:

Since we both cared for our spouses for many years prior to their deaths, neither one of us wants to put the other through that again, so I'm afraid our relationship might come to an end if my memory loss progresses. That is the worst part, quite honestly. (Mrs. V, AD)

Telling [my wife about my difficulties] means then I'd have to admit that I wasn't what I used to be. And, you know, with my being older than her and being her first marriage, maybe she'd regret marrying me, someone twenty-two years older than her. Maybe she'd be upset. (Mr. N, MCI)

RB: Have you ever heard of Alzheimer's disease?
MRS. B: Oh yes. It was mentioned when I went for that test.
RB: Do you remember in what context they mentioned it?
MRS. B: Well, in my context.
RB: Did they tell you that you had Alzheimer's?
MRS. B: Well, I think they implied it.
RB: What do you think about that?
MRS. B: Well, I don't think much of it. I was *really* concerned when they said I wouldn't be able to drive. (female, AD; emphasis in the original)

Well, I like to read and I like to watch good programs on television and I just hope that I can continue to do that because it's enriching to my life and I know what's going on. That's important. So, when I get to the point where I can't remember or do anything—they've got places to put me. I'm comfortable to the point that I realize that there isn't much that can be done. (male, AD)

As was the case with the experience of the neuropsychological tests, people being diagnosed with AD/MCI drew on a variety of strategies to manage the news being delivered and the interactions based on the diagnosis. In particular, respondents utilized humor, asked questions, denied or attributed their memory loss to normal aging, and focused on what could still be done and/or past achievements to avoid being equated with their deficits. For example, when asked to talk about their memory, three patients responded: "They're gone but there's a lot left. I used to be very bright" (male, AD); "I remember things that are important, that I want to remember, that I set my mind to, but if it's insignificant, I just forget it. It doesn't seem too abnormal to me because we don't always remember everything" (Mrs. B, AD); and "I mean I just [forget] those arbitrary things" (male, MCI). When asked if she had any questions, a 70-year-old lesbian being diagnosed with AD responded:

"How long will I live?" and laughed. More elaborate efforts at impression management included:

> I can remember what happened a long time ago but maybe I don't re-member what happened yesterday or the day before. I can recall some of it but because I don't concentrate on it or bear on it [I forget]. Some of the events that have happened in the past are not what I call *real* [emphasis in the original] important so I forget them. Also, I don't look at it as a dis-ease but as being an ornery Swede [laughs] and not remembering some things. (male, AD)

> I say it's a blessing when you can open your eyes in the morning and the sun is shining. It's the start of something different in my ability so I'm gonna hang on as long as I can. You can't put all your eggs in one basket and depend on the medical field to cure you. You have to realize your abilities of what you can think and what you can do and you've got to ac-cept them as such. (male, AD)

> I make a lot of lists and have been hiding it for a long time. My partner said I'm a really good actress but I wonder if that's not something bad to do. I wonder if this may skew things, or make other people think that I'm [actually] better off than I am. (Mrs. V, AD)

Rather than passively taking on the master status of a diseased and/or forgetful person, most people who participated in this research worked to negotiate a sense of self postdiagnosis that was first, favorable and second, compatible with how they had defined themselves prior to their diagnosis. Although the reactions to the actual diagnosis were intense and largely negative, the immediate shock, anger, fear, and other emo-tions were quickly (though not uniformly) replaced with responses symbolic of *living with* Alzheimer's rather than fighting it,[13] as reported elsewhere.[14] Not surprisingly, past perceptions of memory loss, aging and disease, relationships with doctors, and their existential views influ-enced their responses to the news of an AD/MCI diagnosis.

On Being Diagnosed: Short Case Studies

Rather than suggesting that experiences of diagnosis are uniform or generalizable in some way, these narratives demonstrate the unique, idiosyncratic dynamics at work in clinical interactions. The following cases depict distinct interpretations of and reactions to the diagnosis of AD/MCI. Clearly, the person-specific factors these excerpts portray affected the extent to which the individuals assumed Alzheimer's identities. While the first woman was fiercely independent and did not have what she referred to as "blind faith" in doctors, the second gentleman was somewhat skeptical of medicine yet quite eager to get the necessary help diagnosis affords him. The third case study portrays a complex picture of a man who, while being fit and a proactive health seeker, was far more concerned with the loss of status associated with MCI and how it might affect his relationship with a much younger woman than the diagnosis itself. These three types of responses can be seen as interpretations of AD/MCI as "not personal/problematic," "deeply personal/problematic," and "interpersonal/socially problematic."

"Not Personal/Problematic"

Mrs. B was a petite 81-year-old retired housewife whose husband had died a few years prior to our meeting. As she brought me into her studio to show me her art, it was clear that her ability to do what she found fulfilling—sculpting—provided her life with satisfaction. Despite her stellar health and staunch independence, she was brought into the clinic by her daughter, the only one of her four children who lived locally. In our follow-up interview, just weeks after being diagnosed with Alzheimer's, she appeared to have few reservations about her memory loss. The following excerpts provide a glimpse into her personal context:

> I've always been very healthy. I've been lucky. I've gone for a check-up once a year, otherwise only if it is something alarming do I go to the doctor.

> I'm 81 and I just have this sense that my life is winding down. My life is very simple. There are certain things that aren't worth storing away

[remembering] and the things that are important I usually manage to retrieve. And it's also normal for old people not to remember everything, I think. There's a lot to remember when you're 81.

I was a little bit surprised at the result [being diagnosed with AD]. It never occurred to me that I was really losing anything seriously. Maybe it's so gradual that I don't notice that there's a change in anything that I do. I seem to still do the same things. Of course I put things and I can't remember where I put them, but that is not so strange.

I've managed to accomplish just about every goal I've been able to set for myself. I'm a happy person, very satisfied; I've had a good life. I'm just going to enjoy what is here at the present. I don't feel hindered at all by my memory or this diagnosis.

Mrs. B had lived a long, healthy life free of medical problems, unlike a number of her close friends. Having survived all of her immediate family members, she had no remaining contemporaries. She felt fortunate to have the life experiences she had and was accepting of her own mortality. As someone for whom medicine was not an organizing framework, her life was naturally and gradually slowing down, which was neither upsetting nor problematic, and an Alzheimer's diagnosis (or at least the so-called symptoms associated with it) was just another part of the aging process. While the fact that her Alzheimer's diagnosis was not personal or problematic for Mrs. B was clearly a counternarrative, this outlier case also sheds important light on the variation among respondents and perhaps demonstrates keen insight into the nuances of the "entanglements of dementia and aging" anthropologist Margaret Lock claims result in "the Alzheimer conundrum."[15]

"Deeply Personal"

In stark contrast, *Mr. D* was 84 years old and had gone into early retirement over twenty-five years prior to our interview. A short, stocky bachelor, he had a warm, larger-than-life presence. As a very proactive health seeker, his home was literally filled with medical bulletins, journals, and books, which he said he spent the majority of his time reading to be informed about any ailments he had or might someday have. He wasn't anxious per se, but rather wanted to be well-informed; it almost felt more like a hobby. Immediately after being told he had MCI, he asked the clinician "Is there a pill?" (He was prescribed Aricept, which he had been taking for the two months since his diagnosis but had not noticed any changes.) He assigned a sense of imperative to the situation not observed in Mrs. B's case despite his not technically being given a diagnosis. Somewhat atypical for his generation, Mr. D was a lifelong consumer of complementary and alternative medicine. Although he was suspicious of traditional medicine, he strategically utilized its diagnostic ability to seek alternative treatments for his many allopathic conditions:

Sometimes we get wrong information from doctors. It's surprising the mistakes they make. Some doctors just routinely see patients and say, "Take an aspirin" or "You're getting older." That's one thing I can't stand is when they tell me, "Oh you're just getting older."

I look up a lot of things myself and I learn a lot. In fact, any prescription the doctor gives me I look up in my odd books and make sure what they are giving me I understand. I want to speak up—the doctors should learn about alternative medicine—they don't have to go to school to learn—the books are good on it. All the new studies that come out every month are in that magazine [Life Extension]. So the whole point of that is—they think it was a good study, they don't wait until the AMA decides it was right. They give you enough details and I'm sold.

I called your organization [Brain Clinic] and I got an appointment about seven months later. Now that is what I'm complaining about. I have a problem and it's gotten worse. It's gotten worse in those seven months. That's one of the things I wanted to talk about. If they don't have enough people, my god, get enough people to take care of clients.

What I got from the neurologist that talked with me was that they are going to try to figure out what is causing it and "if we find we have a new medicine for it you'll get it and if we don't you'll just wait until we get something" and to me that's why I thought I better go back to my alterna-

tive medicine doctor. And I have to go back in two months to see the neurologist and by then I guess he'll have a better idea what the problem is
and if they have a medicine for it. See, doctors either have a medicine for
it or they have surgery for it. Nothing else and I've gotta get a third thing.

I'm not embarrassed about [my memory loss]. It is just a problem I am
having and I take help wherever I can get it.

From Mr. D, one sensed urgency in his situation with his memory (and
perhaps all medical ailments). As someone for whom medicine was a
primary socializing agent, he thought his memory loss was abnormal
and reversible, he intended to do everything he could to fend off any further progression, and he would readily admit his shortcomings insofar
as it aided him in getting help. For Mr. D, a model of neoliberal public
health efforts at preventative medicine who nonetheless pursued primarily holistic remedies to health problems, MCI was "deeply personal/
problematic."

"Interpersonal/Socially Problematic"

A tall, thin gentleman, *Mr. N* was 76 years old with a wife over two
decades his junior. He was a smartly dressed, charming, well-educated
man who had been working as a docent at a museum in San Francisco
for many years. He strongly identified with being healthy and fit and
had few interactions with medical doctors as a result. His wife of almost
ten years felt that his memory loss was markedly worse when he drank,
though he disagreed. His narrative of life with memory loss (MCI) felt
remarkably different from the others:

I always prided myself on the condition of my health.

One of my biggest concerns is the fact that, from my perspective, I do
forget things. And it changes things for both of us [him and his wife].
Especially it upsets her. It's not a major thing, I mean we've had little tiffs
but we work through it. But because of this, we now, between the two of
us we now go to three different therapists.

> Given the circumstances that have existed [memory loss], I don't want
> to tell her [when I forget something]. Telling her means then I'd have to
> admit that I wasn't what I used to be. . . . maybe she'd regret marrying me,
> someone twenty-two years older than her.

For Mr. N, his symptoms are not a problem; his major concern was his
relationship with his wife. His potential inability to be an equal partner with his wife was particularly bothersome as was the possibility of
burdening her. The negative effect of his memory loss on their marriage was his biggest fear. Since the experiences he was having with his
memory were changing the dynamics of his relationship in ways that
were upsetting to him, the diagnosis was largely "interpersonal" or a
"social problem" for Mr. N.

What is most telling about these three stories—and the narratives in
this study broadly—is the way in which similar news can be interpreted
and used very differently. Whereas Mr. D willfully accepted an Alzheimer's identity even without a diagnosis of it, Mrs. B recognized her deficits
but saw no utility of incorporating them or her diagnosis into her self-
concept, and Mr. N was far more concerned with how his memory loss
would affect his relationship with his wife than the label itself (or even
what it might in the future mean for him personally).

Conclusion: Experiencing an Alzheimer's Diagnosis

The agency and impression management strategies observed during
cognitive evaluation were also present in the experience of and reaction
to the diagnosis of AD/MCI itself. People seeking medical attention for
their memory are keenly aware of the pejorative societal perceptions
of Alzheimer's disease as an alleged tragedy that robs people of their
autonomy and inevitably results in complete dependence and have varying levels of faith in the power of medicine to treat memory loss. For
these reasons, respondents combated some of the perceived negative
experiences by deliberately presenting themselves in a way they found
more consistent with their personal identities and less interpersonally
threatening. During the delivery of diagnosis, study participants noted
detached clinicians who sometimes used a negative tone, did not provide sufficient and/or accessible information, or gave a bleak portrayal

of the future. I am arguing that consequently respondents asked questions, used humor, denied memory loss or attributed it to normal aging, focused on what could still be done or on their past achievements, and highlighted medical uncertainty as strategies *to avoid being conflated with and relegated to the (lower) status of their new diagnosis*. Some respondents willingly, and often light-heartedly, self-deprecated in order to solicit compassion whereas others simply employed the potential disease label in such circumstances.

The social death,[16] or marginalization, accompanying certain diagnoses, and arguably dementia, engenders a situation where (pathologically) forgetful people potentially embark on a career or trajectory[17] of becoming an Alzheimer's patient. By employing the terms trajectory and career, I follow a long trend within the qualitative arm of medical sociology in studying illness narratives to understand the subjective aspects of the *illness process* and the ways in which people attach *evaluative meanings* to the typical sequence of movements constituting their path to becoming a patient. Illness careers and trajectories are characterized by critical turning points, or status passages into the next phase, which requires a redefinition of self. While this book generally investigates how an individual's identity as a forgetful person is shaped through interactions with biomedicine, what is most central here, however, is that some interpretations mirror biomedical ideology and others counter it. These narratives underscore the importance of a person's outlook on and prior relationship with medicine for their interpretation of the diagnosis. Those individuals for whom medicine is a central organizing principle in life are more willing to assume the status of an Alzheimer's patient (even when they are not technically diagnosed with it).

For people seeking medical care for their memory loss, the transition from experience to symptom requires a redefinition of forgetfulness as a problem. The diagnostic process, then, may serve as a legitimating force for atypical experiences (or assumed symptoms). Respondents vacillated between fully assuming the master status of Alzheimer's patient, simply exploiting such terminology when necessary, and completely normalizing their memory loss. The interactional tensions created by the assumptions of clinical practice required diagnosed individuals to engage in processes of identity management. The utilization of such tactics by study participants demonstrates an ability to manipulate one's interactions that counters the public perceptions of incompetency by highlighting the agency of individuals diagnosed with Alzheimer's. In practice, then, the social function of diagnosis is an important element of Alzheimer's identities.

The variation among respondents demonstrates that the social context in which aging, memory loss, and disease exist as well as personal aspects of one's identity influence the acceptance of clinical diagnoses as a master status to be adorned. Beliefs on the aging process, previous interactions with medical doctors, and the purpose of life as well as traits such as outlook, reaction to bad news, or resilience were crucial in determining how a person reacted to a given diagnosis. Consequently, the identification as sick or needy is not the only response to the news of an AD/MCI diagnosis. The reality of these data is that taking on the status of an ill person is certainly not instinctual or even the predominant reaction to a diagnosis of AD/MCI; it is far from a master status immediately following diagnosis.

Instead, this chapter argues that the process of developing into a person with Alzheimer's, which starts with cognitive evaluation but officially commences with diagnosis, involves the intentional application of this medical label only as deemed necessary. The processual nature of becoming an Alzheimer's patient demonstrates the fluidity of management strategies and the ways in which identity evolves over time. The experience of having been diagnosed served as an integral stabilizing force for some people who could not otherwise explain their behaviors (and also allowed them to avail themselves of services). Clinical processes, of course, are in turn shaped by potential patients who work to foster counternarratives resisting biomedical presumptions of incompetence or at least manage interactions that are awkward due to the institutional logic and environmental dynamics of specialty clinics. More broadly, medical efforts at earlier diagnoses also generate the advent of articulate and potentially proactive individuals diagnosed with memory loss who need to be accounted for and incorporated into the discourse of clinical practice. If the story of this resistance reaches the lay public, thus revolutionizing the ways in which people with Alzheimer's are represented, it will accomplish an equally important political task by offering people an alternative framework for understanding the meaning and course of their illness. This could well provide an important corrective to a singular (biomedical) story about cognitive impairment.

Chapter 6 explores the experiences of everyday living with memory loss postdiagnosis. By engaging core sociological debates concerning structure and agency, it will show how the employment of disease status is consciously utilized as deemed necessary[18] rather than strictly superimposed upon individuals by definition of the condition with which they have been diagnosed. Therefore, in concert with other sociological work highlighting the nuanced ways in which various marginalized populations have promoted their own self-interests and awareness in spite of potential consequences to them,[19] people accept—to drastically different degrees—the label of AD to the extent to which they think it aids them in certain realms or harms them in others. Individuals with clinically relevant memory loss navigate their way around the diagnostic label ascribed to them by the medical classification system. Rather than medicalization being a process whereby individuals are forced to participate in their own subjugation in a top-down manner, many of the potential and current patients in this study are active accomplices in subsuming Alzheimer's identities. This conduct is emblematic of what critical scholars call the "new biomedicine."[20]

6

Everyday Life with Diagnosis

The New Normal

At the moment, I feel just fine. I intend to live the remainder of the years God gives me on this earth doing the things I have always done. I will continue to share life's journey with my beloved Nancy and my family. I plan to enjoy the great outdoors and stay in touch with my friends and supporters.
—President Ronald Reagan, "Alzheimer's Letter," 1994

Mrs. W, a 72-year-old recent widow, had been diagnosed with Alzheimer's almost one year prior to my meeting her at the monthly support group she attended. Beneath conservative attire and a petite stature, was a contagious enthusiasm for life. Her informal mantra represented a theme common to most study participants: "I'm still the same person I've always been. *It's just that now I'm* me *with Alzheimer's.*"
—Field notes, emphasis in the original

The advent of being evaluated and diagnosed with Alzheimer's/mild cognitive impairment have been depicted as necessary turning points, or status passages,[1] legitimating the incorporation of experiences of memory loss into the everyday lives of affected individuals. Based on in-depth interviews with forty individuals who had been diagnosed with MCI or early-stage AD between two months and four years prior, this chapter examines the mechanisms through which the medical label is employed to normalize continually worsening difficulties, to justify socially awkward behaviors, and to garner support when deemed necessary in the months and years following diagnosis. Simultaneously, however, respondents still refused to blindly take the second step of accepting the demented label necessary in the process of becoming an Alzheimer patient; thus they struggled to avoid being assigned the master status"[2] of demented person so often associated with the label that we saw in chapters 4 and 5, and strategically worked to avoid such degradation. Both the late President Reagan and Mrs. W above echo the sentiment that, ultimately, they want to be seen for who they are, not for the disease they have. Yet there were only a few exceptional people in my study who did not buy into the medical version of their experiences, and thus did not seek out support groups or even actively resisted the medical label ascribed to their forgetfulness; that is, they never took the second step of adorning their label.[3]

The final step in the process of becoming an Alzheimer patient, joining a subculture, was initiated by attending support groups or participating in research studies. The vast majority of respondents in this study attended support groups sponsored by the Alzheimer's Association or held at the Brain Clinic or Health Center, which promote biomedical interpretations of memory loss, signaling Howard Becker's third and ultimate step in assuming the master status. The fact that nearly all the participants ascribed medical labels to their forgetfulness attests to both the success and potential consequences of offering exclusively biomedical solutions to memory loss that characterizes the contemporary social construction of Alzheimer's disease and the individuals with the condition.

Medical anthropologists have long addressed the role played by stories people tell about their experience of illness in informing both medical discourse and personal life.[4] Such illness narratives, or first-person accounts of illness, focus on suffering, healing, and the human condition[5] to demonstrate the importance of distinguishing between illness and disease. Accordingly, illness addresses things that traditional medicine does not, in fact *cannot*. Building on this, medical sociologist Arthur Frank's *Wounded Storyteller* is not a diseased person; rather s/he is an individual living with and through a disease.[6]

Sociologists depict a *moral career* or process of *becoming* a patient that commences upon receipt of a diagnosis.[7] In this view, individuals embark on a career as a sick person after being assigned a medical label. Accordingly, ill individuals are not immediately accepting of their label, but instead must *learn* how to become a patient in keeping with their diagnosis. The achievement of this objective solidifies a career in that vein and involves various moments of significance throughout the process. For instance, sociologist David Karp elucidates how diagnosed persons often find themselves in an interpretive dilemma of trying to navigate between rhetorics of biochemical determinism and a sense of personal efficacy.[8] Subjective accounts of disease, particularly a person's moral career as a sick person or a patient, provide important insights into understanding the sociocultural meanings of health and illness.

Social and behavioral researchers have long been interested in the relationship between illness and identity.[9] Within identity studies, social constructionists and symbolic interactionists note that the construction of one's social identity is a lifelong process.[10] Moreover, because identity changes over time, managing one's identity is a process involving the employment of various strategies. As such, identity is formed, maintained, and altered through interaction and experience. This is particularly the case with illness. Illness often fosters transformations of identity, sometimes drastic ones, but it need not do so in an exclusively negative or deterministic manner. Insofar as the term relates to identity, illness is part and parcel of personal narratives. In contrast, disease is a biomedical condition that is prescribed by medical professionals rather than "storied" by those most intimately affected.

Medicine, as an institutional structure with sets of knowledge and practice, identifies an etiological explanation for the disease process, thus theoretically allowing individuals to integrate their behaviors and experiences into their everyday lives. The process of retrospectively reconstructing one's past behaviors as symbolic of a recent diagnosis allows for an insertion of present experiences into one's existing identity rather than reconstituting a self that has been changed in permanent and foreign ways. As such, normalization of symptoms helps minimize what Michael Bury long ago coined the biographical disruption and medical anthropologist Gay Becker called disrupted lives.[11] Critics of the assumption that illnesses roundly present individuals with intense crisis, thus potentially requiring a radical redefinition of self,[12] argue that the biographically embodied self in conditions of late modernity[13] make it possible for illness to lead to "biographical reinforcement," "biographical flow," and even "narrative reconstruction."[14] Either way, while the clinical constructs of AD/MCI originate from medical knowledge and practice, they permeate other realms of life in ways that are psycho-socially significant.

While much of the research attention in the area was initially devoted to acute and terminal illnesses, more recently the focus has shifted to chronic illnesses. Since chronic illness requires various adjustments to one's identity,[15] if roles that are deemed characteristic diminish or disappear the sense of self must be actively reconstructed.[16] Chronic illness also brings up issues of temporality that require those who are chronically ill to live in limbo or spaces of liminality[17] because they cannot predict whether it will be what medical sociologist Kathy Charmaz calls a "good day" or a "bad day."[18] The uncertainty that can arise, especially if one has an invisible or concealable illness such as chronic pain, fatigue, or an autoimmune condition involves a deliberate and recurring "unmasking"[19] that requires interactional work on top of managing the symptoms of the illness itself. Joseph Dumit refers to these ailments as "illnesses you have to fight to get."[20]

Unlike episodic or acute illnesses, where recovery identities can be attained,[21] chronic illnesses like multiple sclerosis, pain/fatigue, or even AIDS are often lifelong. Likewise, the persistence of memory loss engenders obstacles for people with dementia.[22] Rather than being able to speak as survivors of their condition, individuals are instead forced to deal with constant changes over time and from one day to the next,[23] requiring continual negotiations and management strategies.

It was long ago demonstrated that specific images of identity remain despite the barriers to maintaining a diseaseless self—indicating a fundamental concept of identification.[24] Overall, illness narratives concerned with subjective experiences of medical conditions highlight an enduring sense of identity and the use of diverse strategies for achieving such ends, which this chapter engages through the diagnostic categories of Alzheimer's and mild cognitive impairment.

After first delineating the types of experiences that lead people to notice that "something just wasn't right," I examine the various changes following diagnosis and methods of management implemented to regulate these transformations. Next, I explore the benefits, as perceived by respondents, of being diagnosed. The chapter closes by analyzing potential justifications for and implications of the clinical management efforts explicated in chapter 3. Throughout the chapter, I highlight the social and emotional effects of facing this illness and the subsequent threat to human interactions.

Although in this chapter I predominantly report on the first-hand accounts, or narratives, of people diagnosed with AD or MCI who attend disease-based support groups, I utilize information elicited from family members of those diagnosed where applicable.[25] The forty respondents drawn on in this chapter had been diagnosed between two months and four years prior to involvement with this research, with an average time since diagnosis of one year. The vast majority of study participants were deemed by clinical staff to have only minor memory loss.

Something Just Isn't Right

Respondents noted a number of things that had originally made them suspect that something was wrong with their memory (or the memory of a loved one). Although sometimes these incidents had gone unnoticed for months or even years, typically there was a very specific episode, or turning point,[26] signifying the magnitude of the problem. Even if it was a vague recollection by the time they participated in this study, all respondents eventually acknowledged that something "just wasn't right." Mr. C, from the previous chapter, for example, did not recognize his daughter's long-time fiancé at a formal gathering. For Mr. S, a flutist who had traveled with big bands, the following incident signaled a fundamental problem to him:

> I go quite a number of years back in terms of worrying. I'm trying to remember, it's something like five years or six years ago I had what I now look upon as sort of a performance anxiety. I was playing at a music camp. I play the flute, and two things happened. One of them was very easy. I just missed, I couldn't [read the music]. And I had not had that happen before. And I got really worried. (male, MCI)

Likewise, these two wives corroborated that both they and their husbands had noted clear turning points:

> He came out one morning and he was trying to figure out from his IRA his required minimum distribution, and he couldn't add up a column of

figures. This is a man who would never use a calculator. He didn't like them. (husband diagnosed with AD)

At one point [my husband] said, "What's this green stuff on my plate?" It was broccoli. That was kind of bad, but he hasn't done it anymore. So it's just a series of ups and downs. (husband diagnosed with MCI)

Experiences such as these and sometimes pleas from loved ones eventually led all respondents to seek medical attention for their memory and to subsequently receive a diagnosis of AD/MCI. The most common reactions to diagnosis mirrored those discussed in chapter 5, ranging from disbelief to sadness or relief, and highlighted similar variation.

Despite the different reactions to diagnosis, study participants reported strikingly similar types of experiences regarding living with memory loss since being diagnosed, perhaps best encapsulated by Mr. F, a retired fireman diagnosed with MCI, when he said: "[Memory loss is] like a little obstacle that I can't really get around." Others elaborated further that what they struggled with the most were routine tasks like driving, making the bed, and recalling names or numbers. An exchange between two members attending a Bay Area support group for mild cognitive impairment demonstrates this:

R1: I don't drive any more. Things I used to do I'm not doing, and probably will not be doing any more. And I don't exactly get lost, but there is a memory problem even somewhere you've lived all your life. Even though there are places I know, sometimes I find I've forgotten the name of a specific street. (male, MCI)
R2: I have the same problem. You know you know it, but you can't grab it. You can't find it in your memory. (female, MCI)

This was further supported in data from individual interviews:

I have a problem trying to make up the bed. It takes forever to do it. And things I did, you know, without giving it any thought, now is a big chore. And it takes a lot of doing to get the job done. Sometimes I'll just have to call [my wife] and say, "Come up here and give me some help." (male, AD)

I find that remembering people's names is very difficult. I mean I can't remember my best friend's name sometimes. It just blanks out. I can remember two service numbers from World War II, but I forget my phone number, which I use every day. I mean I just . . . those arbitrary things. (male, MCI)

What was most noteworthy about their experiences was the marked change from what life had been like prior to the onset of memory loss. Although there was variation in terms of length of time since diagnosis, the actual diagnosis, and the reaction to the diagnosis, common themes reported included changes in activities, roles, and relationships, which were discussed repeatedly throughout interviews and focus groups. If roughly half of those who screen positively for dementia in general practice "refuse subsequent diagnostic evaluation because of concerns about harms associated with a diagnosis such as losing health insurance coverage, driving privileges, or employment; anxiety and depression; stigma; and effects on family finances and emotions,"[27] then my data suggest their fears are well founded.

Consequences of Diagnosis: Interactional Tensions

In concert with prior claims that a diagnosis of dementia "affects identity . . . roles and relationships within the family and in wider social networks,"[28] study participants reported that significant transitions had occurred in their lives since they were diagnosed with AD/MCI. In particular, two kinds of changes were perceived to jeopardize their identity as competent individuals and thus required significant impression management efforts. The first pertained to the activities and roles that they had performed prior to diagnosis and the second related to how their relationships with other people were altered by the diagnosis. These changes required deliberate efforts to resist relegation and handle relationships as two key aspects of their strategy to manage life with memory loss.

Resisting Relegation

Respondents perceived a general decrease in the activities and roles of their daily lives since being diagnosed. Some noted specific tasks that they were no longer able or allowed to perform which used to be important parts of their lives, such as driving or cooking. Driving symbolizes independence and spontaneity for many Americans and cooking is a core aspect of identity for many women of this generation. The following focus group excerpt reveals the perceived losses that accompany the inability to drive a car:

> R1: As for driving the car, I used to like to. We were getting somewhere. But now I have to get in a car with someone else and tell them where I want to go. Or I go where they're going. (male, AD)
> R2: That's so frustrating too. It really is. (female, AD)
> RB: What's frustrating about it?
> R1: You can't do what you want. You have to do what somebody else wants. They have to do it for you.
> R2: You can't just do it yourself. You have to ask. So you have to adjust your schedule to someone else's. I guess the best word for it is that it is somewhat humiliating to be in that position when you're used to running your own life.

Likewise, for these two women with AD who prided themselves on their ability to provide food for their husband and children, difficulty with cooking was a complete assault to this prized identity: "I had somebody helping me [with] cooking for a while and that really bothered me. It made me feel less than myself. I learned how to cook when I was 12 years old"; and "Even when I worked I came home and fixed dinner. Now I go to do it and I'm an absolute blank how to make that dish. I mean, it's gone. It's gone just like everything else."

On top of their admitted shortcomings, their previously held perceptions of themselves as independent, autonomous, and capable people were often questioned by others as a result of the diagnosis, which significantly complicated everyday life and often reversed social roles such as parent, nurturer, or partner. These two men with AD were typical of the general remorse and frustration expressed by respondents: "I think the disease itself is enough problem but the constrictions that they [family members, doctors, etc.] place around you. You can't do this, you can't do that. You can't drive. You end up being extremely frustrated"; and "We are treated differently obviously. We have to be because there are certain things we can't do, and they have to do them for us. That's the one that was hardest to give up . . . independence."

Closely related, living with AD/MCI meant a potential loss of privacy and freedom, leading to significantly more constricted social lives. This conversation between a woman and man attending an AD support group reveals how this is often framed as a choice by these respondents: "I don't very often go out on my own. I don't feel very secure all by myself. You know, well, what if I forget where I'm going? What if I forget where I've been?"; and "Well, I've reached that stage too in that I really can't go anywhere unless somebody takes me and brings me back." The following sentiment expresses a feeling of infantilization commonly reported by my study participants, regardless of whether they were diagnosed with AD or MCI:

> [B]efore when I was free to go, I'd go take a walk around the block rather than blow my stack. By the time I got back my feet hurt so that I quit worrying what I was mad about. You can't get away from everybody now. Your husband will go with you, and that doesn't do it. Your neighbors will stop and talk to you, just for a minute. Then they'll say, "Well, I'll walk around with you." And I wish I'd never told them I have it because it took away my freedom. (female, AD)

A general decrease in activities since being labeled with AD/MCI was almost uniformly reported. Typically, these tangible losses, such as the treasured roles of a retired academic, were troubling: "I used to teach classes, I used to edit a journal. I used to do all kinds of things I'm not doing now. I used to go to workshops, and I'm not doing any of those things. And I really, really miss them" (female, AD). Others simply no longer have the energy or interest to continue doing what used to be so meaningful to them, like these two men with MCI who have lost their passion for languages, music, or writing:

> I was always very interested in languages because I learn languages easily, and music, I had a good ear for music so I could play a few things by

ear, but I noticed that actually as time has gone by that I've lost interest in doing those things. And I sort of blame it, have a tendency when I think back to think that it's because of memory loss. (male, MCI)

I do find the hardest thing is to become stimulated in doing something. I used to become stimulated in writing or a musical instrument or something like that. And I don't have any interest there right now. But when I find something that interests me, then I start to go. But to maintain that interest and enthusiasm is not so easy. (male, MCI)

In addition, perceptions of being deemed compromised led many respondents to express feelings of aggravation. The loss of roles and activities was of great concern to the individuals in this study, who although they acknowledged their shortcomings, emphatically pleaded that they not be conflated with them.

In corroboration with first-hand accounts, the spouses of people living with AD/MCI also noticed differences and were particularly distressed about the losses they observed. The role of change in the equation was common, as seen by the husband of a woman with MCI and the wife of a gentleman with AD: "It's like he is slowly just vanishing. It's like his mind is shutting down"; and "It's really a sad thing to watch somebody who was very sharp just go down to where they can't speak, they can't dress themselves, they can't do anything." More explicit accounts of the unpredictability and loss of control involved in dementia were also reported:

I find that I'm having to do more, or at least more of the detail stuff, and I get angry. I try not to, but I do. I don't like what I'm seeing. I'm scared. There isn't a whole lot more I can do except try to, please god, have patience. I feel like [my husband] isn't cooperating and so I get angry. I mean he has the puzzle books, he has other books, the things he's interested in, but he doesn't do it. That book hasn't been opened! You have to keep at it. And I guess I get angry if he's not going to help himself, I get angry. It has to be a two-way thing. (husband diagnosed with MCI)

All of a sudden I have seen a tremendous drop in his mental ability and I am so scared. Because I don't know now, I did know, I knew exactly what

I could count on and I had everything, more or less in balance, the help I needed, but now I don't even know what I have, and so I am frightened. And this is a period of sizing up. I'm simply beside myself. I'm having a hard time. I'm trying to be calm and take it one day at a time, but if I go any further then one day I get dizzy, really dizzy. Because of the ambiguity of this stuff. The ambiguities are just awful. (husband diagnosed with MCI)

The fear and uncertainty of these two women whose husbands were diagnosed with MCI—not even AD—echo that of those diagnosed themselves. Both parties are aware of and rightfully concerned about the changes that have transpired.

The decreased roles and activities that individuals with minor memory loss experienced and their spouses corroborated typically led to more restrictive lives since being diagnosed. Although many respondents willingly noted the need for additional support in certain realms, few felt comfortable with the connotation of being less than competent or needy that accompanied their diagnosis and no one spoke without remorse about their newly tarnished identity. Study participants acknowledged that their previous identity was threatened by their present condition. This situation required negotiations with others and a management of one's identity on a far more conscious level than had been necessary before being diagnosed.

Handling Relationships

In addition to living more restricted lives, another important change requiring impression management concerned their relationships with others—as the quotes above indicate. Individuals suggested that interactions with their families and friends had been altered by the diagnosis. One of the most compelling examples of this came from 81-year-old Mrs. O, long ago widowed and the matriarch of her large family. Her long gray pigtails hanging halfway down her back, her sparkling blue eyes began to tear up as she told me the following account:

My family members' relationships [with me] changed as soon as they found out that I was "no longer competent." The things that I say seem to be a lot more subject to question than they used to be. It's as if I can't possibly know anything anymore. At least that's the way I feel. I'm very irritated. [Laughter.] I realize that I forget things and that I'm not always completely with it, but I feel like I still have enough intelligence, you know, *to be a person, and not just someone you pat on the head as you go by* . . . . I guess maybe I'm a bossy person by nature, but I really resent being bossed around and being told how I should do something when I know I know how to do it. It's devastating, and *it takes away your sense of self*. And I find it very hard to deal with. . . . It is important to me because I feel like I'm still a person and my wants and desires should at least be considered before decisions are made. (female, AD)

Another man, Mr. F, told me that he and his wife had grown apart since his diagnosis six months earlier: "I think that what happens is that you do some things yourself instead of doing things together" (male, MCI). In contrast to prior studies suggesting that couples are involved in a joint career of managing memory loss,[29] this finding may provide evidence that prior relationship status or differing reactions to the diagnosis may influence whether couples "do things together" and maintain an "us identity" or not.[30]

Perceived changes in relationships as a result of diagnosis created a situation whereby individuals felt they needed to manage not only the symptoms of their disease but also had to vigilantly negotiate their everyday interactions. Respondents felt their diagnosis had caused increased tension over the management of self and others. This in turn caused interactional problems and required further management, producing a *spiral of dilemmas*. Although the processes through which individuals extricate themselves from this messy and dangerous situation are idiosyncratic, some patterns are identified in the following section on methods of management.

The families of people with AD/MCI also talked about how many of the negative changes resulting from memory loss were difficult to watch and sometimes put a strain on the relationship between themselves and their loved one. Wives of men with AD were particularly vocal about the changes that had transpired in their marriages, especially when cherished traits or aspects of the relationship were now compromised: "One thing that really attracted me to him was his mind. I was attracted to that more than anything else. And it has been hard for me to see this [memory loss], because our conversations have diminished and his executive abilities are all practically gone"; and "I miss the lack of sharing more than anything. There's less intimacy, which I deeply miss. Less fun, but still lots of pleasure." The wife of a man with MCI expressed similar concerns: "It has affected our relationship because sometimes he accepts the help and sometimes he doesn't want it. As I see the situation, there is absolutely no planning on his part and it's very hard for me to have to think of everything else that needs to be done, for his safety as well as for mine."

As these data demonstrate, an AD/MCI label significantly affects both those who are diagnosed and their loved ones, often leading to feelings of loss, anger, uncertainty, and frustration, as reported elsewhere.[31] Arguably, many of the changes that occurred were based on assumptions of (at least pending) incompetence from those with whom they were interacting, including clinicians, Alzheimer's Association staff, and family members. Nonetheless, both diagnosed individuals and spouses reported significant changes and often framed them as losses. Since social interaction requires constant negotiation, such restrictions created the need for active impression management on behalf of individuals diagnosed with memory loss on top of dealing with the physical and functional realities of their condition.

Assessing the Positive Aspects

Although contemporary assumptions regarding the changes accompanying a diagnosis of AD/MCI pertain to loss, many people with dementia and their spouses also noted positive aspects of the diagnosis. Importantly, these included the ability to travel, to spend more time with loved ones, to focus on those things that brought enjoyment, to appreciate what one still had, and to plan for the future. For example, "[Since the diagnosis], we're taking advantage of everything that comes our way that we can afford to do" (female, MCI); and "I think we're doing more things together as a result of it because you don't know what's going to happen down the street" (wife diagnosed with MCI). While the previous quotes revealed a certain outlook or perspective per se, others were more task-oriented: "I think I have a very different view about how long

I'll be around, or when life will come to an end, or when I'll be incompetent, than I did before the diagnosis. No question. And I'm getting rid of things at home. . . . There are all sorts of decisions of that sort and I didn't used to think about death before but now I do" (male, MCI); and "I'd like for him to write [his stories] down to go into the computer for the kids because he's got a lot of good stories to tell and I don't want them forgotten either. I'd like him to do it before his memory gets worse, looking into the future" (husband diagnosed with MCI). Mirroring the findings from chapter 5, after the initial shock abated these respondents were often relieved at the news, glad to be able to identify it as some known entity, and empowered to do something as a result.

These data suggest that individuals diagnosed with memory loss often felt they were socially disenfranchised as a result of being diagnosed; beyond physical and functional limitations, the social and emotional effects of the diagnosis were evident. Despite the tangible consequences of being diagnosed, however, there were also positive aspects of the label. For many respondents, the potential to have an input in their final years and medical care that would not have been possible if they were diagnosed later in the disease trajectory, or with any condition of sudden-onset, was framed as a benefit. Importantly, both negative and positive changes accompanied a diagnosis of minor memory loss for these study participants, each precipitating the need for various identity management strategies. In stark contrast to the exclusively negative framings of AD in the media and medical arenas, these data offer a counternarrative that includes the perceived benefits of being diagnosed. Thus, both positive and negative aspects of a diagnosis influence the paths, or careers, of Alzheimer's patients.

Methods of Management: Interactional Tensions

Since the framing of AD in the public media and biomedicine is overwhelmingly grim, study participants echo the sentiments of the late President Reagan when he said, "Unfortunately, as Alzheimer's disease progresses, the family often bears a heavy burden. I only wish there was some way I could spare Nancy from this painful experience,"[32] in reporting fears of how their memory loss will harm those they love. Given this neoliberal framing and the concrete changes that had transpired since their diagnosis, individuals with memory loss implemented various methods of management or ways of adjusting to the changes they noticed, to normalize their experiences and minimize threats to their existing identities. Such efforts generated, arguably inadvertently, a shift in identity as well as a sense of community belonging for the group of individuals attending AD/MCI support groups. Their methods of management included focusing on the positive, accepting help, attaining serenity, employing humor, and being proactive.

Focusing on the Positive

The desire to remain positive appeared to be a basic tenet of all support groups observed. One particularly common strategy was to focus on what could still be done rather than on shortcomings or what had been lost. Many people reported the importance of trying to continue doing what they had done before the diagnosis, including an inherent optimism, personality traits, and treasured identities: "I forget a great deal. It's annoying. I think this is the kind of thing we just have to deal with. We have this problem and we can't change that, but we can improve our lives by not letting it just bring us . . . unhappy twenty-four hours a day. Make the best of it and do the best we can" (female, AD); and "I feel good. I try to do everything that I normally do: walk and watch television and go out for dinner and things like that. [I try] to make it just go as even as possible" (male, AD). Likewise, two men with MCI, one a retired small business owner and the other a retired academic, remind us of important aspects of their identities through the following claims: "The cognitive ability, the thinking, is slower I think, but still there. I can still make a contribution at the office, although it takes me longer and so use it or lose it" (male); and "Yesterday I got the page proofs from another article, a very scientific sort of article, of which I'm sort of the lead author because I put it together. But there are four other authors, and it is being published in an important journal. So suddenly I'm on cloud nine." (male, MCI)

This effort to maintain the norm or balance between equals seemed to be especially important to the spouses of people with AD/MCI, who wanted their partners to be involved. For example, "It's really important that [people with memory loss] have a sense of some doing" (wife diagnosed with AD). More elaborate explanations include the following:

> It's very interesting because I slip back and forth on this, but I feel until he cannot do for himself he has to take ownership of the disease. So that I don't want to be overprotective. I feel he needs to be doing and having some responsibilities. I think that makes him better, because he has a reason for being around. And if we do everything for them what's the point? Until they are unable to do it. (husband diagnosed with AD)

An overarching theme throughout the data was the need to remain positive, to appreciate what remains, and to resist the corrosive rhetoric of loss of self. As reported elsewhere, people with AD/MCI were able to do this especially well when their spouses interpreted their memory loss similarly.[33]

Accepting Help

Other respondents spoke of the advantage of being open and honest about needing assistance and accepting help from others. This also came from data with both the diagnosed individuals and their spouses: "I certainly think that it's important to let family all be aware of one's problems. Not to the extent of complaining and complaining, but this is what it is and I have to deal with that. I wouldn't deny it ever" (female, AD); and "[My husband] uses [the term] memory problems and he finds it very comfortable to tell people. If he gets stuck with a word, instead of struggling with it he just says, 'Just a minute. I have memory problems, and I'll get it in a minute,' or 'I'll think of something else'" (husband diagnosed with AD). Mrs. O makes a similarly compelling plea for appealing to people's basic humanity to elicit help as needed:

> RB: How would you explain what you are experiencing to someone else?
> MRS. O: I would say, "I have trouble remembering things. Sometimes you'll tell me something and I'll forget it and you'll have to tell me again." I'm a very direct sort of person. But that's the way I would talk to my grandchildren, or anyone actually. You know, "I listen to you.

I hear what you're saying, but I won't always be able to remember it, and you might have to tell me again." I find being direct is usually the best way to handle things like that. (female, AD)

As reported with countless other medical conditions, admitting short-comings granted the support that respondents sometimes required and, ideally, garnered empathy from those with whom they were interacting. Accordingly, being communicative and accepting help were seen as important methods for managing difficult circumstances by the diagnosed individuals and their spouses alike.

Attaining Serenity

In addition to focusing on the positive and accepting help, many respondents demonstrated a general serenity when talking about their condition that echoed the mantra of other self-help movements, particularly Alcoholics Anonymous,[34] whose cherished motto borrows from Reinhold Niebuhr's well-known poem:

> God grant me the serenity to accept the things I cannot change;
> courage to change the things I can;
> and wisdom to know the difference.
> Living one day at a time;
> Enjoying one moment at a time;
> Accepting hardships as the pathway to peace;
> Taking, as He did, this sinful world
> as it is, not as I would have it;
> Trusting that He will make all things right
> if I surrender to His Will;
> That I may be reasonably happy in this life
> and supremely happy with Him
> Forever in the next.
> Amen.

The views expressed by study participants diagnosed with AD/MCI echo a similar sense of serenity: "I have a clear picture, more and more I have a clear picture of what I can and what I can't do and I accept it" (male, MCI); and "It's [memory loss] been going on for several years. It didn't come on suddenly. It sort of grew. I'm just accepting it. There's not much else I can do" (female, MCI). Another woman, exhibiting a common dissatisfaction with the term disease, nonetheless demonstrated extraordinary serenity: "I just hate the term disease . . . I have a great lack of ease with not remembering things. Oh god, it drives me crazy . . . but we have to accept what we can't change" (female, AD). More detailed accounts reveal the strength of character that is required/can evolve from taking a stance of serenity:

> I've improved in the sense that I'm more able to accept the fact of what is happening to me, and that it's not getting better, that I am losing my memory. And so at first I would become sort of angry or a little upset, but now I'm beginning to accept that and be able to adjust to that, and I do see there's a certain amount of compassion that people show, and that makes me feel good, and also reminds me that I should feel the same way because, although they may not have the same problem that I have, they certainly are human beings like I am. So that's an adjustment that is making me feel good about myself. And it makes me feel stronger, as far as being able to handle it. (male, MCI)

While it does seem to come quite easily for many respondents to accept their forgetfulness, it seems that some of this may be related to being part of what has been called the last great generation—people who lived through world wars, depressions, and other socioeconomic hardships. The story of Ms. R, an 83-year-old woman living with AD, demonstrates a clear acceptance of her condition that involves her making an implicit comparison to others who have been less fortunate:

> What have I got to, excuse me, bitch about? Because there's nothing big in my life that's happened that's really horrible. I don't know anyone who's had as good a life as I had, despite the fact that I have this problem now.

With a sense of altruism, she continues:

> I'm glad I have this problem instead of one of my family, someone in my family, because that would absolutely, all day long I'd think about it every

night. I think I'd suffer more if someone I loved had this problem than if I have it myself.

She sums up with the role of religion in her life:

Now if that's not the Lord taking care of me, I don't know. I really do appreciate that, and I tell Him every night. . . . I just had the best life I've ever known anybody ever had. And I'm still having it now [that I've been diagnosed]. (female, AD)

While spirituality/religion were not overarching themes in these data, I have reported elsewhere on the significant role such positive modes of coping can play for people with memory loss and their loved ones.[35]

Comparisons between groups like Alcoholics Anonymous, where the narratives of self loss as an alcoholic are prevalent, and other disease-based support groups like those for Alzheimer's, AIDS, or cancer are useful. Importantly, the realization of the identity of alcoholic, while spoiled,[36] provides both internal biographical continuity for individuals and external social cohesion with other group members. In particular, conceiving of alcoholism as a disease generates "a sense of consubstantiality or kinship" among members of Alcoholics Anonymous.[37] The sense of fighting for a common cause and of hope for the future commonly pervades the rhetoric and daily discourse in these types of support networks,[38] as the fight is against the disease and not the person with it; that is, the person is not the disease. Such framing signals both the initiation into joining a subculture, the necessary third step to Becker's career model, and the accomplishment of the hybrid patient/research subject/support group member that Keating and Cambrioso claim is part and parcel of the bioclinical manifestation of modern medicine.

Even with conditions for which diagnostic processes are ambiguous or treatment regimes are emergent, such as Chronic Fatigue Syndrome, infertility, depression, or AIDS, research demonstrates that support groups serve a unifying and legitimating function.[39] Thus, even (potentially) spoiled identities can achieve solidarity in the company of people in the same situation. Such circumstances play a crucial role in uniting members of various health-related social movements (as chapter 7 will discuss) and both legitimate the condition and unify individuals in their processes of incorporating Alzheimer's identities.

Employing Humor

Humor was another strategy used by many respondents. Humor and joking have long been considered mechanisms of social control,[40] implicitly or explicitly communicating ideological assumptions while displaying social identity. However, humor is also an important resource for managing conflict during emotionally laden experiences,[41] and for encouraging a sense of community among members dealing with common contingencies.[42] Humor can also be used as an act of resistance against dominant paradigms, here the loss of self. DeShazer uses the movement to make breast cancer scars visible as an example of what she calls rebellious humor to deflate the culture of optimism that renders invisible (or marginalizes) the pain and suffering in the moment as well as those deaths that do result from the condition.[43] In other words, humor is a tactic whose results are at least twofold, that is, it is a mechanism for both elaborating and controlling conflict.[44] The following support group excerpts demonstrate how humor operates both as a coping mechanism and as a means through which social bonding is produced:

RB: How long have you been experiencing memory loss?

MR. T: Well, it's certainly been at least ten years, I'd say. Maybe I just made that up [laughing]. (male, AD)

R1 [to R2]: Do you think I have Alzheimer's disease? (female, AD)

R2 [to R1 and R3]: Yeah, both of you have it. (male, AD)

R3: [Exaggerating for effect] I resemble that remark! (male, AD)

R1 [to R3]: And all this time I thought you were faking it all. (male, AD)

RB: How would you describe what you experience [with memory loss]?

R5: [In a jokingly pedantic, academic tone] What's on my record is that the distal end of my central nervous system is not up to par.

RB: How about more specifically?

R5: [Rolling his eyes] It's a pain in the neck. (male, AD)

Likewise, jokes were a common thread in all my interviews and humor permeated the support groups, which may have alleviated some of the pressures of being confronted with their memory loss. For example, three men with AD made the following jokes: Regarding forgetting one has dementia, "That's the good side of memory loss"; [when asked about current activities] "I just try to avoid trouble. You know, fly under the radar"; and [in reference to wandering] "They ought to tie me down." Such inclusionary putdowns[45] serve to minimize negative experiences by sharing the distress with others who can relate to such incidents. In this way, humor and joking establish boundaries of membership while simultaneously allowing group members to candidly discuss what they are going through. The use of humor was a central characteristic in support group, interview, and observational data.

Being Proactive

While fully cognizant of their increasing shortcomings, participants believed they had, or could have, control over at least their response to being diagnosed. What they did *after* the diagnosis was up to them. Consequently, the method of management that was by far the most frequently expressed in the support groups was being proactive and doing something in reaction to the label. The utility of being purposeful immediately following the news of a terminal illness is well established in the social science literature.[46] Arguably a mechanism for attempting to normalize what were often described as unpredictable behaviors and atypical experiences, discussion of medications, alternative therapies, and recent medical findings were customary in the support groups. For respondents, knowledge was empowering, and especially in the eyes of these three men with MCI, medical information was central: "Dr. Weill was on last night on Larry King and he says to do the turmeric, so, I'm going to try that. What the heck. There's nothing to lose [and there] may be something to gain"; "I think the more you know, the more you learn about MCI and Alzheimer's and dementia, the more you learn the better able you're going to be to make a decision when the issues start. . . . So the more you read the more you understand, and the more of us talking to each other, the better decisions we can make"; and "They [researchers] are saying more and more that we should start earlier and earlier on medication. Then of course they're going to begin saying soon that actually anybody from age 50 on should take NSAID's or anti-inflammatories."

As these quotes suggest, many people endorsed biomedical discourse when they spoke about how important it was to be informed and active in learning about what was going on and keeping up with new discoveries. Although these types of reactions are perhaps more closely related to the sample population of affluent, highly educated, Caucasians accustomed to self-advocacy than to a general adaptation to the diagnostic label or experience of memory loss, study participants demonstrated a clear enthusiasm for being proactive about informing both their families and medical personnel of their needs and experiences. For example, this woman with AD and man with MCI make strategic appeals: "If you don't get out there and make yourself known and heard, make yourself heard, and you really need to. . . . I need to have the knowledge that I'm doing what I can"; and "If you put yourself out there and identify who you are, what your problem is. And say, 'Let's talk about what's happening and what we can do about it.' It's not enough to just curse the darkness. We need to get some light on the subject." Similarly, an 89-year-old retired physician reports actually feeling better as a result of his concrete effort to be proactive:

> I'm feeling better recently because the more knowledge you can get about it, that helps just get through the day and to begin to put things back in perspective again. And I'm a realist, that there is no cure . . . but I keep reading and studying and saying [to family members], "Hey, come in here and read this." So to be informed. And I think it is the issue here. Who you turn to that will listen to you or work with you or help you to work through the problems. (male, MCI)

The attitude of these information seekers resembles the process of becoming professional patients that interactionists have noted comes with the uncertainty infusing the illness trajectory of cancer.[47]

Notions of staying mentally active were observed regularly and the adage "use it or lose it" was employed repeatedly by both individuals with memory loss and their spouses alike. For example: "I don't think we should let the Alzheimer's eat us up. If you like to play checkers, play them!" (female, AD); and "It struck me it's like physical exercise. If you don't get any physical exercise your muscles get tired and you can't do it anymore. If you don't exercise your brain the same thing would happen" (male, MCI). While these sentiments undoubtedly reflect a neoliberal emphasis on self-regulation, they simultaneously bolster a sense of agency. The hope for a fix, of course, is also present in many statements, such as: "I think that we may be passing up ways of solving, of fixing it, the Alzheimer's. . . . Because I think all of us can have a vocabulary, and I may be wrong about that, but most adults our age have a good vocabulary. It can be spoiled, though, if we don't find a use for it" (male, AD). Nonetheless, spouses also reinforce this rhetoric and arguably gain a similar sense of security from it: "I've been watching [my husband] really working hard at exercising his brain. I don't know where he gets the motivation, but it really is nice for me because I can see him doing whatever he can to keep things functioning" (husband diagnosed with MCI). In fact, the proverb "use it or lose it" appeared to be an informal mantra of the support groups I observed. Since a similar theme characterized my in-depth interviews with diagnosed individuals, it appears that the role of being proactive rather than passively letting the disease attack was a crucial organizing principle for study participants, especially those attending support groups where such logic was touted.

These findings demonstrate that respondents used various methods to manage their interactions and identities after being labeled with AD/MCI. Although the management strategies obviously differed among participants and in accordance with circumstance, impression management was as common a phenomenon for the individuals observed in this research as has been demonstrated with AIDS and cancer.[48] These efforts helped manage the uncertainty both of being diagnosed with an unknown and incurable condition and of contending with behaviors that were often erratic. However, management strategies such as focusing on the positive, accepting help, attaining serenity, employing humor, or being proactive, can also have unintended consequences and the strategies may be perceived differently depending on the context in which they are used.[49]

Opportunities for Diagnosis

Despite the impressive surge of research on the subjective experience of dementia within the social and behavioral sciences, there is a general paucity of data exploring the psychosocial outcomes of *being labeled with* AD/MCI. While receiving a diagnosis, arguably itself a strategy for identity management to rule out psychiatric problems or "illnesses you have to fight to get,"[50] respondents noted that an important function was the ability to avail themselves of certain services and opportunities that they might not otherwise have known existed. The two primary resources highlighted were support groups and research studies, both of which served important purposes for the individuals diagnosed and their loved ones by simultaneously offering them a sense of collectivity and agency.

Utilizing Support Groups

Support groups were, not surprisingly, unanimously praised for the guidance and friendship they offered to individuals dealing with memory loss. While not everyone attends support groups, as there is a significant selection bias, the sense of community that emerged from these meetings appeared instrumental for study participants in much the same way as has been documented with other support (or self-help) groups.[51] The benefit of these forums was indisputable for both those with memory loss and their spouses. For example, there were personal benefits, such as: "I had the idea that I was the only one that has it [AD]. I knew that wasn't true but when you actually see other people [it helps]" (male, AD); "[Support groups make it so] you don't feel like you're in it alone" (male, MCI); and "[It reminds me that] there's plenty of other people in the same situation. It's just a small thing, but it's very important. And I'm not alone" (male, AD), as well as social advantages "Talking to other people with shared experiences is unlike talking with your friends and family, no matter how great they are" (female, AD). Spouses again corroborate the feelings of diagnosed individuals: "[Support groups] have worked out beautifully because it's the one place where [my husband] has been able to talk about, accept, and hear about other people. . . . It's important to him to be here. He goes and he knows he has Alzheimer's" (husband diagnosed with AD); and "I really feel that it [the support group] has done a lot for me having courage, I guess. It's easier to have courage when you know other people are doing it too. I think about that when I'm thinking 'this is scary'" (husband diagnosed with MCI).

Given the encouragement they received in these groups, it is not surprising that many respondents championed the meetings as integral to managing memory loss. Support groups were also seen as a forum in which to present and discuss upcoming media coverage, research results, and general questions or information on AD/MCI, which was shown earlier to be an important strategy for individuals trying to manage the changes they were experiencing. Support groups were perceived to provide obvious benefits for members.

Beyond the stated incentives to those who participated in support groups, however, such involvement has some hidden consequences. Since the groups observed in this study tended not to be staged, that is, they met together regardless of where along the disease trajectory they resided, members were often keenly aware of what the future had in store for them. For some respondents, this was a distressing reminder of inevitable decline. It was not uncommon for members of the support groups to express their sadness that eventually they would all be transferred to support groups directed at advanced Alzheimer's (or worse, a day care setting). Alternatively, tragic stories about individuals known by a single participant or represented in the media might be seen as a strategy to lessen the anguish of all members; "seeking reinforcing comparisons"[52] might make their own situations seem more bearable.

Given that the groups were offered either by research centers (such as the specialty clinics where they had been diagnosed) or the Alzheimer's Association, the support group environment tended to have a strongly medicalized culture. As such, group members might have felt pressure to enroll in various affiliated projects, including research. More importantly, while a few study participants tried and stopped coming and fewer never tried, those who chose not to be a part of the groups because they were not comfortable with talk therapy or what sociologist Susan Ferguson has termed psychological gentrification[53] often had few other channels of formal support or information. Consequently, alternative understandings of aging and memory loss needed to be periodically if not wholeheartedly disregarded by members—at least during the support group meetings themselves. If individuals with memory loss must consciously navigate between the everyday experiences requiring innovative and fleeting management techniques and the stationary, technical jargon and explanatory frameworks of biomedicine, then a rift can appear between tangible events and emotional sense-making. Despite the indirect negative results of support group involvement in theory, that is, that they function as what postmodern theorists refer to as a technology of self whereby we act in ways that self-regulate us, in daily life respondents considered such groups an instrumental aspect of living with AD/MCI.

Participating in Research

Closely related to the above, the second resource diagnosed individuals and their families perceived was participation in research. Many respondents felt that being involved in research allowed them to do something (i.e., be proactive), to help advance science, to benefit future generations, and to possibly even receive some personal benefit. Individuals with a family history of dementia seemed particularly eager to be involved in research and none of the respondents noted an unwillingness to participate if offered the alleged opportunity to do so. For example: "My mother had Alzheimer's and my sister was recently diagnosed with Alzheimer's, and that is the main reason I got into the research. Not that I thought I had any symptoms, but then as time [went] on, [I was] more aware and conscious of the fact . . . when I got it" (female, MCI). The following support group excerpt is also instructive:

R1: After the diagnosis I got into a project that was really helpful. For about three years I was on this project, and during that time I was simply like I always was. So, I've really had a lot of [help] because I've had these different people who advised me or suggested things or gave me the opportunity to be in the project. It was a drug trial. And it was really interesting to do. The trial was wonderful because they had such excellent people. We did a lot of things. I think anyone who has an opportunity to get in and see how some of these things can be done, it helps you very much. (female, AD)

RB: Would others of you participate in a drug trial?

R2: I would do it if it were offered. (male, AD)

R3: I think I would if it looked like it promised something to come. (male, AD)

R4: I think I would be willing to do a trial because I'm always interested in innovations and I'm always interested in anything in the medical field. (female, AD)

R5: I have been in one or two drug trials and I would certainly do it again. I mean, they aren't going to give you something that would hurt you, and who knows, it may help. (female, AD)

According to study participants, the perceived benefits of being diagnosed with AD/MCI were noteworthy. In practice, the price to pay, unfortunately, was that one often had to undergo more of the impersonal and degrading tests depicted in chapters 3 and 4, which typically left a person feeling increasingly deficient. Also, since research participation is limited, many people suffered angst over not having access to studies they hoped could assist them or their loved ones. The inclusion criteria for research also reflected the trajectory of AD, as individuals eventually became too impaired to participate in a given study or they became eligible for one that signaled cognitive decline. Such involvement is arguably a reminder of the social degradation of AD/MCI.

Although study participants were experiencing a reportedly harrowing condition, they relied on support groups and research studies to discuss their emotions, to garner information, and to seek refuge. Support groups and research participation were tangible expressions that respondents were doing something. Had their memory loss never been diagnosed, they likely would not have had access to these resources that allowed them to experience a sense of community and agency. Accordingly, support groups and research participation were also concrete strategies employed by the respondents to manage their identities and interactions. As such, with guidance from clinical and research staff, support groups and research participation were mechanisms through which individuals diagnosed with AD/MCI and their families normalized otherwise foreign and disorderly experiences. It is important to note that these were, in fact, the only options made available to people with memory loss. The diagnostic process, then, commenced what had the potential to be a lifelong dependence on biomedical solutions and answers; alternative approaches for managing memory loss were clearly marginalized. The lives of forgetful people become medicalized into those of Alzheimer's patients by offering them exclusively biomedical solutions to problems that are personal, social, and medical.

Conclusion: Being Socially Labeled

A fundamental interest of qualitative sociology is to understand the types and qualities of interactions people have with one another and the effect of these exchanges on their sense of self. Interactionists highlight processes of meaning-making that are not static but continually modified through negotiation. Accordingly, our understanding of the world and our self-concept are always potentially shifting. Roles, and therefore the interactions based on them, are fluid.

Threats to personhood can occur in many contexts, including institutional settings like prisons or mental asylums, sites of degradation and torture in enslavement or detention/prisoner-of-war camps, and perhaps less obviously, with the assignment of various labels, medical or otherwise, that connote second-class citizenry. Viktor Frankl's *Man's Search for Meaning* is a compelling account of a Holocaust survivor's realization that human life is never without meaning. In fact, the hopelessness of the situation, according to Frankl, "did not detract from its dignity and its meaning. . . . [Rather, we should be found] suffering proudly—not miserably—knowing how to die."[54] Being deprived of one's humanity in any setting can destroy a sense of social belonging and render individuals seemingly obsolete. Classifying individuals as criminal, sick, or subhuman has been used to control unruly populations or groups of people perceived to be in need of coercion, if not brutal force, to comply. Ritual acts of insubordination are demeaning and derogatory strategies of social control.[55] Further, the forced suspension of time and everyday life that can contribute to a diminished sense of self for prisoners,[56] can extend to those with particularly debilitating chronic illnesses. Ironically, such a complete assault on a person's identity can *rob individuals of their unique attributes* while at the same time *serving to solidify the group identity* of those sharing common circumstances.[57]

The process of becoming an Alzheimer's patient is neither linear nor facile, but involves many junctures or phases. This chapter has shown that there is a complex trajectory or continuum of AD/MCI experiences. It has elsewhere been claimed that there is a moral career of successful prison gang membership,[58] which includes five phases: pre-initiate, initiate, member, veteran, and superior.[59] Likewise, the process of becoming a patient involves many phases. It is perhaps not surprising, then, that upon diagnosis respondents referred to AD/MCI as a death sentence (see chapter 5), yet interviews years later depicted individuals who were struggling to present themselves in ways that specifically disproved this very sentiment. For these respondents, the process began with the advent of the diagnosis and included various turning points—or steps: being evaluated, getting a diagnosis, accepting the diagnosis, and joining a subgroup—before culminating in an identity as *an Alzheimer's patient.*

Rather than being instantly relegated to the status of a patient or impaired person, as clinical management strategies might imply, individuals instead balanced the diagnosis by incorporating it into their pre-existing identities. Normative expectations of beliefs and behaviors are in fact remarkably difficult to manufacture and sustain in the practice of everyday life. In many ways, individuals diagnosed with AD/MCI embarked on a process of normalization—or the making familiar—of memory loss, which involved a delicate balance between both biomedical facts and personal beliefs. This effort to avoid being relegated to the status of a diseased or sick person was the consequence of a situation whereby respondents felt they had experienced a clear transition (i.e., regression) in the way they were perceived by others since being diagnosed. These data depict views and values of an outside world that require the creative management of social interactions.

One significant departure, or point of resistance, between management strategies and phenomenological processes of normalization lies in the common belief that some memory loss naturally accompanies aging. Thus, the diagnosed individuals were forced to incorporate this tension into their new identities as people living with a brain pathology resulting in forgetfulness. This debate seemed to permeate support group conversations and often prevented respondents from seeking out research studies; frequently individuals would express themselves in a contradictory manner at different times. A conversation that transpired between people diagnosed with MCI speaks to the divergence between group members and a general confusion regarding past conceptions:

> RB: Do you think that what you're experiencing is a disease?
> R1: Yes, I think it is a disease. (male, MCI)
> R2: You do? Or is it a stage? I don't know, maybe it's just a stage. (male, MCI)
> R3: It's probably not a disease because it's something that's going to be with you for the rest of your life and diseases aren't. (male, MCI)
> R4: I think it's a disease. A disease or a malfunction of the brain somehow because there was certainly nothing that I knowingly did to try to get this and then when it did come I didn't recognize it anyway. (male, MCI)
> R5: [When I was younger and before I was diagnosed] I thought all those people who couldn't remember anything couldn't remember because they were old. . . . It was not an accident or an illness. It was a situation that you have to go through when you get older. You forget. Period. (female, AD)

The lack of consensus over what comprises normal, age-related memory loss was the most significant point of contention in the incorporation of the disease-identity for the individuals in this study. As with the data from clinical evaluation, perhaps this resistance demonstrates a keen understanding of the entanglement of dementia and aging.[60] Those diagnosed with Alzheimer's or mild cognitive impairment intuitively resisted the undisputed biomedical labels ascribed to them, thus requiring consistent reminders that *their* memory loss was indeed pathological. Although some of these reminders came from medical clinicians, Alzheimer's Association staff, and family members, the excerpt from the MCI meeting above suggests they also come from within the group itself; members prevent each other from falling off the proverbial wagon and thus losing so-called insight into their deficits.[61] In this way, members socialize one another into biomedical interpretations of their memory loss.

Most importantly, individuals with minor memory loss managed their symptoms by devising concrete strategies to combat biological, social, and personal losses. Respondents had become responsible impression managers of an identity inscribed with the label "demented." To aid them in the challenge of managing a newly spoiled identity, such strategies literally became necessary resources of self-preservation.[62] In efforts to avoid the master status of a demented person, study participants endured the potential threat to their selves by utilizing methods of management reflecting an identity that is constructed and reconstructed over time; identity persists as a fundamental characteristic.

Thus, respondents sought out resources to aid them in their endeavor to understand memory loss and integrate it into their lives without completely compromising who they were prior to the diagnosis. For study participants, after the initial reaction and emotions attached to the diagnosis began to subside, every effort was made to continue living; the focus was on what could be done and not what might have been or would in the future be lost. These individuals especially wished not to surrender the activities, roles, and relationships they had enjoyed prior to the diagnosis. Accordingly, with a supportive environment, dementia becomes what Jenny Knauss called her early onset AD: a manageable disability.[63]

Through participation in things like support groups and research studies devoted to AD, diagnosed individuals further embark on the process of incorporating Alzheimer's identities. While retrospectively reconstructing past behaviors to normalize their diagnosis, people participate in things like research projects and support groups for strategic reasons, which include managing uncertainty, making space for the new diagnosis within their existing identities, and garnering expert help despite the circumscribed scope in which these services are offered. But both support groups and research involvement also afford respondents dealing with memory loss the chance to feel connected to others in a similar situation, help others, and be proactive—a motivation for taking the third step in the process of assuming the master status: membership in a subgroup. The next chapter discusses the role of the Alzheimer's Association, the national voluntary health organization devoted to the cause, in the incorporation of this new voice and its effect on the process of becoming a person with AD.

Rather than obediently adorning the label of a demented person, however, the moral career of my study participants involved (aims) to reconstitute the power relations between themselves and other able-minded people, including clinicians and social others, by continually negotiating their identity as competent people. Their adaptation to the purported symptoms of memory loss and resultant social relations can be seen as a new interactional strategy whereby the diagnosis becomes a resource utilized to get through the day. In spite of the many frustrations and heartaches accompanying the condition, respondents fought to avoid having their lives reduced simply because they had been diagnosed with memory loss. They moved forward and continued living their lives by accounting for and controlling their experiences the best they could. Rather than being passive recipients of a diagnosis as depictions by the pharmaceutical industry, public media, and bench science suggest, these narratives suggest that participants employed the label both as a resource to help them manage the changes in their lives and as something that needed to be taken into account to deal with the recent affront to their social and personal selves.

7

Advocating Alzheimer's

Biomedical Structures and Social Movements

In 1982, President Ronald Wilson Reagan designated the first National Alzheimer's Disease Awareness Week. Ironically, just over a decade later he delivered a speech disclosing his own Alzheimer's diagnosis. His openness and his wife Nancy's active involvement in the cause offered great promise for promoting a more accurate understanding of the condition and a fuller inclusion of affected individuals into the Alzheimer's social movement. Yet this did not happen. Why did their courage, optimism, and activism not promote fundamental social change? Based on in-depth qualitative interviews with twelve staff members from the U.S. Alzheimer's Association, the first and most visible national advocacy organization devoted to the cause, as well as participation and observation at dozens of academic meetings and inter/national conferences sponsored by the Association, this chapter explores how individuals diagnosed with memory loss are envisioned and served by the voluntary sector within the United States. This chapter begins with a background of the Alzheimer's disease movement, specifically the Association's role as the primary social movement organization (SMO) fueling it. Next, I trace the history of the Association and its contemporary contexts and philosophies. Using the perspectives of staff at local and national chapters and the image portrayed on their official website, I will outline the Association's organizational identity and institutional logic. Drawing on organizational theory, my central argument is that the founding ideals of biomedicine are so deeply ingrained within the Association that cause and cure research and treatments to help caregivers cope with the presumed problem of having a loved one with AD are the focus of efforts rather than the inclusion of people with AD themselves, or a care focus.[1] Recent scholarship supports the claim that a contentious issue that has plagued the

Association since its inception is the existence of two related but ultimately conflicting goals: one, to rid the world of AD through a cure or medications to effectively treat the condition, advanced by the medical community, and the other focused on helping people currently living with the condition manage their daily lives, advocated by those providing support to people with dementia (and, more recently, diagnosed individuals themselves).[2]

I will argue that an additional tension also exists between caregivers as the primary constituency and the lived experiences of those with AD/MCI themselves, since the latter is far beyond the scope of biomedicine. If caregiver needs are both historically embedded within the Association and can be easily served through basic science solutions (i.e., pharmacological treatment of behavioral and psychotic symptoms of dementia, or BPSDs, and the presumed stress and burden associated with being a carer), then the well-being of people with Alzheimer's is secondary. The original role of people with AD in the Association was limited to being research subjects and passive recipients of care, which has created what Max Weber referred to as an iron cage for the Association. Consequently, *the social justice aims of combating the negative social constructions of people with AD contradict the organizational identity of the Association.*[3]

I compare the AD movement and more traditional Health Social Movements (HSMs) that rely on medical definitions and simultaneously challenge the authority of scientific knowledge and the practices based on it,[4] which the AD movement has not historically done. Recent mobilization efforts from the on-line community known as DASNI (Dementia Advocacy and Support Network International), the Alzheimer's Foundation of America (AFA), and Dementia Alliance International (DAI) will be outlined to analyze counter or resistance narratives that have sprung up within the movement in response to the Association's perceived inability or unwillingness to be critical of biomedicine or to focus on aspects of care. While the comparatively radical and vocal approach of such narratives of resistance has the potential to change the Alzheimer's disease movement and even its most powerful SMO, the chapter reveals persistent myths[5] that will have to be debunked before goals as lofty as social change can begin to be realized.

Background of the Alzheimer's Movement

Robert Butler, gerontologist, physician, psychiatrist, and Pulitzer-prize winning author, was named the founding director of the National Institute on Aging (NIA) in 1974. He coined the term ageism and is credited with establishing the causal link between senility and Alzheimer's, which redefined the former as no longer an inevitable aspect of aging. Butler quickly established Alzheimer's as a National Research Priority for NIA. In the late 1970s, a disease-based social movement started to coalesce around Alzheimer's and began providing support to family members. With the help of several families attending support groups, another key actor, Jerome H. Stone, founded and became the first president of the Alzheimer's Association after meeting with the NIA in 1979. The Alzheimer's Disease and Related Disorders Association was incorporated on April 10, 1980. That year, the National Institutes of Health (NIH) invested $13 million in Alzheimer's research. The establishment of first the NIA and then the Alzheimer's Association signaled a clear response to views that services and information on the condition were inadequate. The movement's formation was based primarily on the redefinition of senility as a biomedical classification (Alzheimer's disease), which by including cases of people over 65 years of age rendered it the fourth or fifth leading cause of death virtually overnight and thus made it well-deserving of public attention.[6] The subsequent "Alzheimer's Industrial Complex" began swiftly and has since seen tremendous success.

Compared to other contemporary health social movements, the AD movement has been far less inclusive of its target population and exceptionally slow to identify and promote public spokespersons. In the late 1970s, it was practitioners and scientists working with families affected by Alzheimer's who sought public attention for the condition. When the first voluntary organization was formed in its name, the intention was to direct public attention to the condition and garner federal support for research looking for a solution. The movement successfully framed itself through the promotion of AD as a significant social, not simply an individual, problem, transforming senility from a private family matter into a medical epidemic demanding public concern.

Like all social movements, external structures and internal dynamics shaped the maintenance, principles, and outcomes of the AD movement and its organizations. The Alzheimer's Association, with concerted effort from (primarily) bench scientists and affected families and (more recently) people with AD, has been a catalyst for the lobbying initiatives of the Alzheimer's movement. Given its biomedical focus, the Association has been very effective in seeking monies to fund research projects. Attempts to give voice to the perspectives of people with AD, however, have encountered considerable obstacles.

As with other marginalized groups such as children, those with developmental disabilities, or the mentally ill, proxy interviews with carers have historically been seen as the best way to understand Alzheimer's, both reflecting and reinforcing pejorative assumptions that people with dementia are deficient or, worse, irrelevant. This view often stems from the belief that people with AD cannot learn or communicate in a meaningful way, do not want to do so, or would be harmed by the interaction. Such assumptions created by and situated within a society that glamorizes a youthful, fit body and mind further weaken people with AD's ability to assert their interests. In practice, such presumptions of incompetence[7] insinuate that people with AD cannot advocate for themselves, speak effectively in civic realms, or serve as leaders of the social movement claiming to represent them, regardless of their aptitude or aspirations. Ironically, the conundrum is that the most salient barrier to challenging negative perceptions is precisely this lack of visible and credible spokespersons to portray the condition.[8]

In the United States, the rise of activism in other arenas has proven that structural trends change when patient advocates become visible, often forging new types of clinical research and practice.[9] The laudable efforts of the AIDS and breast cancer movements both criticized and galvanized biomedicine. These movements had large and ambitious groups of young, savvy, at-risk activists, including charismatic spokespersons who generated urgency and support[10] and could be effectively targeted for education and prevention.[11] In contrast, the AD movement was not initiated by or originally intended for people with the condition. Further, since cognition is compromised with Alzheimer's, people are less likely (both presumptively and in reality, as the condition progresses) to pursue public speaking and/or advocacy.

Historically, while the AIDS movement kept a local grassroots focus on individual needs, the AD movement's more macro national approach easily converted into an interest group aimed at making policy changes from within existing social structures.[12] The AD movement has not made concerted efforts to challenge medical authority or knowledge, which arguably correlates with the enormous amount of monies earmarked for finding a cure, or what renowned political economist Carroll Estes might call the Alzheimer's Enterprise.[13] In contrast, AIDS activists demanded drug trials and alternative therapies when no efficacious medications existed. The distinctions between these movements include the targeted populations (and their perceived competence) as well as their relations with and expectations of biomedicine.

The U.S. AD movement has been far more similar to the mental health and disability movements in terms of its approach to biomedicine than to the AIDS or breast cancer movements.[14] Despite a constituency comprised of people with stated conditions, considerably less criticism of biomedicine and its implications have surfaced in the mental health and disability movements relative to the AIDS or breast cancer movements. Arguably, this is due in part to the stigma and historically contested legitimacy of certain conditions (e.g., mental illnesses) as a disease and/or the moral accountability often associated with physical disabilities (e.g., genetic deformities or weak immune systems). In addition, the perception of such people as vulnerable engenders an embittered struggle against assuming the stigmatized identity of a mentally ill/disabled person. Yet the mental health and disability movements have both made enormous progress in their efforts at inclusion. The goal of being heard so feverishly achieved by these other movements remains in the elementary stages for people with AD. If the AD movement has constituents who question the biomedical model of Alzheimer's, then it will be important for them to challenge the historical foundation of the Association in order to advocate for people with AD.

The bench science and care provider underpinnings of the Alzheimer's Association—the countrywide powerhouse behind much of the movement in the U.S. media, public discourse, and the research community—have yielded an impressive commitment first and foremost to cause and cure research and to a lesser extent caregiver issues and long-term care policies. Diagnostic advances, including early and even preclinical identification, result in people currently experiencing AD being able to articulate their positions more clearly than when the

Association was established. One result of this biomedical trend is that the movement has been forced to account for this phenomenon. It has responded by trying to incorporate these voices instead of relying solely on the viewpoints of carers. The Association started altering its objectives as previously unheard perspectives emerged, including addressing new realms pertaining to quality of life, experiences of memory loss, and meeting the individual needs of a clientele that is now both young and old. However, as attention shifts, traditional initiatives such as basic science, fund-raising, education, and family support are in direct competition for resources. As the largest and until recently the only social movement organization aimed exclusively at dementia, the Association remains the most influential U.S. player in the AD movement. Discovering the factors influencing the activities of the Alzheimer's Association is essential to understanding what has frustrated the stated intentions of including people with AD.

Part of the obstacle to incorporating these perspectives may be due to the relationship between social death,[15] or marginalization, and social worth. Research on dementia suggests that those who suffer from prolonged terminal illnesses, who are very old, and who are believed to experience a loss of personhood as a result of their condition are often relegated to the status of inanimate objects.[16] The symbolic liminality between life and death presumed of people with dementia risks rendering them socially obsolete. Such existential demarcations exacerbate the likelihood of societal disadvantages[17] engendered by social constructions of AD as the "never ending funeral" and a "living death."[18] The "competence-inhibiting support"[19] implied by the surplus of manuals geared at formal and informal providers of care signifies how easily those caring for people with AD become the object of attention and how often they are perceived as the second, if not the *real*, victims.

Although early attempts to incorporate the voice of people with dementia into research[20] did not gain much momentum initially, an impressive number of both first-person accounts of Alzheimer's[21] and social and behavioral research with people who have AD[22] have now emerged, including two noteworthy sociological articles coauthored by people with dementia.[23] While this impressive surge of studies has begun to reverse the trend of viewing people with AD solely as deficient, which pathologizes their behavior[24] and effectively silences their voices in public life, it has not yet made its way into the Association or reached the point of initiating social and structural change.

If the objectives of the Association correlate with how members are defined and treated, then understanding the interface between media, politics, and medicine and the efforts of social movements and their organizations is crucial. Societies that ascribe worth on the basis of age, or place higher value on citizens who are youthful, both reflect and reinforce structural forces that act to stereotype, devalue, and exclude old people regardless of any SMO's intentions. Likewise, the hegemony of biomedical principles in modern American society also gives preference to cause and cure over care.

The remainder of this chapter will investigate the ideological resources fueling the Alzheimer's movement's central advocacy organization and the environment embedding it. Many social factors influence social movements, including ideological differences, sociohistorical conditions, politics, and constituency resources. Biomedical definitions normalize, or name, diseases, thus making them a household word and legitimating their existence; that is, naming illnesses potentially unites members of disease-based movements. Shifting the definition of Alzheimer's to include dementias of all ages circa 1975 greatly increased the number of reported cases and led to its being perceived as a significant social and health problem. Yet the relationship between science, politics, and cultures of disease has profound consequences for members of health social movements, including the formation of collective identities, minimizing the blame-the-victim mentality, influencing policy changes, procuring research monies, and increasing awareness of targeted conditions.

The dynamics of the Association affect not only people with dementia who may or may not be involved in the movement, but also any implicated actors[25] as well as to their significant social others. An examination of the Association's origins, goals, and tactics can begin to address why incorporating this voice meets such resistance.

The Association and Obstacles to Inclusion

As the previous two chapters have revealed, respondents with AD express a resounding willingness to become more visible and vocal in the dialogue surrounding dementia. Voicing their concerns satisfied a need to do something during a time of heightened uncertainty and was a valuable management strategy, as shown in chapter 6. Unfortunately, forgetful participants in this study also cited a variety of barriers preventing them from being heard, including the fact that the nature of the condition with which they had been diagnosed pre-empted their ability to advocate in a confident and articulate manner. Importantly, despite these obstacles, at least in theory respondents resisted taking on the purported deficiency perspective[26] as a master status, were eager to inform the movement in their name, and sought inclusion to dispute the pervasive rhetoric of self loss.

Likewise, staff from the Alzheimer's Association unanimously stressed the importance of incorporating the perspectives of people with dementia when planning the programs and policies aimed at them: "There's a real consciousness in the Alzheimer's Association . . . to engage people [with AD] and involve them" (Interim President, National Office); and "[There] is a slowly growing voice [of people with AD] that's invited [to participate]. We want their voice as part of the . . . we want to include them in the Association" (Associate Executive Director, Southwest). Yet when Association staff discussed their perceived ethical concerns regarding the utilization of people with memory loss in public forums, they used rhetoric that reinforced notions of self loss. For example, the Interim President at the time of this research said the following:

> We've had terrible moral quandaries over bringing somebody into a hearing room who was clearly demented, making a spectacle of themselves. And you know, they haven't said okay to that. *They don't even know where they are [emphasis added].* And wrestling with that and saying, "Are we exploiting these people?" and "What's the appropriate thing?" You know, we do that [have them testify at senate hearings] with the full participation of family members and surrogates, and recognize that they're sure there's some risk, but there's a payoff that brings it home.

Rather than take the approach of, say, Michael J. Fox, when he went off his Parkinson's medications prior to his testimony before the Senate Appropriations Subcommittee in 1999, the Association has framed the use of spokespersons from within the ranks of people with AD as exploitative of their symptoms, yet it has done so without explicitly discussing that decision with those affected. That is, the Association arguably made this choice based on assumptions that suggest infantilization or paternalism.

In addition, various competing organizational needs conflict with the stated objective of including people with AD. Some of these dynamics are within the Association itself and others are external factors similar to those confronting many voluntary organizations. The staff I spoke with were personally motivated in the struggle to help people with AD and their loved ones, as most had the condition in their own families. They highlighted the importance of including people with memory loss in the realm of research, policy making, and service delivery. Yet, most centrally, they spoke of the benefit of putting a face on the Association itself and thought that the most effective way to do so was by encouraging spokespersons from within the ranks of those living with memory loss. Many, including the interim president, saw increased public awareness as the primary benefit of these efforts: "This is a disease that is so devastating that many people have some experience with it in their families, but when you personalize it—[when] you show somebody who looks like them, it has [an] enormous effect." Others spoke more specifically about "demanding better care":

> [T]here are people who . . . don't want people to know but there are just as many people who . . . don't mind sharing their stories to get the word out. [W]hen you're more visible . . . people become more vocal about demanding better care, . . . more money for research . . . [and] making sure that the families and friends that they know get the care. (Development and Communications, East Coast)

At least one woman had the admirable and pioneering goal of challenging negative stereotypes and assumptions of self loss that could result in meaningful social change: "We will . . . somehow . . . change the face of Alzheimer's disease to show these people who are able to speak for themselves, who are healthy, who work out every day, who take care of their dogs, and who work on their computers" (Executive Director, Northwest).

Despite this staff member's vision of the potential of people with Alzheimer's to combat pejorative framings of AD, however, most Association staff depicted the purpose of their inclusion as more instrumental: to be public spokespersons for the condition (and thus the Association). When this study was conducted, caregivers were the only spokespersons used to lobby policy makers for more research monies to fund biomedical research and spoke at designated points[27] to federal and local agencies, practitioners, and potential private donors. Perhaps due in part to pleas from people like the executive director quoted above, those with the condition were beginning to demand inclusion by serving on various committees within the Association, thus allowing them to inform the very practices and programs aimed to serve them. In 2006, for example, the Early Stage Advisory Group was established to utilize diagnosed individuals in "helping the Association provide the most appropriate services for people living with early-stage Alzheimer's, raise awareness about early-stage issues and advocate with legislators to increase funding for research and support programs."[28] After extensive deliberation, the first person with early-stage Alzheimer's was appointed to the Board of Directors in 2008. But people with Alzheimer's were dissatisfied with the roles that staff envisioned them playing within the Association. When I asked staff what capacity people with dementia could serve in the Association, it became clear they felt that diagnosed individuals could help primarily through quality control and policy efforts:

> I think one of the strongest things a person with Alzheimer's can do is help make sure the services are the right services. You're doing them for those people, and admittedly their needs are going to change as they advance in this disease, but you always want to go to the people who are affected and have them involved in designing the system. (Interim President, National)

> [There is a] role [for] the person with the diagnosis in advocacy for changes in Medicare, Medicaid, etc. . . . . [The Association] holds a Public Policy Forum each year [and] there are more and more people with the disease who not only are invited to come, but are invited to be part of the congressional testimony. The educational role that they played in [this] forum was invaluable. . . . I think they perform a community education

role [as well], either with people who have or may have the disease as well as with concerned family members. The advocacy by people with the disease makes it more likely that we will be able to keep building the prevention side of the spectrum, or the management side. (Public Policy, Midwest)

In contrast, some staff underscored a potential for self-advocacy through "peer support and education" and the importance of going to the source for answers: "I think we are moving to a point where we understand that we need to and have to listen to persons with Alzheimer's disease because they know what we need to be doing to help them" (Vice President, Programs and Public Policy, Southeast). Others elaborated this point:

Education [and] peer support. Educating the public at large, but educating other people within their [support] group or even in the early stages. I think there can be opportunity for peer support. The Association can be a liaison between people who are already involved in the Association and people who may have just received a diagnosis, who want to talk to somebody else about the disease. It's different if I sit down and talk to somebody about their diagnosis versus somebody with the disease talking. (Regional Director, Northwest)

Unfortunately, the initial Advisory Group complained that their role was largely symbolic and there was no real change or authentic voice in the Association.[29] The perceived roles for spokespersons with AD were seen to serve the immediate needs of the Association far better than the larger issues of social change upon which the movement is based or the microlevel experiences of diagnosed individuals.

While the Association's recent interest in persons with the disease might be a form of what social movement scholars call cooptation (e.g., to increase public knowledge of the condition, and subsequently the organization itself), many chapters are now encouraging people with AD to plead their cause by recruiting advocates from the more than 4,500 Association-sponsored support groups across the nation. Facilitators of these groups are ostensibly able to hand-select lobbyists reflecting the image the Association wants portrayed. Since the (biomedical) knowledges and practices informing the Association's activities and official policy positions are often at odds with the subjective experiences of individuals with AD, however, these efforts appear to first and foremost aid the Association in procuring more attention and funding; putting a face is also a strategic maneuver:

> When we talk about how to get the policymaker's attention, they've heard from the 80-year-old caregiver who lost her husband. Part of the judgment to do this [have people with AD testify] was a judgment that tactically we needed something fresh. . . . I think from a strategic point of view, we needed a new voice. The guys on the Hill were kind of getting used to us. "Well here you are back again. Don't have to tell me your story. You told me last year." And when Congressman or Senator [name] had to sit with a guy he went to law school with who is his exact age and who he knows, who is a person with Alzheimer's disease, it was shattering to him. It blew his little mind. So I think strategically we were ready for, we need new faces, we need new voices. We're not getting through. . . . Strategically the times demand that we do something more. (Director, State Policy and Advocacy, National)

Inclusion of people with dementia has largely been framed by staff as a good business decision.

Another important strategy was to encourage celebrity involvement. American sitcom actor and comedian David Hyde Pierce, for example, has done extensive advocacy for the Association since 1998. Princess Yasmin Aga Khan, daughter of the late Rita Hayworth, has also served on the Association's Board of Directors for many years. The Association's most recent efforts to this end, however, have come from their "Celebrity Alzheimer's Champions," a growing list of actors and athletes who make philanthropic donations and compete in contests such as "Who Wears Purple Best?" to raise Alzheimer's awareness. Hyde Pierce, Aga Khan, and designated "Champions" cannot, of course, provide firsthand perspectives on the condition, but instead represent what social movement scholars refer to as symbolic gestures. Despite the ardent intentions of the staff I spoke with, efforts to include people with AD are frustrated by the internal dynamics of the Association, external factors, and overarching features.

Internal Dynamics

On April 10, 1980, representatives from five family support groups and staff from the National Institutes of Health and the National Institute on Aging cited two primary objectives in forming the Alzheimer's Disease and Related Disorders Association, Inc.: increasing public awareness and the search for a cure. By 1988, dropping the "and Related Disorders" solidified a constituency and clearly demarcated the organizational objectives of the Alzheimer's Association. This single-disease orientation is still evident today in the organizational identity of the Association provided on its website:

> As the largest non-profit funder of Alzheimer's research, the Association is committed to accelerating progress of new treatments, preventions and ultimately, a cure. Through our partnerships and funded projects, we have been part of every major research advancement over the past 30 years. The Association is the leading voice for Alzheimer's disease advocacy, fighting for critical Alzheimer's research, prevention and care initiatives at the state and federal level.[30]

Since the Association was primarily established through input from professionals trying to eradicate the condition and families trying to cope with the stress and burden associated with what was commonly referred to as the disease of caregivers, vast contributions have been made in both areas. Diagnostic efficacy has greatly improved, allowing for much earlier diagnoses, and there are now five FDA-approved medications for treating AD.[31] Significant research on caregiving within the social and behavioral sciences[32] has translated the perspective of care partners into both the Association's efforts and public policy. When I asked about the Association's mission, the tensions between cure and care, or hope and help, were evident: "Our objective is obviously to help find a cure. But in the meantime, to provide services and programs" (Communications Coordinator, Midwest); and "Well, [our mission] is twofold. To cure, to prevent this disease, do research. And to enhance care and quality of services for persons with the disease, their families, and the health care community" (Chief Executive Officer, Southeast). A more detailed elaboration underscores "help and hope":

Our ultimate objective is to be out of business. That said, we know we have to be in business for awhile, so we also work very strongly on care issues. To me, the mission of the Alzheimer's Association . . . is about help and hope; help for people with Alzheimer's and their families today [and] hope that through research it's over. (Director, State Policy and Advocacy Programs, National)

Interestingly, only one respondent noted that a choice was involved in deciding what to emphasize, "You can put the care or the cure first, depending on which chapter you are, but [The Association's mission] is to eliminate Alzheimer's disease through the advancement of research and to enhance care and support for individuals, their families, and caregivers" (Associate Executive Director, Southwest).

Since the founding ideals mean that people with the disease and their perspectives are often overlooked, staff noted that the long-standing history of a caregiver-based organization had only recently begun to shift. When I asked about the biggest change in their time at the Association, most noted efforts to include people with dementia, "In the 80s the research was clearly on caregiver burden, caregiver stress . . . the caregiver's support groups. In the late 90s we began to turn the corner and look at the person with the disease" (Regional Director, NorthBay); "The Association has, for probably the last decade, but very strongly in the last six or seven years, been shifting its focus from being primarily caregiver driven to much more of a balance, looking at the needs of individuals" (Interim President, National); "The most interesting thing in the last three years has been the emergence of persons with Alzheimer's into full membership, if you will, in the movement" (Director, State Policy and Advocacy Programs, National); and "[The Association] was set up by the families to support the families. In the last five years there has been slow movement where the voice, a voice would come up here and there of a person with dementia . . . there is a slowly growing voice that's invited" (Associate Executive Director, Southwest). While staff estimates varied regarding how long the trend to include people with AD had been going on, most said it had started around the turn of the century. Critics suggest that efforts to include people with AD are far from being realized, and some staff clearly had yet to begin turning the corner at all. When I asked about the objectives of the Alzheimer's Association, a few showed clear caregiver priorities, "Basically to be the primary resource for families, caregivers, and the people who are in the environment of the individual with the disease" (Executive Director, Washington, D.C.); and "We want to be the number one, primary resource for the caregivers" (Chapter President, East Coast). A decade and a half after the move to include people with AD began, it has not been achieved.

Although participants noted various reasons for the shift toward incorporating people living with Alzheimer's, they primarily attributed it to scientific progress, namely, earlier diagnosis rather than the human rights or social justice aspects of inclusion—demonstrating the biomedical hegemony: "Some of that is that the science has changed. There are things that you can tell people now. And so there is a different relationship" (Interim President, National); "It had to do with people receiving their diagnosis earlier. The medical professionals became more aware of the disease and had better criteria. A knowledge base was gained, so that the disease was being processed earlier, and so people were being given the diagnosis at a stage where decision making could be made" (Vice President, Programs and Public Policy, National); and "For years and years when both the diagnosis and family public acceptance of that diagnosis occurred so far down the line in the disease course, the likelihood that people with the disease would be engaged in self-advocacy was pretty cut off. It was a little too late. But the science has improved and the visibility of the disease has improved. We consequently open up the opportunity for people to be acting in their own best interests" (Public Policy, Midwest). In concert with the last line in the previous quote, one staff member, who revealed progressive views in prior quotes, mentioned the emancipatory potential of inclusion: "With the earlier diagnosis now comes the opportunity for people to be their own spokespeople" (Regional Director, Northwest). These data demonstrate variation among Association staff.

Yet despite scientific advances and the designation of AD as a spectrum disorder that can now allegedly identify people decades before they show clinical signs of dementia—which offers the potential for inclusion of individuals simply at-risk and thus removes some of the ethical concerns—there are factors within the very Association itself that have prevented the incorporation of people with AD. The salient features of the Association's organizational identity presenting the largest obstacles include habits, survival, and structure.

Organizational Habits: The Slow Wheels of Change

Chapter 2 highlighted the complex environment embedding AD. Combined with basic science and family-support underpinnings, staff suggested that these dynamics obstruct the incorporation of diagnosed people into the debate even within the Association itself:

> We're like all organizations in that we've been doing things in a certain way and it's hard to change. And the people that we serve [now] are the people with the disease. . . . That's changed since I've been with the Association, but it's been emerging over the last decade. (Interim President, National Office)

> The strength of that history as a families helping families organization may make it hard for the leadership, which is made up of people who have had family experience and people who are vendors of all kinds of services, [to] focus on the person with the disease. (Regional Director, Northwest)

> The primary barrier [to incorporating people with AD as spokespersons] may simply be working through habits. . . . That kind of conscientious consideration of the role of the person with the disease in our advocacy work, in our leadership, is just work that hasn't been done yet. (Public Policy, Midwest)

This reflects what organizational theorist Phillip Selznick long ago argued happens when policies and practices become so deeply embedded within an organizational culture that they are mistaken for goals.[33] Accordingly, organizational habits, or what Meyer and Rowan called institutionalized rules and rationalized myths,[34] aimed at finding respite for families were consistent with the curative focus of the founding scientists. Even though they took a back seat to the search for a cure, efforts to detect and treat the stress and burden of caregivers as well as manage allegedly difficult behaviors and depression in advanced cases of AD were well within the realm of medical science at that time and important psychopharmaceuticals have resulted from that work. Despite the fact that diagnoses now happen far earlier, when many people are only mildly impaired, the primary organizational habit at both the policy and practice levels remains a biomedical (even pharmacological) focus, including the allocation of over $315 million to bench science since 1982 (this is up from $150 million in 2005).[35] The constraints of the biomedical "iron cage"[36] encouraging conformity (by not deviating from institutional norms) were corroborated by staff: "We are the largest private funding organization in the world for Alzheimer's research. And caregiver support" (Director, State Advocacy Policy and Advocacy Programs, National); and "Even at the chapter level, ultimately, the research funding at the federal level is our number one goal. I think nationally, state and local, that's our number one focus. A lot of what we do at the policy level in the state is try to deal with current family caregiving situations" (Public Policy, East Coast). Unfortunately, both these factors potentially impede the inclusion of people with AD despite the avowed aims of staff.

The Association's founding ideals of cause and cure are also evident in the medical and scientific underpinnings of the organization's objectives. Staff at the Association reveal an entrenched biomedical focus through their framing of at least three key issues: differentiating AD from mental illness, distinguishing dementia from normal aging, and defining mild cognitive impairment (MCI) as preclinical AD.

An important decision made by the Alzheimer's Association was its deliberate attempt to distinguish Alzheimer's from any sort of mental illness. Staff members reinforce medicalization by emphasizing the legitimacy of Alzheimer's disease lest it be conflated with mental health concerns for which, unfortunately, far less sympathy is thought to exist. Recall that chapter 2 demonstrated that what most distinguished the 1906 discovery of Alzheimer's was the *observation* of plaques and tangles that removed the condition from the realm of psychiatric conditions. When asked to define Alzheimer's, staff reinforced efforts to medicalize memory loss as well as the psychiatric/neurologic divorce that were the impetus of the Association, their subsequent drawbacks being based perhaps in the fact that bench scientists were involved in the Association's founding (that is, neurologists and biologists rather than sociologists and psychologists). Some opted for general descriptions, such as: "To a lay audience I would say that it is a disease that has a reality in changes in the brain, and as an aside to you, the reason I would do that is because so many people think of it as a mental condition" (Chief Executive Officer, Southeast). Others, however, were far more explicit:

> It [separating Alzheimer's from mental illness] is a complicated issue. . . .
> I know there was a problem, actually when I first started. Something went
> out from the Association that said, "Alzheimer's disease is not a mental
> illness." I think it was shortly after I came here [circa 1990], and I didn't
> know any better. And obviously others didn't know any better. But it be-
> came clear to us not to draw that line very fine. There's research fund-
> ing from NIMH [National Institute of Mental Health], there's psychiatric
> services—there's a whole lot of services that we thought we would surely
> be allowed to access through Medicare but we weren't because what was
> happening was that the carriers—if you got the Alzheimer's code, there
> were a number of Medicare carriers around the country that were de-
> nying people mental health services, occupational therapy, you know, a
> number of services that were allowed under Medicare. But the idea is
> if you have Alzheimer's you can't benefit from those, so they were be-
> ing denied. We brought the researchers in saying, "Your information is
> no longer relevant. Research shows people can learn, and lots of benefits
> come to people with dementia." And it took us almost four years, but
> we got the rule changed. It's now a policy that's distributed throughout
> the country. Having an Alzheimer's diagnosis cannot be used to deny
> any services. But one of those services is mental health services. (Interim
> President, National)

While the Interim President attributes at least some responsibility for this problem to the Association, others saw the issue as far more systemic and financially motivated:

> I think the folks that were trying to say that Alzheimer's is not a men-
> tal illness didn't want our folks to get caught up in a dysfunctional sys-
> tem. Also, you've got the great divorce that goes back fifty years between
> neurology and psychiatry, which we still suffer from to this day. And I
> think there is a lot of evidence in the late 80s that state mental health
> departments took efforts that this population would not be on their tab.
> My home state of Massachusetts, California, and New York, and others,
> adopted policies that said, "We are not going to be the primary payer for

somebody who has psychosis due to an organic cause such as Alzheimer's or related dementia." So I think there were some proactive efforts by state officials to kind of keep this costly population off their books, if you will. So that's why there was a lot of that "Alzheimer's is not mental illness" stigma. (Director, State Policy and Advocacy Programs, National)

So long as people with Alzheimer's were afforded their necessary rights under disability regulations, the Association appeared to prefer employing the medical categorization of Alzheimer's *disease* rather than risk the stigma of a condition that was deemed a mental illness. This was arguably a political decision to allow their constituents to benefit from the rights granted to the disabled without identifying with them. Similar to the process of assuming an Alzheimer's identity outlined in chapters 4 to 6, there is also an evolving organizational identity for the Association similar to that discussed within other social arenas.[37] While I will outline the organizational consequences, these efforts to remain distinct from mental illness also have significant social and individual effects. The Association resides in a tenuous space of allying with but remaining separate from the realm of mental health, a struggle social movement scholars suggest signals goal displacement in the process of niche development at the Association.

While noting its strong reliance on the disability movement, the Interim President posited that the Alzheimer's Association was not the place for radical activism like seen in the disability movement: "We've been working with the disability community for—well, I started . . . in 1987. And we've been working hand-in-glove—we have very good relations with the disability community." He went on to elaborate:

> If you look at the disability community as a model, you could argue, "Gee, people chaining themselves to Senator's desk, refusing to leave their offices"—could get results. . . . We have gauged that as we've gone along. Every few months we sort of ask that question, are we being militant—as militant as we should be? Are we pushing as hard as we should be? What's appropriate not only for the outcome we're seeking but for the people we represent? It's an association that has a culture and has people that have sensitivities about—they don't want to do Act Up kinds of things where they get out and lie down in the middle of the street.

If our environments shape us, then the context within which social movements exist matter. As demonstrated with the senior rights movement[38] for SMOs trying to serve a diverse clientele, such as AARP, activism often takes on an admittedly more innocuous process of lobbying policy makers for concrete things rather than fighting for the larger social justice issues, such as preventing agism and negative perceptions of people with the condition. As with the Gray Panthers' role in that movement, the Interim President of the Association felt there were more appropriate groups aiming to combat issues of justice, particularly web-based forums sharing information on dementia and posting editorials: "In the Alzheimer's web-based international group [DASNI] there are some people that are much more sort of militant and demanding and they're getting people to pay attention and mostly within the Alzheimer's movement as opposed to effecting legislation. But I think that's a sensitive action in general." So, while seemingly not opposed to the intentions of these "militant groups," the Association "has a culture" and "people that have sensitivities." Much like AARP, rather than seeing themselves as a potential catalyst for social justice, the Interim President sees the Association resembling more of an organization or company first and social movement participant in a supportive or secondary capacity (if indeed at all).

The second aspect within the Association that reinforced biomedical knowledge was the persistence and urgency with which staff distinguished dementia from normal aging. Such distinctions may have been necessary when the Association was founded, but are now dated. When asked to describe Alzheimer's, however, staff echoed biomedical tenets and still vehemently demarcated this divide: "That it is a disease process; it is not normal aging. That it is different from a memory impairment that can be age associated" (Vice President, Programs and Public Policy, Southeast); and "We distinguished it from senility. We said this was a disease. It was not a normal part of getting older" (Regional Director, Northwest). More alarmist descriptions included: "I would say it's a disease that's not a normal part of aging, or it's a disease where you lose bits and pieces of who you are. . . . It gets worse and worse until you can't take care of yourself. People say it's a normal part of aging but it's not" (Communications Coordinator, Midwest). Here the Association both reflects and reinforces narrow pejorative biomedical constructions of

AD insofar as the very definition of the condition is presented as self loss "where you lose bits and pieces of who you are," and involves social death whereby "you can't take care of yourself." These data suggest a similar perceived need for the Association to clarify that memory loss is atypical as chapter 3 revealed it was for clinicians diagnosing it in the first place. Without such differentiation, after all, the very existence of the organization is questioned. Since there is something that can be done to treat dementias, the Association performs a vital service. Therefore, biomedical principles bolster the legitimacy of the Association.

Although Association staff viewed these historical and biomedical factors as potential barriers to diagnosed people seeking services, they routinely substantiated these myths[39] in their own materials, support groups, and training. In light of their need for consumers, compliance with biomedical practice maintains security.[40]

The final example of what Clarke and her colleagues call the new biomedicalization[41] is shown through the staff depiction of mild cognitive impairment, a rare categorization (even more so at the time of this study) used in specialty clinics, as simply the earliest stage of Alzheimer's disease. This was done despite the fact that the medical community did not officially designate it as such until 2011—years after I completed this study. Yet staff spoke with frustration regarding those who did little to make it clear to people that they were on their way to AD (which would ideally usher them to the Association):[42]

> I got really pissed off when they came out with the mild cognitive impairment crap and I'll tell you why: because it gave people a reason to be more in denial. And I was hearing things like, "Well, we're not sure if this is going to *turn* [emphasis in the original] into Alzheimer's." And I'd be like, "Yo! It IS, what is this it is not going to *turn into* [emphasis in the original]." It gave people more of a reason to be in denial. . . . I constantly get people, especially adult children, asking me clear questions about a real progressive dementia and then they'll say to me, "Oh, but my father doesn't have Alzheimer's disease, he has MCI." But the questions they will be asking me are clear-cut dementia and somebody somewhere along the line, probably because they couldn't treat it anyway, said, "Oh, I think it's MCI." I understand its place but it seems to be misused. (Education/Support Group Manager, East Coast)

The astute Director of Policy and Programs at Headquarters in Chicago echoes the concerns about MCI laid out in chapter 2, but is concerned for very different reasons:

> DIRECTOR: For my two cents, mild cognitive impairment is early Alzheimer's disease. And it's bullshit to dress it up.
> RB: Why do you think it is being dressed up?
> DIRECTOR: Well, I think it's hard to deliver a sentence of Alzheimer's disease. I think it's a lot easier for even our best physicians to say, "Well, it's just some mild cognitive impairment. Down the road it might turn into Alzheimer's disease, but we really don't know." It's a buffer. I think it's a buffer for the health care professional. I'm kind of with John Morris in Saint Louis, who says MCI is bullshit. It's a research term. And it is. If you look at where MCI came from, it came from something we don't have in this country, National Data Set Analysis in Canada. . . . It's a retrospective term of art from population-based research. I don't know that, I think that clinically it's used to soften the blow. And it confuses the public. (Director, State Policy and Advocacy Programs, National)

Noting the medical futility—"because they probably couldn't treat it"—and lack of hope—"it's hard to deliver a sentence of Alzheimer's disease"—MCI is interpreted as a buffer for doctors and as giving "people a reason to be more in denial." In this way, the Association relies on medical experts to identify pathological memory loss and *at least* inform people of their diagnosis so potential consumers can avail themselves of the services being offered. The tension between the Association and the general medical community (as opposed to memory clinics) being relied on to diagnose AD was evident throughout the interviews. Without clear diagnoses, potential constituents will not seek out Association-sponsored programs, make donations, or otherwise identify with Alzheimer's.

Organizational Survival

As a nonprofit agency, the Association relies heavily on private donations. This affects the inclusion of diagnosed perspectives vis-a-vis the public image portrayed and the allocation of money. As a voluntary organization, the Association realizes that certain things sell better than others and has not always encouraged favorable portrayals of people with the condition.[43] As with childhood conditions or those striking young mothers, pulling on the heartstrings and depictions of pathetic victims are essential tools for fund-raising, despite the fact that this is no longer the (only) picture to portray.[44] Along with epidemic projections, notions of a complete annihilation of self have historically served the Association well in garnering sympathizers (i.e., employing fear to advance resources).[45] As with the habits of the Association, such initiatives are institutionalized:

> The Memory Walk is a prime source of not only income but visibility for us. There is something very powerful about seeing a large group of people in T-shirts walking down your street saying, "We're dealing with the disease" and "Get ready, you might be dealing with it too." If you have an early-stage celeb come out, who is in the prime of life and says, "This is what happens." I think that is going to scare people. (Development and Communications, East Coast)

Some staff explicitly referred to the potential of genetic testing to produce spokespeople for the condition, despite criticism that biomarkers or "genetic tests for late onset AD make no sense at the individual level"[46] given the massive uncertainty when dealing with susceptibility genes.

> When I get my hands on a person who's 30 or 40 years and says, "Nothing's happened to me yet, outwardly, but my brain is beginning to deteriorate and over the next 20 years . . ." At first people won't take that person seriously . . . but the more they hear from that person, and, of course, it won't be one person. It'll be hundreds of thousands of persons. And you'll have CEOs saying it, and you'll have athletes, and you'll have teachers and sanitation workers, and you'll have neighbors . . . and it will be all around you. And still a lot of the four million people with Alzheimer's are hidden away [but] it won't be that way when it's people who don't have symptoms, but have the disease. They're out there. There are lots of 30 year olds with Alzheimer's, but they are 20 or 30 or 40 or 50 years away from symptoms and they don't know it. (Public Policy, East Coast)

Whereas AARP has been accused of including younger and younger people to market old as sexier, the Association endorses apocalyptic demography[47] and metaphoric images of scientific progress as combat to unify members and help elicit support under the common goal of disease eradication despite the resultant tensions. Yet staff understand the double-edged sword involved:

> It creates an interesting dilemma for us. The more you emphasize that people have rich lives and should have and should play more of a role . . . but think about the flip side of that: "Oh, Alzheimer's isn't so bad. Look at all the creativity, and look at how wonderful . . ." it's fraught with complications. How do you reconcile with the need to tell people that this disease is awful, and that we should get rid of it. That it isn't a good thing to live with this disease. So you're constantly juggling . . . if you allow one picture to dominate, you get a distorted view. (Interim President, National Office)

This "interesting dilemma" leads some to highlight the human rights issues:

> What we have to do is make sure we're protecting human rights at the same time we're letting the world know how awful and ugly and destructive the disease is. Separating the human, the person, from the disease is a trick because you need the person to exhibit the disease. (Public Policy, Washington, D.C.)

Like many nonprofit organizations serving vulnerable constituencies, in an effort to combat the perceived contradictions they face vis a vis "human rights," the Association orchestrates the need for public awareness and education because its members and staff believe, based on medicoscientific fact, that a disease exists which demands attention.[48] Demographically, financially, socially, and personally, the problem is portrayed as devastating and warranting resources matching its prevalence, thus echoing the Association's ethos and the scientific investigations behind it. The complicated and mysterious nature of the disease also aids the Association in its efforts to excite adequate monetary and human investments in the cause. Its website has shown this employment of ambiguity for over a decade, where cure is always just around the corner. In 2004, the website reported:

> Hope, formerly nonexistent, is growing. Scientists are slowly solving the disease's mysteries. . . . Within five years treatments could be available to delay or prevent the disease.[49]

A decade later, the Association boasted:

> The race is on. Alzheimer's and related dementias research is a dynamic field, and momentum builds each year. . . . The Alzheimer's Association has been involved in every major advancement in Alzheimer's and related dementias research since the 1980's and is a leader in the global fight for a world without Alzheimer's.[50]

Similar to clinicians employing ambiguity in chapter 3, the Association draws heavily on a rhetoric of hope and scientific progress. Reminiscent of the Nixon era's War on Cancer, predictions of cutting-edge breakthroughs combined with catastrophic projections are effective means of creating hype for investment.[51] Yet such representations also have unrecognized consequences for people with AD that fragment the face of the social movement in irrefutable ways. For example, depicting AD as a complete annihilation of self arguably prevents potential members in the early stages from joining the social movement or seeking services from an organization that makes such one-sided portrayals. Such derogatory public portrayals and lack of genuine inclusion of people with dementia have led to outcries from and arguably even the foundation of more radical groups, like Dementia Advocacy and Support Network International (DASNI) and the Alzheimer's Foundation of America (AFA) since the turn of the century as well as the 2014 establishment of Dementia Alliance International.

Regarding resource allocation, most funding comes from private philanthropists who have family members with the condition. Thus, staff noted that funds tend to be earmarked:

> Most people when they're asked what we should be doing say, "You should be doing more research." That's where the general population

thinks we should be investing all of our time. The caregivers they couldn't care less about. The people that care about the caregivers and those issues are the families that are dealing with it. (Development and Communications, East Coast)

Therefore, discrepancies exist between where patrons and the general public, and perhaps even Association staff, think monies should go (i.e., programs vs. advertising or care vs. cure).

Association staff perceived a lack of adequate funding to devise and implement new objectives, including the inclusion of people with AD.[52] Many chapters do not seek foundation funding and few, if any, obtain government support. Respondents postulated that financial constraints result in encouraging those services that reach the most people, are the most cost-effective, and are fundable. That is, a tension exists: "There's the whole utilitarian thing of do I try to help the most people a little or a few people a lot? I try to help a lot of people at least a little and you hope it helps some of them a lot, but you at least go for the broad effect" (Public Policy, Washington, D.C.). An organization historically addressing the needs of families requires substantial reorganization to first identify and second, meet the needs of this new clientele. Accordingly, the Interim President astutely observes that the Association must begin by answering the question of who its client is and then either redirect or expand its efforts accordingly:

There are a lot of organizational issues here. Who is the client? and what is the role of the client in defining what an organization does? The organization isn't the movement. There is a much bigger thing going on out there. The organization is obviously the most visible part of it in some ways, it plays a leadership role [but] what are some of the organizational issues?

Thus, since "the organization isn't the movement," efforts to reconcile the Association's history with the changing dynamics of its constituency serve the institutional goal of ensuring stability first and foremost. In a market economy, not only are individualized services costly and beneficial to fewer people than standard caregiver-based or group programs, but the Association is already well-equipped to serve these latter needs. A middle ground between a largely biomedical focus and a more social-psychological one has yet to be realized.

Organizational Structure

Another internal obstacle to incorporating the voice of people with AD is the decentralized structure of the Association itself. While it is represented in all fifty states and claims to reach millions of people affected by Alzheimer's across the globe through the national office and more than 75 local chapters, the number of chapters has steadily declined since 1993, when there were 221.[53] Decisions directly relevant to the population each chapter serves are made at the local level. Although the Association has an impressive web presence and a clearinghouse where all chapters can review protocol for programs used in other regions, the individual chapters within the organization have differential access. The devolution of services suggests there is little infrastructure unifying the chapters more broadly, which may create a lack of cohesion on the issues of advocacy and inclusion:

> We [chapters] are affiliated with the national office in Chicago but they really can't tell us what to do. We are our own 501c3 with our own board of directors, by-laws, etc. so boards, through the years, have made distinctions over how they wanted to structure their organization. Right now I would say that 90, 85–90 percent of all the chapters are like this one where they don't have a good handle on the programs for the individual. (Chapter President, East Coast)

> It [incorporating people with AD] is probably more prevalent in the metropolitan chapter areas. . . . It's only us because we have a long-standing history with early stage, but in the other offices [it is] not so much. I think that's probably pretty typical. There are chapters that don't even have support groups for people with the condition. (Executive Director, Northwest)

Since there is no official Association policy on such endeavors, some chapters are pioneers in their efforts to incorporate people with AD, but most "don't have a good handle" on it because they lack the resources, savvy, or impetus. The focus of local chapters on individual communities potentially obfuscates the unification of Association staff on the larger social justice issues upon which the movement is based, despite their potential for furthering efforts aimed at specific people with AD.

Institutional theorists argue that organizations will adopt inconsistent, even incompatible, practices to gain external support and stability.[54] If the Alzheimer's Association—like all formal organizational structures—is comprised of rationalized institutional rules, then the framing of AD as an epidemic, as devastating and yet constantly on the verge of a cure, is a *myth* incorporated in rule-like ways to gain and maintain legitimacy from the medical community, resources from donors, and thus enhanced stability and survival prospects. Accordingly, parent organizations, regulatory agencies, and financial sources create an iron cage encouraging and rewarding conformity,[55] in this case to the strictly biomedical framings of AD and the associated pejorative assumptions of life with the condition. The organizational habits, survival, and structure of the Association remain so deeply entrenched in biomedicine that the pursuit and politics of that worldview have become goals in and of themselves.[56]

External Factors

Conflicting ideologies within the Association itself are further exacerbated by the external factors confronting the Association, including public perceptions of aging and AD, the role of science/medicine, and client characteristics.

Public Perceptions

Depictions of Alzheimer's remain skewed if not overtly pejorative, as a general cynicism pervades the discourse on topics of aging and AD despite the Association's founding thirty-five years ago (in 1980). Association staff attributed much of the struggle over inclusion to larger issues of ageism: "I think that probably the bigger problem is ageism and that age is still discounted to some extent. You know, old people get sick and they die" (Education/Support Group Manager, East Coast); and "I fear that because of a level of ageism in public life and in private life that what gets public officials' attention more is the person who is still in his or her working years. It makes it all the more, 'My god! This could be me'" (Public Policy Director, Midwest). Some staff even demonstrated an understanding of the misrepresentation of AD:

> I believe that the dominant perception of Alzheimer's among just average folks who haven't had much contact with people with the disease would be a prototypic 80-year-old person who is no longer able to communicate, who is incontinent and who is drooling from the side of the mouth (which they don't). (Public Policy, Midwest)

Ageism universalizes aging experiences and conflated all AD with the end stages, which is inaccurate despite the latter being helpful in terms of garnering sympathy. As an organization in the voluntary sector, various dilemmas regarding appeals for support are encountered. Considering demand side client characteristics,[57] the Association serves people who are both personally and socially disenfranchised. Accordingly, personal disadvantage occurs when the ability to communicate is deemed impaired. As people with AD allegedly require others to act on their behalf, professionals and families of people with AD historically served as proxy interpreters of their perspectives. The social death upon which these assumptions are based marginalizes people with AD, thus silencing their agenda.

My data with diagnosed individuals corroborate the concern that the general public holds a number of misconceptions about the condition and the people with it. If many people believe that AD is an old person's disease, then the decision to unite the rare early-onset strain of the condition with the relatively common state of senility exacerbated this inaccurate conflation. While the vast majority of people are over 65 years of age, less that 4 percent of current AD cases are people diagnosed with early onset AD in their forties and fifties[58] as with the initial categorization of the disease over a century ago. Many people also consider it normal to have some memory loss as people age, and hence they conflate aging and disease.[59] As the prior quote showed, another common portrayal is that of a sudden onset and a catastrophic outcome, or universalizing the condition to one stage: the late-stage. In reality, AD is a gradual process with significant variation in the ensuing eight to twenty years during which people typically live with the condition. To a large degree, Association staff attributed many of the public misconceptions to (past) media portrayals of people with dementia as old, defective, and destitute or with otherwise inaccurate projections of memory loss: "If you look back fifteen years at any television documentaries on Alzheimer's what they focused on was the person in the fetal position" (Vice President, Programs and Public Policy, Southeast). Again, a public policy representative shows a nuanced grasp of what sells in the media:

> What the press tends to pick up about Alzheimer's issues falls into two categories, I think. One is the breakthrough drugs, there are lots of stories about, "Well, they've finally found out what causes and cures it, and all we have to do is go through seven more years of clinical trial and we'll know for sure." There's always a story about that. And then the other is of the special care unit in the nursing home where people are ballroom dancing. Between those two poles of Alzheimer's experience, there's not a whole lot of press. (Public Policy Director, Midwest)

Noting the lack of attention to daily life with AD, or what is "between these two poles," the media is framed as doing a disservice to diagnosed individuals and the Association alike. Although participants were hopeful that this was beginning to reverse, the negative media projections were perceived as potential barriers to getting people with memory loss to even seek a diagnosis, let alone avail themselves of the services offered by the Association. While staff said they were critical of the media coverage of Alzheimer's, they did so without interrogating their own role in the portrayal of life with AD[60] or how it serves their institutional interests. Given the iron cage of biomedicine, tragic portrayals of people with Alzheimer's justify the Association's continued need for financial resources from private donations and foundations even as they contradict the personal views of staff. Yet, using fear as a motivator for resource allocation is a double-edged sword for the Association, as this inherent contradiction puts the Association in a tenuous situation whereby intangible social justice issues like adequately representing people with AD become secondary.

Staff also suggested that a general paternalism surrounds the treatment of people with AD. In particular, family members might not want their loved ones to be spokespeople so as to prevent them from potentially being humiliated in public: "There are so many families and individuals where if you go to them and say, 'We'd like you to be a spokesperson,' they won't because of not wanting to deal with the public perception and the stigma or just the unwelcome encouraging words" (Public Policy, Washington, D.C.); "This disease is so *horrible* [original] and so *demeaning* [original] [that] I don't think families want to parade that person around" (Education/Support Group Manager, East Coast). While the latter quote reveals negative portrayals even in-house, others took on more responsibility: "We [Association staff] get a little paternalistic at times and are overprotective of people, and sometimes we have to recognize that persons with Alzheimer's disease have the right to make decisions too" (Vice President, Programs and Public Policy, Southeast). Being overprotective, common among many families, service providers, and Association staff, assumes that people with AD (necessarily) require protection, which critics refer to as a process of infantilization,[61] despite individual notions of human rights and an implicit understanding of this tension.

Poignantly, the type of candidate respondents thought would be most persuasive as a spokesperson posed serious dilemmas. Association staff envisioned someone famous, young, and early-stage despite the statistical improbability. They voiced a collective need for a spokesperson of celebrity status, such as Christopher Reeve or Michael J. Fox. As previous data revealed, younger people with AD (early-onset or even biomarkers) are allegedly more tragic and resonate more powerfully with politicians, particularly in the later stages:

> The challenge is that people in the very early stages look very normal, and sometimes there's a bit of disconnect. They say, "Well, gee, he doesn't look so bad. That person is functioning pretty well." Some of the most effective testimony has been with a person present who is actually fairly far advanced in the disease, but who is themselves not old . . . when they look at a 58-year-old fighter pilot who's owned his own business and is very handsome and looks much like the legislator sitting there across from him, there's some connection. And when they see that guy sitting there muted by Alzheimer's disease, that's pretty powerful. When your 85-year-old grandmother is going senile [people think], "Well, she's just old and that's what happens." So, I don't think there is the same sense of

urgency as when you look at somebody who's 65 and go, "Oh my god!" (Director, Development and Communications, East Coast)

As chapter 2 noted, however, early-onset AD is extremely rare and has a far more rapid progression and biomarkers are a matter of susceptibility, not predictability. This complicates the ability of individuals with early-onset AD to serve as spokespeople and makes the validity of those with the biomarkers doing so questionable. Therefore, groups with early onset or biomarkers are both poorly situated to accurately represent AD experiences. Yet staff highlighted preclinical cases, including genetic predisposition, biomarkers, and what at the time was a relatively recent emergence of mild cognitive impairment, as promising far more compelling spokespeople yet raising ethical quandaries surrounding debates on diagnostic efficacy, genetic testing, and the Human Genome Project. Therefore, although both the Association and the movement benefit from the expansion of classification systems,[62] it engenders medical and public uncertainty and exacerbates ethical dilemmas. Similar to AARP's role in the senior rights movement, the Association's decision to delay or forgo taking a stance on issues that might alienate (parts of) its constituency jeopardizes the objectives of the larger social movement.

The Role of Science/Medicine

While both basic science and biomedicine have played profound roles in the Alzheimer's movement and its leading SMO, staff members envision general practice physicians constituting a major barrier to the Association's ability to employ the voices of people with AD. As chapters 2 and 3 demonstrate, there is considerable scientific controversy surrounding a unified definition of dementia and debates persist about whether or not AD is qualitatively different from normal aging.[63] Since Alzheimer's cannot be definitively determined premortem, the accuracy of diagnostic procedures varies, sometimes widely. As people age, it is even more difficult to discern pure cases of AD, since few are without comorbidities. For those diagnosed, there are no magic bullets to cure AD and there are no "survivors" as there are with other health social movement constituents, which amplifies the obstacles to self-advocacy.

All these issues confound the diagnostic process in clinical practice. In support of the clinical data from chapter 3, Association staff accused general practice doctors of a particular lack of education regarding the Association's services and AD more broadly: "The biggest barrier [to including people with AD] I see is lack of knowledge on the part of physicians, which also leads to them not identifying it [AD]" (Public Policy Director, Southwest). While this staff member framed it as lack of knowledge, others ascribed more intentionality:

> Doctors study their whole lives to cure things, or to at least be able to treat things, and only in recent years have we even been able to *treat* [original] this and I find doctors often don't even give them clear a diagnosis. I find they want so much to give them hope, and I'm not criticizing the doctors because I think they want so much to give them hope, but then people come to me either in my support group or my early-stage group or here [chapter] and they don't even have a clue of the progression of the disease. . . . And they're saying to me, "Well, it won't get any worse than this, will it?" which is so pitiful. Up until very recently, we couldn't do *anything* [original] and I think doctors feel so hopeless about that and I think that's why they don't know what to say. (Education/Support Group Manager, East Coast)

Despite focusing on how doctors "don't even give them a clear diagnosis," including the effect of this on her interactions with diagnosed individuals, she was empathetic. Others, in contrast, noted how doctors failed to refer to the Association:

> [Relations with doctors] have always been a challenge. We know that physicians don't refer families. We're hearing that physicians say, "Yeah . . . yes, I think you have Alzheimer's disease." So they don't complete the diagnostic process. And they give them a medication like Aricept or Excelon and think that they've done everything and they send them on their way. Or they know that the diagnostic process is complete and the diagnosis has been confirmed, but they don't know exactly what to do, so they give them a pill and they send them on their way. . . . Basically it comes down to time. They don't have the time to talk from time to time about the Alzheimer's Association. They don't have the knowledge of the

Alzheimer's Association. They don't know we're here. They don't know what we're doing. If they know we're here, they don't know how we can help. I don't think a lot of it is deliberate on their part. I think it's just lack of time and ignorance, frankly. (Regional Director, Northwest)

While the above respondent was somewhat sympathetic to the institutional constraints under which doctors operate, namely time, others were less charitable:

A lot of families, unfortunately, have less than positive experiences where [the doctor] will say, "We suspect your husband has Alzheimer's, here's some pills, good luck," and the family is kind of left hanging. They are cared for on the medical side, the physical side, but the emotional, mental, financial, legal, with all of those things they are left hanging. And if the physician doesn't know enough to say, "Call the Alzheimer's Association and they will get you into a support group and they'll hook you up with an elder law attorney, etc." If they don't know to do that, what is a family to do? (Communications and Development, East Coast)

To try to reduce the number of families being "left hanging," the Association had numerous physician training efforts under way:

[There is a] terrible disconnect between the medical system, which is to me what's happening when doctors aren't saying, "There's an Alzheimer's Association. Here's some community resources you might tap into," and so forth. . . . You ask people where do they get their information and they say their physician. . . . You have to create a culture [of referral] within the physician community. To try to educate physicians [is] really tough because how do you get them, and why should they care what the Alzheimer's Association says? (Interim President, National Office)

In contrast to the prior quotes that place the onus on doctors or "a terrible disconnect," this woman framed it as a matter of educating consumers better:

In every training I have done in the last eleven years the issue of physicians has come up: they don't know enough, they don't diagnose, they

don't treat, they don't refer. . . . There's not an awful lot of law or regulation
or public programs that can change physician behavior . . . the only thing
that is going to change physician behavior is equipping the consumer to
get more out of that physician visit. (State Policy and Advocacy Program,
Washington, D.C.)

Despite earlier diagnoses, when people *could* talk about their condition
freely, doctors were allegedly not channeling people to the Association
quickly enough, if at all. Rather than acknowledging the concerns of
physicians regarding over and mis-diagnoses, the lack of efficacious
medications, and difficulties arising from time constraints, emotional
burden, and jurisdictional issues,[64] Association staff again echoed the
sentiments of clinicians in specialty clinics. In this way, Association staff
viewed doctors as both the problem and thus the potential linchpin to
solving some of their internal obstacles: "I think getting physicians to
refer people to us. We have to get that. I mean if our goal is to get to
people early and support them through the journey, we have to partner
with physicians, or physicians have to partner with us. I think that is the
huge barrier" (Executive Director, Northwest). Given the Association's
biomedical tenets, attributing this discrepancy between diagnosing and
referring people to a lack of knowledge on behalf of the doctors "conve-
niently recreates the authoritative position"[65] of biomedical *solutions* as
opposed to their being part of the cause. Efforts to educate consumers
(people with AD and their families) arguably have the same effect of
assigning blame due to lack of information.

Client Characteristics

There are also characteristics specific to the Association's clientele that
potentially reduce the inclusion of people with AD and the visibility
of their perspectives. Staff felt seniors were less comfortable speaking
about personal experiences to their doctors: "The cohort of people who
are that age [in their 80s] are kind of shy about this advocacy business.
Generationally, you just didn't speak about these things" (Public Policy,
Midwest). Yet others predicted a sea change: "I think there's the beginning of a cohort effect, where you've got people who are more willing
to talk about this. Older generations may be a little more shy about it,

even if they could do it" (Interim President, National Office). Staff members were confident that times would change with the aging of the baby boomers. In fact, many presented the boomers as a solution to the problems with doctors outlined above: "The baby boomers are saying, 'We're not going to put up with this. We are going to question our doctor, we're going to figure out what's wrong, and we are going to come out in the open'" (Education/Support Group Manager, East Coast); and "The social reform is going to happen on its own because this next generation of people are the generation of people who are the most likely to question their diagnosis and question their doctor and want answers and they are not going to tolerate a doctor saying, 'Well, you have dementia. Goodbye.'" (Chapter President, East Coast). Interestingly, most of the staff I spoke with were roughly in the baby boomer generation, so when statements like the last line below were made, they came with strong conviction:

[C]learly with the boomers aging our way of looking at aging is changing and is going to continue to change. [They] don't buy that they have to be decrepit and are less likely to say, "Ah, that's just aging" and accept it. I think that the boomers are more likely to ask their . . . physicians questions and to seek alternative medicines if the medicine doesn't help them. . . . *They'll fight. They're not going gently into that good night* [emphasis added]. (Associate Executive Director, Southwest)

Unfortunately, accepting such factors as inevitable or beyond the control of the Association also prevents a more critical stance that would advance the aims of the larger movement and aid inclusion efforts.

Another client characteristic perceived to obstruct the incorporation of first-person perspectives was the sheer variability among people who have AD. Reflecting concerns expressed in chapter 2 about the lack of uniformity in the neuropathology of AD, staff noted this conflict: "Because it varies from person to person and it has so many different effects on everybody . . . there are so many different layers. It's hard to pinpoint one thing for them to look after [i.e., advocate] when it just varies so much" (Communications Coordinator, Midwest). Accordingly, the different layers complicated the Association's ability to serve the wide range of client needs:

> [If] [e]very case of Alzheimer's is a new case of Alzheimer's, [then] . . .
> take that new case of Alzheimer's to a family, which all families are dif-
> ferent with their own dynamics, so there's another new situation and so I
> don't think there's any [one] thing. . . . A little bit of extra finances would
> help but the financial is not the, it's just one of many, many burdens in-
> volved with this. (Chapter CEO, East Coast)

Such heterogeneity in demographics, comorbidities, disease progression,
and stage of the condition threatens to preclude a sense of cohesion, a
group identity, and a unified public image—all things that fuel social
movements and social change—and also makes choosing a spokesperson
difficult. Organizational theorists Meyer and Rowan might argue that
the biomedical policies and practices have become so ingrained within
the Association that they have become ends in themselves. Abiding by
the institutional rules of biomedicine, like an iron cage,[66] has become
the overarching organizational goal of the Alzheimer's Association.

Thus, factors such as public perceptions of aging and disease, the role
of science and medicine, particularly doctors, and various client characteristics are framed as the main obstacles to the inclusion of people with
Alzheimer's as spokespersons by the Association. This seemingly un-
questioned buy-in to biomedical interpretations of memory loss by the
leading advocacy organization makes the AD movement significantly
different from other traditional health social movements.[67]

Historical Context: An Overarching Obstacle

Another crucial factor related to conveying the perspectives of people
with AD is the pathology of the disease itself, which exacerbates both
internal and external barriers. The dilemmas the Association has
encountered in trying to change its image and orientations from a singular focus on families to one that includes those with the condition
have important ramifications. Health social movements often work for
the benefit of carers, whose activism is crucial to building SMOs. Now
that people with AD are diagnosed far earlier in the disease trajectory,
remnants of families as the real victims mentality severely fragment
the movement. Unfortunately, the site of pathology engenders assumptions of incompetence based in Western views that brain functioning

defines humanness. The etiology itself also confounds the situation, since traditional deficiency perspectives[68] view symptomatic forgetfulness as an impediment to communication. In a hypercognitive society, where people envision the fundamental essence of themselves as located solely in the brain,[69] this conflation between personhood and the mind/brain reflects and reinforces constructions of diseases as threatening a person's core being in the world. Similar to mental illness or childhood conditions organized around proxy advocates, a history of family advocacy is particularly difficult to combat even when articulate people with the condition emerge.[70] Despite the increasing availability of people with AD to engage, the social construction of AD obfuscates efforts to debunk suppositions of ineptness.

Further, learning to incorporate a new constituency is laborious. The efforts devoted to branding a personal face for AD so clearly advocated by Association staff are also hindered by historical factors. The (past) social construction of the disease as a condition where people were often diagnosed without any awareness of their situation led to many of the (present) views that people with AD cannot advocate for themselves. The current availability of people in the earliest stages renders a large group of people who are high-functioning and will live far longer with the condition. As a result of this dynamic, the Association has yet to reach equilibrium with the diagnostic advances allowing for, if not demanding, such incorporation. Although related to the external factors of both public perceptions and the role of science/medicine, these views are largely the result of the protracted translation of science to the public. Finding spokespersons from a group of people with a progressive degenerative disease poses dilemmas for the Association:

To use an awful term, when you're "branding," my hunch is you can't brand as easily and as quickly for someone who is going to go away. . . . So, to be perfectly cold and blunt about it . . . you know their day will come sooner, when they can't—no matter what their drive, they physically and cognitively won't be able to anymore. (Public Policy, Washington, D.C.)

[We wanted] to have a representative from the early stage [support] group on our program committee [as] the liaison [but we decided] to have it be a time limited position, and so what we chose was six months, at which time we can renew that. But by being very up-front with the person . . . we didn't have to face the issue of how do we delicately and with dignity and integrity ask the person to leave [when they are no longer capable]. (Regional Director, Northwest)

Accordingly, "branding" would be difficult since it is unpredictable how long a given person's ability would last or how they might be feeling on any given day. Therefore, advocates who have a shorter window of time are seen as less efficient and effective than unimpaired care partners or celebrities. The intersection of disease pathology and the Association's mobilization strategies is thus critical. The historical and social constructions of AD further confound the internal and external barriers to assigning spokespersons from within the AD community.

Overall, elements both within and beyond the Association as well as the environment embedding the condition must be acknowledged. The disparities between what Association staff want and what is organizationally feasible are noteworthy. While we may begin to see spokespersons utilized earlier in the course of illness when the symptoms are less visible and/or they are more receptive to pharmaceutical treatments than in the past, the current climate provides a tremendous disincentive.

Narratives of Resistance: Lessons from Outlier Cases

While most of my respondents were patients of specialty clinics, and the majority accepted biomedical interpretations of their memory loss, which is clearly a sampling limitation, both Mrs. B and Mr. C from chapter 5, in particular, tell us something important about the possible variation within clinics but also how the majority of people who are receiving diagnosis (from PCPs) might experience the condition. Readers will recall that both were put off by the tests that they felt focused on their shortcomings and the overly reductionistic tone of being diagnosed with AD and MCI, respectively. Neither employed medicalized notions of memory loss, so while admitting their difficulties, they were not comfortable with the identity options being offered. They saw clinicians who were fatalistic and looking for deficit. When Mrs. B asked me,

"How sure are they that this isn't just about age?" and Mr. C inquired what the technical difference was between MCI and the early stages of Alzheimer's, they arguably reflect a nuanced understanding of the Entanglements of Dementia and Aging.[71] There are no doubt many more people like Mrs. B and Mr. C who never seek evaluation for their memory loss in the first place and/or do not visit specialty clinics.

In terms of the social movement, by around the turn of the century various groups were beginning to coalesce in reaction to the perceived inadequacies of the U.S. Alzheimer's Association. The primary short-comings identified mirrored the power struggles that arose in the found-ing years of the Association,[72] including conflicting interests of bench scientists and caregivers, between Alzheimer's and related dementias, and more recently between the needs of diagnosed individuals and care-givers. Critics complained that the Association was too focused on cause and cure research at the expense of supporting people currently living with the condition, that preference was given to Alzheimer's over other dementias despite the difficulty of distinguishing pure cases, and that the perspectives of people with the condition were marginalized or alto-gether ignored. While the AD movement followed a grassroots model[73] in the formative years, contemporary divisions have led some to suggest that the movement is currently more representative of an interest group model.[74]

In 2000, the Dementia Advocacy and Support Network International (DASNI) was created as an on-line forum to promote discussion among and support for people dealing with dementias of all sorts. As of 2005, the organization reported having 200 members *with dementia*. Cur-rently, they boast that one-third of the affiliates are living with dementia, the other two-thirds being comprised of "those involved with our well-being," including primarily sympathetic others such as family members as well as more radically minded academics, service providers, and even neuroscientists. According to their website, DASNI's principles, beliefs, and values include:

> We are autonomous and competent people diagnosed with dementia,
>   and our loyal allies;
> We believe that shared knowledge is empowerment;
> We believe our strengths provide a supportive network;

We are a voice and a helping hand;

Our purpose is to promote respect and dignity for persons with dementia, provide a forum for the exchange of information, encourage
support mechanisms such as local groups, counselling, and internet
linkages, and to advocate for services.[75]

In stark contrast to the advocacy efforts of the Alzheimer's Association,
the DANSI motto declares: "Nothing About Us, Without Us!" Not
surprisingly, then, rather than lobbying Congress, DASNI members
worldwide make presentations at Alzheimer's Disease International
(ADI) conferences (arguably the most progressive international organization devoted to the cause) as well as national and local meetings, and
launch far more attempts to promote social change. Members also pub-
lish books, give TV and radio interviews, and write academic and lay
articles on the subject of diagnosis and living with dementia. The existence and strong presence of this group speaks to the desires and unmet
needs of people with dementia to be included in the associated debates.

DASNI is clearly a more radical group within the movement, who
advocate for the full inclusion of people with Alzheimer's and *all* dementias in the debates that so intimately affect them. A good example
of their grassroots efforts is when I published an article on this topic in
2004 and the then president sent me an email expressing dissatisfaction that I had failed to reference their organization. Coincidentally, a
few years later I was later involved in publishing an article with Jenny
Knauss, a DASNI member with early onset AD, and her husband who
had recruited study participants predominantly from that organization
and elicited my help analyzing and writing up the data. In off the record
conversations, a number of DASNI members told me that the Association's efforts to include them (as of 2008) felt like a "dog and pony show."
At that point, involvement from people with dementia had been along
the lines of speaking about their experiences at various Association-
sponsored conferences and events. Along with the Alzheimer's Societies
of Canada and the United Kingdom, a few seminal social and behavioral
scientists are credited with being DASNI Supporters on the website, including American sociologist Phyllis Braudy Harris, psychologist Steven Sabat, and British psychologist Linda Clare (and her colleagues),
some of the first academics to study narratives of dementia. Studying the

impact of developing a shared social identity, Clare and her colleagues reported the "Collective Strength" of DASNI through interviews with members. DASNI gave people with early-stage dementia a needed sense of belonging, identity, purpose, and positive value. Most significantly, "belonging to DASNI helped to counteract the challenges to self and identity posed by developing dementia, thus significantly affecting the experience of living with dementia, and creating the possibility of effecting social change."[76] In short, the shared social solidarity among members provided hope and space for resisting the dominant negative framing of dementia allegedly reflected and reinforced by the American Alzheimer's Association.

Unfortunately, a number of the charismatic leaders of this particular SMO are no longer actively participating in the forum, presumably due to either death or more advanced symptoms of dementia. Since many of the original members were people affected with early-onset AD or other progressive dementias, the website seems to have lost its momentum and doesn't appear to have many recent postings.

Also around the turn of the century, another major resistance organization, the Alzheimer's Foundation of America (AFA), was established in New York City in reaction to a perceived inadequacy of existing services (read Alzheimer's Association) to meet the needs of diagnosed individuals and their families. AFA's celebrated motto is "Caring for the Nation—one person at a time," and it urges people to "Reach Out For Care." With its stated mission being "to provide optimal care and services to individuals confronting dementia, and to their caregivers and families—through member organizations dedicated to improving quality of life,"[77] this SMO was established as a "consortium of organizations to fill the gap that existed on a national level to assure quality of care and excellence in service to individuals with Alzheimer's disease and related illnesses, and to their caregivers and families."[78] As a result, their goals were far more focused on meeting the everyday needs of affected persons and families by increasing public awareness and education than on finding a cure, and they clearly demarcate themselves as grassroots: "Help remove the fear and denial surrounding Alzheimer's disease and related illnesses, Lead to early detection and proper treatment, Prompt greater utilization of community resources, and Ultimately improve quality of life."

The establishment of Dementia Alliance International (DAI) in 2014 appears to share many of DASNI's core objectives. A nonprofit group of people with dementia from around the world, they are "an advocacy and support group, of, by and for, people with dementia."[79] The professional looking website touts "We can all live well with dementia," and an all-encompassing mission statement:

> To build a global community of people with dementia that collaborates inclusively to:

1. Provide support and encouragement to people with dementia to live beyond the diagnosis of dementia.
2. Model living beyond the diagnosis to other people with dementia and the wider community, and living with purpose with dementia looks like.
3. Advocate for people with dementia, and build the capacity of people with dementia to advocate for themselves and others living with the disease.
4. Reduce the stigma, isolation and discrimination of dementia, and enforce the human rights of people with dementia around the world.[80]

Unlike DASNI, only people with dementia can be members of DAI. The Alliance is also in partnership with Alzheimer's Disease International, both referring to themselves as "the global voice on dementia." DAI's social justice aims are evident on its website, including pieces entitled "I Repeat: Please Don't Call Us Sufferers," "It's Time to Redefine Dementia," and "People with Dementia Still Have Capacity," and a stated vision of "A world where a person with dementia continues to be fully valued."[81]

As a result, the organization has initiatives like Quilt to Remember, the nation's first dementia-related quilt that "pays tribute to all those who have passed or are living with dementia, and their families, so that others can recognize the reality and enormity of this disease, and acknowledge that we stand united for optimal care and a cure."[82] This quilt is comprised of donated memorial squares covering over five Olympic size swimming pools and has been traveling the country for almost ten years. Another noteworthy aspect of the organization is AFA Teens, which "seeks to mobilize teenagers nationwide to raise awareness of Alzheimer's disease and to engage, educate and support teens and their families."[83] These actions stand in stark contrast to the biomedical underpinnings of the Alzheimer's Association, both in terms of the decidedly more innovative and arts focus and the intergenerational grassroots structure.

As of 2015, the organization touted more than 2,300 member organizations who were "dedicated to meeting the educational, social, emotional and practical needs of individuals with Alzheimer's disease and related illnesses, and their caregivers and families . . . all resulting in better care for those affected by the disease."[84] An outgrowth of AFA, Alzheimer's Foundation International currently includes member organizations in Canada and Israel.

While the relatively recent addition of these three SMOs bolsters the AD movement's overall strength in theory as well as the breadth of affected individuals who can be reached, neither DASNI, the more radical SMO, nor AFA, the more middle ground one (in terms of stances taken or commitment to bench science) have nearly as much political power as the Alzheimer's Association. It is too early to determine what impact DAI will have on the landscape. In many ways, the AD movement mirrors the role of SMOs within the senior rights movement generally, and the relative strength as well as shortcomings of its most powerful organization, the AARP.[85]

Conclusions: Despite the Best Intentions

Drawing on organizational theory, I argue that biomedical ideals are so deeply ingrained within the Association that they serve as an iron cage whereby they become ends in themselves. Since the institutional thought structure of the Association is a clinical one, following rules that abide by a distinctly biomedical framework has become a goal in itself. Thus, social constructions of Alzheimer's as an epidemic and a disease are the organizing principles of advocacy within the Association at the risk of further marginalizing the very population for which it is named.

The Alzheimer's disease movement is given credit for encouraging the emergence of AD as a social problem that recast the disease from a relatively rare phenomenon to the fourth or fifth leading cause of death in the United States in just one decade.[86] The mobilization of resources that advanced and organized the AD movement occurred within a context of structural and psychosocial conditions that contributed to the creation of a movement necessary to cultivate the presentation of AD as a significant global health concern. Engaging the age-old structure-agency debate, tracking how the AD movement has responded to and affected the voice of those with AD might begin to bridge micro experiences and larger structural forces by examining how health social movement organizations influence illness experiences, and vice versa.

Although biomedical constructions of AD serve as a unifying force within the Association, the increased sophistication of diagnostic technologies yielding vast numbers of people far earlier in the disease process has not had the effect of bringing to the forefront personal accounts of the condition. This is arguably because the Association, and the movement upon which it is based, elevates certain goals (e.g., cause and cure) at the expense of others (e.g., quality of life, social justice, or care). As with other single-agenda organizations,[87] the Association neglects potentially competing concerns; the biomedical ethos impedes an understanding of the many ways people live with and experience the disease. Such rival ideologies are impediments both to micro level aims such as serving people with AD and their loved ones and the macro level social change agenda of the movement.

While external funding allows for the provision of more, often badly needed, services, monies can exert strong pressures on SMOs to organize in ways consistent with funding sources. This may result in an organizational focus on providing more programs and sponsoring more biomedical research at the expense of policy initiatives and more innovative changes. The situation is confounded by the fact that the majority of financial resources come from individual donors earmarked for finding a cure and improving services for family members. Thus, there is a tension between the wishes of individual staff, family members, donors, and people with AD/MCI and the organizational needs of the Alzheimer's Association.

Despite the availability and willingness of people with AD to speak about their experiences, both they and Association staff perceive various barriers to this integration. On an organizational level, organizational routines, the pursuit of funding, and a decentralized organizational structure prevent the incorporation of people with the disease. Regardless of intentions, inherent biases favor biomedical aims and caregivers as the primary clients. Beyond the Association, external factors, including public perceptions, the role of science/medicine, and client characteristics further obstruct these efforts. An overarching factor encumbering the Association's ability to incorporate these perspectives is the disease pathology itself. Both the social construction of AD historically and Western links between personhood and brain functioning encourage organizational habits of paternalism. More first-person accounts promise to help reverse assumptions that people with Alzheimer's cannot effectively organize and campaign, yet the conundrum is that the perspectives of people with AD are not integrated into the philosophy of the Association. Arguably this is a result of the perception of an AD diagnosis as social death. Despite the fact that encouraging more people with AD to speak publicly can benefit the Association's efforts, the incorporation of personal spokespersons for the AD movement suffers from the same biomedical and caregiver biases as does Alzheimer's research and practice. Although diagnostic advances aid the Association by offering access to people in earlier stages of the disease, biomedical, social, political, and economic forces continue to generate significant obstacles. Given the perception that people with AD are incompetent, barriers may relate to the biomedical foci of the organization itself that do not address such misconceptions about affected individuals. Future attempts to bridge the gap between the biomedical/caregiver focus and the perspectives of those with AD will prove crucial to the Alzheimer disease movement and as the trend toward earlier diagnosis continues, it might become vital to the survival of the Association itself as well.

The Association's efforts have resulted in its conformity with certain biomedical agendas, presumably at the cost of more emancipatory efforts such as combating the conflation of aging and disease or Alzheimer's and social death. Such diffusion risks transforming a social movement into an interest group working for moderate reform from within existing sociopolitical processes and structures. If the Association appears to be a formal, professional organization working for reform via conventional methods, then it is not surprising that obstacles to including people with AD are so pervasive.

My data highlight the difficulties of incorporating the narratives of people with AD into biomedical structures and the social movements based on them. Despite the considerable potential to recruit advocates from support groups to lobby as members of the social movement, that so few chapters currently do so is likely a result of the contradictions within the Association itself. Presently, the recent advances in including the perspectives of people with AD only exacerbate the Association's already severe schism between achieving biomedical and client objectives.

This chapter discusses the history and the biomedical underpinnings of the Alzheimer's Association, particularly the institutional rules championing a biomedical framework and promoting a distinct (narrow) view of AD. In practice, the Association channels patients into research subjects and support group members. While DASNI, AFA, and DAI, the three groups that more recently came onto the scene in response to the Association, or others like them, may someday offer an alternative framework for the movement and affected individuals, recent strategic decisions to highlight 1980s sitcom pop idol Punky Brewster[88] rather than people with dementia themselves, have had the unfortunate effect of diffusing the American Alzheimer's Association's potential for creating meaningful social change despite the stated intentions to that end of many of the staff.

8

Forget Me Not

The Future of Alzheimer's

Alzheimer's was first diagnosed in 1906, well over a century ago, yet the cause remains unknown, disputes over how to classify it persist, and definitive diagnosis can only be made postmortem. Since the 1980s, when the National Institute on Aging and the U.S. Alzheimer's Association were established, Alzheimer's has included both people under 65 as well as those (the original AD, now called early-onset) 65 and over (referred to as typical or late-onset and comprising over 90 percent of cases, but previously considered age-related senility). Fueled by medical and political interests, the decision to unite the two categories rendered AD the fourth to fifth leading cause of death seemingly overnight, launching what critics call the "Alzheimer's Industrial Complex" that, with projections of $638 million National Institutes of Health dollars allocated in 2016, is still going strong.[1] The NIH research portfolio devoted to AD corroborates what scholars of the political economy of aging such as Carroll Estes might predict: the primary area of federal investment in AD research is the development and enhancement of diagnostic tools to identify the condition as early as possible, including bio- and preclinical markers and pharmaceutical treatments for behavioral problems. This is despite claims that "[e]xpanding the diagnosis of dementia mostly increases profit for corporations and industries involved with developing screening and early-diagnosis tests, and pharmaceutical and complementary medicines marketed to maintain cognition in old age."[2] Among the more than $500 million allocated specifically to AD research by the NIH annually, there are very few projects devoted to the psychosocial aspects of Alzheimer's and none that rely on the subjective experiences, or narratives, of diagnosed individuals themselves. As a result, the lion's share of time and money has gone into drug trials and developing techniques to identify pathological precursors of

AD. Yet thirty-five years after uniting senility and what we now call early onset AD, we still do not have efficacious medications or consensus on what is causing the condition. While we currently have five medications, no major pharmacological discoveries have been made in the past decade and, according to most scientists and clinicians, the medications that exist at best plateau decline for a year or so. We don't even know what causes Alzheimer's. Well-intended, highly esteemed scientists have devoted entire careers to it and certainly tens of billions have been spent on finding a cure. Yet disagreement about whether the characteristic tau or beta-amyloid are the cause persist, and recent developments suggest a third, entirely new, causative agent known as TDP-43—a gene most commonly associated with amyotrophic lateral sclerosis (ALS) and frontotemporal dementia (FTD).

Despite the new diagnostic guidelines proposed in 2011, a number of potential problems arise with increasingly earlier diagnoses, including a lack of scientific consensus and increased uncertainty among practitioners, (potential) patients, and the lay public alike. As the NIA and U.S. Alzheimer's Association aligned in yet another medicopolitical move to add both a presymptomatic phase (SCI) and make what had been considered a potential precursor (MCI) a bona fide stage of AD, Alzheimer's joined the growing list of spectrum disorders, demonstrating a classic case of what sociologist Peter Conrad calls "diagnostic expansion." Diagnosing people at a point when they are aware of the disease trajectory and representations in the mass media, however, also opened the door to exploring how medical efforts to detect an AD diagnosis affect the individuals being diagnosed and how patients might in turn shape practice, both of which were among the goals of this study.

Medical sociology has a long history of investigating the meaning and social construction of various medical conditions and technological innovations. Building on the rights movements of the mid-twentieth century, there has been a rise in health social movements and increasing attention to patient/consumer experiences drawing on illness narratives. Studies in this area have shown that various factors constitute the social worlds of biomedical science and its technologies on the one hand, and people seeking medical care on the other.

My data suggest that the deficit-based biomedical focus of specialty medicine generates a process that by design questions the narrative coherence of individuals being evaluated for memory loss. That is, their competence is de facto questioned by the act of seeking evaluation (even though the vast majority initiated contact themselves and did so to establish a "baseline"). Consequently, the diagnostic process serves as a harbinger socializing potential patients into Alzheimer's identities. When diagnosed individuals seek out the Alzheimer's Association, another important transition occurs; individuals become a model of the afflicted through interactions with socializing agents touting a strikingly similar biomedical ethos. The Association's explanatory framework for interpreting AD is strictly medical despite the persistent scientific disputes, lack of consensus, and strong internal commitment to care aspects. In particular, involvement with support groups and research studies—welcome sources of camaraderie for the newly diagnosed—are also crucial steps in solidifying Alzheimer's identities. As a social constructionist and symbolic interactionist, in my view a major social consequence of being diagnosed with Alzheimer's is the resulting interactional tensions in addition to the very real symptoms of disease associated with the condition. These tensions are especially distressing in a modern capitalist, arguably ageist, society.

Given the narrow biomedical interpretations of illness, that is, the lack of alternative frameworks or ways to interpret AD, and scant attention paid to context and/or psychosocial aspects, people diagnosed with Alzheimer's are forced to navigate their way around medical labels and institutions. And they do so in an attempt to maintain their pre-diagnosis sense of selves and to combat what Erving Goffman would have called their newly spoiled identities. My respondents demonstrate keen stigma management strategies when they push back—albeit often subconsciously—against what they see as the restrictive and demoralizing structures associated with their label. The people with AD who participated in this research resist the exclusively negative framing of the condition and their perceived relegation to second-class citizenship resulting from it. But they do not do so easily or without cost.

Theory Generation: Incorporating an Alzheimer's Identity

The sample level theory that my data have generated suggests that an AD diagnosis launches a social process that requires diagnosed individuals to incorporate the label into their lives and balance the threat it presents to cherished identities. Diagnosis is the first major turning point and involves negotiating everyday forgetfulness, converting forgetfulness into so-called symptoms, and eventually embarking on the path of Alzheimer's. The diagnostic process, then, serves an important social function and for most respondents begins the transition to the process of incorporating an Alzheimer's identity. Yet living with Alzheimer's involves interactional tensions that necessitate the employment of various strategies to manage them. One of the most surprising things to me is that their efforts at impression management draw from a decidedly optimistic repertoire, including focusing on the positive, accepting help, attaining serenity, employing humor, and being proactive. After being diagnosed, interacting with the Alzheimer's Association is the second crucial turning point in socializing individuals to see themselves as persons with a disease rather than simply forgetful, and the majority of my respondents do so. Despite the important resources afforded as a result of being diagnosed, including time to plan, medications, and services such as support groups and research studies, however, individuals with mild memory loss do not naively, willingly or fully adopt the label of an AD patient.

As they actively resist being conflated with their condition and treated as deficient by utilizing various interactional strategies, however, my respondents also demonstrate what Michel Foucault called "technologies of self" (whereby they subconsciously self-regulate) and in so doing they both reflect and reinforce modern biomedicine. Perhaps the best example of this is how reminders of their collective forgetfulness during support group discussions reinforce a biomedical understanding of memory loss. Since lack of awareness is said to be part of dementia symptomology, this support simultaneously legitimates the diagnostic criterion itself. Outside biomedical contexts, however, one-on-one interviews reveal a very different interpretation of their memory loss—one that demonstrates decidedly more resistance, at least in theory, to the perceived consequences associated with their diagnosis. Countless respondents—dare I say the vast majority—were decidedly more nuanced in their understanding of the complexity and multifaceted nature of memory loss during my personal interactions with them than I observed at the clinics or during Association-sponsored support groups.

For example, over a shared cup of tea in her Berkeley Hills home, Mrs. B vehemently rejected the medicalized version of her memory loss offered by the clinic while fully acknowledging the symptoms involved and even her fears that it would progress. Mr. C was clearly more concerned about the social aspects of his MCI diagnosis than the biological ones. Likewise, Mr. N and Mrs. V were predominantly worried about the impact of diagnosis on their intimate relationships rather than themselves. Mr. and Mrs. R sought a follow-up appointment with his primary care provider to seek a second opinion in spite of the grim picture painted for him by the specialty clinician. Both Jenny Knauss and Richard Taylor were diagnosed with early-onset AD at 58 and 65, respectively, and devoted the remainder of their shortened lives advocating for the accurate portrayal of life with AD.[3] These accounts demonstrate the continuum of resistance keenly and actively employed by respondents in my study.

Throughout the empirical chapters of this book, I have discussed the social and institutional conditions that I observed in my study. Drawing on the political economy of aging, which argues that structural forces and processes make important contributions to the social constructions of old age and aging, I note that macro social dynamics, such as the dominance of science and medicine, technological innovations, and diagnostic changes through the NIA-Alzheimer's Association proposed guidelines, surround and shape individual experiences of memory loss. In terms of the seemingly disparate practices of specialty medicine, data reveal that the medical approaches of neurology and psychiatry in practice create experiences that are in fact strikingly similar for individuals undergoing evaluation. Observations of and interviews with clinicians diagnosing AD/MCI indicate that standardization, presumed patient incompetence, and the need for patient management characterize the practices of specialty medicine despite well-intended practitioners. The biomedical milieu of memory loss in general as well as within the specific disciplines of neurology and psychiatry ultimately offered postdiagnostic alternatives that included predominantly pharmacological interventions and research participation.

Various interactional consequences resulting from the conditions outlined above were reported, yet my respondents do not describe their diagnosis or life with AD in nearly the same negative tone that might be expected. The experience of being evaluated is indeed harrowing for many, including the demoralizing, impersonal, and anxiety-provoking exchanges with clinicians. Their reactions to the diagnosis range from disbelief and anger to sadness and fear. At the end of the day, however, the vast majority also report being relieved. Since a diagnosis promises potential order in the presumably chaotic world of memory loss, the vast majority were also happy to learn that they were not "going crazy" and it was not "all in their heads." For respondents, the transition from experience to symptom required a redefinition of forgetfulness as a problem. Although the path of forgetful persons begins long before individuals have something to call it, being diagnosed is a crucial turning point commencing an illness identity. The diagnostic process, then, serves as a potential legitimating force for socializing patients to reframe forgetfulness and atypical interactions as symptoms. That is, an important juncture in becoming an Alzheimer's patient, rather than simply a forgetful person, is giving the forgetfulness a medical name. In practice, the social meaning of diagnosis is an important element to people seeking medical attention for their memory loss.

Upon diagnosis, however, respondents note significant transitions in their lives. Thus, while being diagnosed normalizes awkward behaviors and removes personal blame, it also demands identity management to avoid the self-fulfilling prophecy of an Alzheimer's diagnosis at a time when the "zombie trope"[4] serves as a powerful cultural metaphor. A big part of the problem is that we conflate AD with the late stages, when most diagnosed individuals—like the rest of us—will die from something else long before they forget to breathe or swallow.

Since the consequences of a given situation become the structural conditions for future actions, the experiences of diagnosis influence the subsequent social interactions of study participants in significant ways. To commence an Alzheimer's identity, the second step required accepting a medical definition of their forgetfulness and retrospectively categorizing past experiences as pathological, which the vast majority of my study participants willingly did. An unanticipated result of being diagnosed, however, is that extensive interactional problems must be managed in addition to the already socially and emotionally disruptive experience of degenerative illness. Respondents reported two kinds of interactional tensions: struggles with everyday activities and their relationships with others, both requiring various methods of identity management. Since medical diagnoses, like all labels, involve potential social ramifications, diagnosed individuals are forced to navigate their way around the diagnostic label ascribed to them and the related medical structures. The tension between defining experiences as neurochemical deficiencies and assuming the status of a deficient person risks falsely dichotomizing biomedical determinism and a sense of decline in personal efficacy and self-worth. My respondents rightly perceived the diagnosis as a threat to their self and identity. However, noteworthy positive opportunities resulting from the diagnosis were also reported, and the subsequent resources, such as the ability to order one's life and a sense of both autonomy and collectivity when with others similarly diagnosed, were framed as benefits.

After being diagnosed, many people with memory loss seek information and services from the Alzheimer's Association. Given the Association's organizational identity, the limited alternatives available to individuals diagnosed with AD involve primarily biomedical solutions. Three overarching conditions affect the Association's interaction with AD/MCI patients and ultimately the identities of these individuals. First, there is an inherent bias within the Association in favor of biomedical research and caregivers as the primary clients. Second, both the social construction of AD historically and Western links between personhood and brain functioning encourage an organizational culture of paternalism despite compelling, if recent, data suggesting otherwise. Third, the perception that people with AD are inarticulate or incompetent as advocates, coupled with the biomedical focus of the organization, diminishes the opportunity to address progressive goals such as misconceptions about people living with Alzheimer's. The portrayal of AD as both mysterious and devastating benefits the Association's efforts to increase awareness of the disease and the organization itself as well as to solicit financial support. This orchestration relies on the existence of Alzheimer's as a medicoscientific fact warranting attention and the promise of a cure. Thus, dynamics within the Association, including organizational habits, survival, and structure, obstruct the incorporation of diagnosed individuals themselves, despite the staff's stated intentions to the contrary.[5]

Thus, although diagnostic advances aid both the Association and specialty medicine by offering access to people in the earliest stages of the disease, the sociohistorical context and deficit-based approach simultaneously generate significant obstacles to a fuller understanding of people with Alzheimer's. By neglecting potentially competing concerns, the biomedical imperative impedes an understanding of the many ways people *live with* and *experience* the disease. Also sacrificed are more emancipatory efforts, such as combating the conflation of aging and disease, brain functioning and personhood, or Alzheimer's and social death.

My data highlight the barriers to incorporating narratives of people with AD into biomedical structures and the social movements based on them. The highly structured and routinized character of clinical medicine positions patients (especially cognitively impaired ones) as objects of science (i.e., "cases") rather than partners capable of interaction (i.e., "biographies").[6] The Association's capacity to address the needs of people diagnosed with AD is limited to services within the existing biomedical infrastructure, namely, support groups, research participation, and the occasional opportunity to advocate publicly for funding to do cause and cure research. Further, public policy initiatives have focused on procuring monies for biomedical research rather than reforming long-term care services or financing. Thus, the Association has had little effect on policy that improves quality of life for current clients with AD or the more progressive objectives of the larger social movement. When diagnosed individuals interact with the Association, another important turning point in assuming a biomedical identity occurs, thereby positioning its clients to further embark on the road to becoming patients. Involvement with support groups and research are essential steps in achieving this identity.

Therefore, these data demonstrate that study participants moved between a series of identity turning points in learning to view themselves as persons with Alzheimer's. The various phases in the transformation from a forgetful person to an Alzheimer's patient, which are based on interactions with specialty medicine and the Alzheimer's Association, highlight how biomedicine and the organizations based on these processes affect identity. Although not unidirectional, these junctures include: 1) exhibiting everyday forgetfulness, 2) noting that something just wasn't right, 3) seeking and receiving a diagnosis, 4) initiating contact with the Alzheimer's Association, namely, by attending support groups and/or participating in research studies, and ultimately 5) managing an Alzheimer's illness identity. My data also depict micro (or individual level) interactions that are capable of influencing mezzo practice and macro structures. For instance, medicine creates its own (potential) undoing by generating huge numbers of people who are diagnosed early enough in the process to articulate their (negative) experiences of testing procedures, their views on memory loss (as people who lived many decades before the redefinition in the 1980s), and the increased expectations of practitioners ushered in by the baby boomers. Nonetheless, it perhaps comes as no surprise that so few respondents expressed outright dissatisfaction with the medicalization of AD, since acceptance at least on face value is requisite to receiving access to the limited support that does exist. The only explanatory framework is being a patient—an AD patient at that—which while bad, also potentially elicits sympathy. Those who did question the utility and ethics of diagnosis, however, were a vocal minority and we would be wise to heed the caution these narratives of resistance suggest.

The transformation of forgetful experiences into an Alzheimer's identity involves at least two major turning points: being evaluated and diagnosed and interacting with the Alzheimer's Association and/or participating in research studies or support groups. While the interactional tensions associated with an Alzheimer's diagnosis are significant and require additional impression management on top of the already cumbersome task of dealing with the symptoms of the condition for all respondents, the perceived benefits the Association could offer outweighed the psychosocial costs for the vast majority who ultimately took the second step. For them, the illness trajectory included four aspects: reconstructing and reinterpreting past behaviors in light of new notions of forgetfulness as disease; relating to others based on this news and the subsequent interactional tensions; establishing resultant management strategies; and ultimately finding common cause and hope for the future through participation in support groups and/or research. These four stages are not linear; rather they overlap and interconnect in socially messy ways, which further increases the complexity of the experiences and interactions surrounding them. Furthermore, the small but vociferous narratives of resistance refute any uniformity suggested by a stage-model approach.

In addition, there are also various reciprocal effects between conditions and actions. For example, advanced technologies lead to earlier identification of AD/MCI, which in turn generates potential spokespersons. The latter insisted that the Alzheimer's Association include an early-stage advisory board and people with AD on the board of trustees. Subsequently, the internal dynamics of the Alzheimer's Association, its exclusive focus on biomedical research, and the general perceptions of these conditions were all altered. Likewise, earlier diagnoses inevitably affect the processes of clinical practice as patients, including those who actively opt out of taking on the Alzheimer's identity, are able to speak about their experiences of symptoms, cognitive evaluation, and diagnosis.

Most crucially, this book is a story about individuals diagnosed with Alzheimer's or mild cognitive impairment—especially those willingly adopting an AD identity—who consciously exploit, negotiate, and resist the undisputed biomedical label ascribed to them. While they have to do this if they want to save face or minimize stigma, they also desire the legitimacy and hope for a cure that in modern Western societies only medicine promises them. As a result, the medical label itself is something to be achieved. Since diagnoses are socially constructed, or material/social artifacts,[7] respondents require reminders that their memory loss is indeed pathological. Although most of these prompts come from medical clinicians, Association staff, and family members, they also come from within the support groups; members socialize one another into medical interpretations of memory loss. Thus, support groups, as well as research participation, reinforce AD identities for both patients and families alike. Since AD is a condition that according to biomedicine robs people of meaningful social interaction, my findings call into question the diagnostic label itself. These narratives depict views and values of an external world, including clinical practice, advocacy agencies, and intimates, that motivate people to manage their social interactions. That is, this book traces the processes of socialization through which the majority of my respondents do ultimately become Alzheimer's patients, including both passive and active consumption of biomedical tenets, and in so doing interrogates the perceived mandate to do so. When I, the sociologist and human being, hear the projections of the prevalence or economic cost of Alzheimer's, all I can think about is the angst, the restlessness, the dry mouth, and the racing heartbeat that I felt every single time I observed someone being evaluated and diagnosed. The seemingly palpable silence that followed. And I can't help but wonder, this is all *to what end*?

Contextualizing the Stories

Although a diagnosis of Alzheimer's disease or mild cognitive impairment is in theory treated as a condition of immediate debilitation, now that we diagnose so early it is a circumstance that requires new and often innovative types of interaction. My respondents strove to achieve an identity free of disease despite—or arguably as a result of—being diagnosed with a condition surrounded by a rhetoric of irreversible devastation and the associated assault on their personhood.

As the disease progresses, individuals with AD risk losing the ability to manage their identities in the manner deemed so important by my respondents. As impairment increases, social structure may more readily assign labels despite (past) protests from people in the earliest phases. Although those diagnosed adeptly advocate their sovereignty in this study, further decline will threaten their efforts. In a culture of age-based worth, social interaction is challenging enough for seniors with keen memories. When a society also has strict normative expectations of communication, interaction, and so-called reality, the status of nonperson is ascribed to any individual who is deemed to have a sick brain, not be fully conscious, or otherwise be cognitively compromised. What this book argues is that we, "the not yet demented," as DASNI members refer to us, are the problem. Our own cultural reticence translates too easily into unwillingness to join people with dementia *where they are*. Since dementia represents a particularly horrifying state (we are socialized to believe), the biggest barrier to a meaningful life in spite of dementia is the fear of unimpaired others. Our anxieties, that is, become yet another problem for diagnosed individuals to manage. We would do well, then, to learn from my respondents, like Mrs. W, for whom life—while decidedly more challenging—is far from over.

This ethnography has analyzed the processes through which popular social and medical discourses collude and collide with personal narratives of ostensibly non–age-related memory loss. Although there are perceived social and personal opportunities resulting from being diagnosed, the scientific debate over what constitutes pathological memory loss and subsequent medical efforts to delineate methods of interpreting evidence obscure accounts of subjective experience. Thus, people with Alzheimer's/mild cognitive impairment have experiences which standard evidential methods are not accustomed to (or capable of) managing.

The unintended consequence for clinical practice is that a cohort of worried well have flooded into specialty clinics seeking evaluation. The escalating diagnoses of early-stage AD generates an entire reserve of individuals who can articulate their perspective far more clearly than was the case even a decade ago. While it is beyond the scope of this book, it remains to be seen whether the new diagnostic guidelines rendering MCI a stage of AD are the cause of or a reaction to the exponential increase of people seeking cognitive evaluation. Either way, this creates a new and different clientele for clinical practice and constituency for the Alzheimer's Association.

Since the questions that are asked both in science and in practice influence the possible answers that can be found, people diagnosed with AD/MCI undergo considerable socialization into a medicalized version of their experiences. Examining the social and personal effect of Alzheimer's diagnoses in context elucidates the importance of continuing to engage debates of agency-structure as well as nuanced issues of illness narratives, the social construction/biomedicalization of health and aging, and the interface of people seeking medical care with various practices and technologies. Symbolically, a diagnosis of AD represents what I term a social demotion, whereby individuals labeled cognitively compromised are threatened with circumstances of social death (whether immediate or anticipated). This directly correlates with current constructions that equate brain functioning and personhood. For only when the fundamental essence of self is reduced to the brain can such disenfranchisement of our most deeply forgetful members be accomplished. The stories of medical professionals and advocacy organizations must be further compared and contrasted with illness narratives. Since competing discourses and ideologies exist in a pluralistic society like the United States, it is through a multiplicity of perspectives that social understanding and, when necessary, change can be realized. That is, it is time to admit that "the concept of Alzheimer's is an artifact of value, one which has taken on a life of its own among medical practitioners, the public, and advocacy groups alike,"[8] and ask the difficult questions that follow.

Engaging Theory

This research project analyzed macro processes such as the biomedicalization of forgetfulness, the relationship of medicalization to the identities of forgetful older members of society, and the political and economic mechanisms through which the generation of biomedical knowledges transforms and permeates society. My foremost interest, however, was in the micro accounts of identity management and the patient careers or illness trajectories in daily life. In particular, I wanted to understand how the processes of biomedicalization transform the identities and illness narratives of individuals diagnosed with Alzheimer's disease.

Biomedicalization and its reliance on technoscience have fundamentally shaped the history of Alzheimer's, its conceptualization in clinical practice, its organization in advocacy realms, and its implications for identity management in everyday life. The data reported here engage existing theory on biomedicalization by highlighting two major themes: the perceived potential benefits of medicalization and the reciprocity of biomedical knowledges and practices, that is, the way in which *patients* influence practice. First, rather than medicalization being an exclusively negative experience, as has been the typical presentation, these data suggest that there might be positive aspects to having a diagnosis, including increased social bonds with others so diagnosed and a degree of personal efficacy in their remaining years. This corroborates findings from a handful of other studies on the medicalization of conditions such as alcoholism or Chronic Fatigue Syndrome[9] that report positive aspects of a diagnosis, including validation, a sense of relief, and support. Second, in addition to the opportunities afforded to individuals diagnosed, there are obvious contingencies which restrict the lives of the respondents in my study. The generation of a large group of persons with early-stage Alzheimer's/MCI increases the expectations that biomedicine should take the accounts of these individuals into consideration and that the

Association address this constituency. Although largely theoretical at the present time, these factors have created the potential scrutiny of biomedical diagnoses for which a definitive diagnosis can only be made postmortem and the need to justify the unification of early- and late-onset AD. The bioethical implications of this debate should significantly alter the future organization of practices addressing memory loss.

My data also engage concepts of an illness trajectory or an individual's career as an ill person, which insinuate a process leading to the absolute adoption of a given identity. Research on specific medical conditions has shown that when people are diagnosed they often take on the status of a sick or impaired person or of a patient,[10] at least in the eyes of those with whom they interact, particularly if they have a chronic illness. In fact, the diagnostic label is generally thought to become for people what sociologists call a master status.[11] In concert with work on Holocaust survivors, prisoners, and people diagnosed with AIDS, I challenge the notion that people take on the status of patient or otherwise compromised person in an immediate, complete, or detrimental sense. Instead of fully assuming something like Talcott Parsons's sick role, my data show that respondents fluctuate between utilizing the diagnosis as a necessary strategy of identity management and incorporating AD/MCI as merely one aspect of their identity. In everyday life, respondents manage the changes they are experiencing as a result of memory loss to accommodate the diagnosis of Alzheimer's into their pre-existing identities. Understanding that this subject in formation we call a patient involves a continuum of experience including a normalization of symptoms, an employment of diagnosis as a resource, and the discovery of positive aspects in the diagnosis, challenges and expands existing theory. It allows for the emergence of a path which simultaneously incorporates resistance and acceptance.

Many social theories on identity construction/management imply unidirectionality, if not linearity, of illness experience that was not corroborated in my data. The advent of diagnosis is indisputably a crucial juncture for individuals living with forgetfulness, but after diagnosis noteworthy vacillation between stances and identities occurs. Thus, my data support alternative frameworks suggesting a pendular reconstruction of identity[12] that I argue is artistically crafted. Being diagnosed with AD/MCI clearly involves a labeling process that requires identity management, but individuals also use and manipulate the diagnosis. Identities are processual and so are diagnostic labels and the various interpretations of such biomedical classification systems. It is important to understand the processes through which illness realities are socially constructed. As the narratives of resistance demonstrate, there is nothing intrinsic to the feelings expressed by these respondents that necessarily and inevitably lead to a definition of forgetfulness as a disease. In fact, my data indicate that in order for individuals to take on an identity that involves an illness they must have that identity *reinforced by biomedicine and the structures based on it.*

Perhaps the most important aspect of this study, however, is the finding that individuals diagnosed with AD/MCI are a far cry from the passive victims of disease that we commonly perceive and portray them to be. Whether their efforts to seek help and support indeed encourage technologies of self that involve surveillance and buy-in to the medical model or not, the narratives of resistance (both in terms of the majority who accept but resist biomedical framings and the minority who flatly refuse the medicalization of their forgetfulness) demonstrate the potential for agency. That is, these are not simply cogs in a Marxist medical machine. The predominant narrative of assuming an Alzheimer's identity—as and when they see fit—is a conscious decision. While critics of biomedicine would be correct to argue this is a heavily constrained choice, one that as I've shown comes with clear consequences for the diagnosed individuals, not a single respondent in this study evoked a sense of pity or elicited a deficit-model approach. Not one person.

Since this book argues that Alzheimer's diagnoses rely more heavily on clinical than objective criteria, the fact that scores of people may be diagnosed with MCI who would otherwise have gone unnoticed had they not gone for testing suggests the magnitude of the medical gaze.[13] Alzheimer's, especially in its preclinical (now defined as the earliest) stage, is the quintessential medicalization of our time. We must ask ourselves what early diagnosis means, sociologically speaking, for them and the rest of us as we ourselves age and anticipate ourselves as future old people. If the diagnosis is not reliable, as Peter Whitehouse and his colleagues have argued,[14] and given the psychosocial tensions identified by my respondents, then bioethical discourse must attend to the potential effects of such medical reductionism on the everyday lives of people who may simply be deeply forgetful. It is time we asked: is late-age Alzheimer's really a disease? Would we all get Alzheimer's if we lived long enough? How and why have views on this changed over the years? What is the utility of labeling people with it when no efficacious treatment options currently exist and we cannot definitely diagnosis until autopsy? Do the perceived benefits of the diagnosis outweigh the psychosocial costs?

Moving Forward

The medicalization of memory loss and the sociology of illness narratives, my two analytical anchors, provide insights into a few key contemporary debates. Given the central place of memory in modern Western life, I question whether or not memory-centeredness, and particularly memory loss being seen primarily as a medical problem, is good for seniors or, for that matter, the rest of us. Conversations about memory problems currently taking place in academia and in the public at large are telling about views on aging and the salience of memory in the United States today. My respondents and I are not alone in our skepticism about the expansion of AD diagnoses. Recent provocative books, including *The Myth of Alzheimer's, Forget Memory, Treating Dementia: Do We Have a Pill for It?*, and *The Alzheimer Conundrum: Entanglements of Dementia and Aging*,[15] are lenses through which we can consider the advantages and pitfalls of conceptualizing Alzheimer's as we do in the current biomedical milieu. Bioethicists, social science and humanities scholars, and even a few vocal neurologists, have begun arguing for a reframing of AD that questions the very utility of diagnosing it. Neurologist Peter Whitehouse and anthropologist Daniel George dispute the current social construction of Alzheimer's, especially the decision made in the 1980s to include people aged 65 and over, instead suggesting that *The Myth of Alzheimer's* is propagated by the various institutions and actors who stand to gain the most from medicalizing the condition—or the said Alzheimer's Industrial Complex. They suggest that a strictly medical approach has social and psychological consequences that are not offset by the only minimally efficacious treatment options currently available. Artist and humanities scholar Anne Basting paints an intimate picture of why we should in fact *Forget Memory* altogether and yet cannot seem to do so. Arguing that we need more appreciation of in-the-moment meaning in the lives of all people, including those most deeply forgetful among us, Basting adds to the growing empirical evidence on how the arts therapies can benefit people with memory loss. Accordingly, "arts provide a means to tap into imagination and foster creative expression and meaningful experiences, the essence of which is likely beyond measure."[16] Historian Jesse Ballenger and colleagues' edited volume directly challenges both our cultural obsession with silver bullets and pharmaceutical quick fixes as well as the specific *lack* of efficacious treatment options for Alzheimer's a century after it was discovered and billions of dollars later. Renowned medical anthropologist Margaret Lock aptly states, "No amount of preventive measure and no drugs will defeat aging . . . nor can dementia be 'wiped out' as though it is an infectious disease—aging and dementia cannot be disentangled."[17] By championing experiences of dementia as something larger than tales of tragedy can capture, these pioneers interrogate the Alzheimer's Industrial Complex itself. Joining the ranks of those writing against a defeatist interpretation of memory loss, my work contributes to the growing scholarship highlighting an explanatory framework for Alzheimer's that celebrates the humanity, dignity, grace, and personhood of those living with the condition. In so doing, this book aspires to contribute to the nascent field I envision as academic narratives of resistance.

I argue that by highlighting the social nature of memory and how self is relational, AD can be seen as a singular case of more general and processual social phenomena common to modern Western societies. Not only is the current case of Alzheimer's the quintessential case of biomedicalization, but it is also steeped in deep-seated cultural ageism. Contemporary American views about aging position seniors not as actors or agents in their own right, but as a drain on limited societal resources. Our fear of growing old both reflects and reinforces the current cultural age bias. In stark contrast, sociologist Meika Loe allows seniors themselves to define their own conceptions of aging well. Unlike the successful aging discourse within psychology, *Aging Our Way*[18] demonstrates the resilience and resourcefulness of the oldest old in spite of various obstacles.[19] Drawing on cultural capital and social networks, her respondents strive to age in place rather than crumble under the deficit model attached to aging in a manner similar to that which I have elsewhere argued can happen when diagnosed individuals see AD as a "manageable disability" and/or couples adapt to Alzheimer's by "negotiating the joint career."[20] Many social scientists have highlighted the importance of incorporating the perspectives of older adults into the conceptualization of aging well, yet few have done so empirically. By meeting seniors where they are and learning the lessons that *they think are important* in organizing *what they define as* successful living and aging, we might well begin to reverse the ageist cultural assumptions preventing meaningful intergenerational dialogue. Literary critic Margaret Morganroth Gullette[21] shows how and why contemporary social constructions of Alzheimer's are based on the dominance of cognitive hierarchies across the lifespan, fueled by what she calls the "memory-obsessed media" and American anxiety about decline. According to Gullette, unless we are *Agewise* we cannot even begin *Fighting the New Ageism in America*. To paraphrase J. Eric Oliver's *Fat Politics*,[22] we hate old people (just as we do those who are "fat")—despite the lack of data to support the grim public portrayal of aging—because our fear of growing old both reflects and reinforces the current cultural age bias. When a particular framing of an issue has cognitive resonance, it becomes exceedingly difficult to challenge. In the ways identified here, this book engages these larger debates, especially an understanding of the "ways of aging" Loe so eloquently depicts and an endorsement for striving to be "agewise." By interrogating our societal fear of Alzheimer's and ageism more broadly, and showing more accurate portrayals of life with the condition, I hope the counternarrative offered here advances public and sociological understanding of what has been framed as the most dreaded disease of our times. The cognitive resonance of the "dementia narrative" as presented by the mass media and biomedicine makes it difficult to debunk. Yet, if we want to bring some humanity to memory loss, *and we should*, then it would behoove us to remember what Mrs. W, a 72-year-old widow, told me weeks after being diagnosed with AD: "I'm still the same person I've always been. It's just that now I'm me with Alzheimer's." And at the end of the day, who among us would want to be seen any differently?

This book has traced the processes of medicalization through which cadres of forgetful seniors come to see themselves as Alzheimer's patients, and the (often hidden) glimpses of agency and resistance along the way. Experiences of dementia occur within a cultural context that has expanded, in seemingly endless fashion, the range of behaviors defined as abnormal. Our willingness to interpret forgetfulness, especially in seniors, as disease has increased exponentially. Is it any wonder that we so strongly resist imagining ourselves as future old people? If we continue to proceed without caution, ignoring the context of social conditions and issues of the larger social order that political economists of aging warn against, then we might well find that we have destroyed the precious little space within which we as modern humans can age meaningfully.

APPENDIX A

Interview Guides

(Family members were asked modified versions of these questions.)
- When did you first notice changes in your memory? Can you give examples?
- How did you feel about your memory difficulties at the time?
- When did you share these changes with your friends and family? Who specifically did you share with or who did you choose not to share with, and why?
- Why did you seek medical attention for your memory?
- What was your experience of being tested like?
- Do you feel comfortable discussing your diagnosis?
- How did it feel to hear that you had AD/MCI? What was your first thought?
- How have your family and friends dealt with your diagnosis?
- How has your life changed since your diagnosis or discovery of some memory loss?
- How would you describe your situation to someone else newly diagnosed or a friend who does not understand the experiences you may have?
- How do you feel the general public understands Alzheimer's disease?
- Has seeing your medical doctor been helpful to you, why or why not?
- Have you heard of the Alzheimer's Association? If so, do you interact with it and in what capacity?

II. CLINICIANS
- Background: What is your training and how long have you been in the field?
- What are some of the typical reactions to diagnosis?
- Do you find that families or patients themselves seek diagnosis?

- What are some of the experiences that lead people to seek diagnosis?
- How do you (or your team) inform people of their diagnosis?
- What resources are available to people once they are AD-diagnosed?
- What are some of the barriers to making a definitive diagnosis?
- How has the role of geriatric assessment impacted formal diagnostics?
- How has the role of diagnostics/pharmaceuticals/other technology changed since you entered the field of AD?
- How would you describe the etiological process of AD to a layperson?
- What exactly is "mild cognitive impairment" and the current information regarding using it as a diagnostic category?
- What is the biggest effect of diagnosing people early?
- How has this changed clinical practice? Research?
- Are there any potential negative effects to diagnosing people earlier in the disease trajectory?
- How do you think AD fits into the long-term care system more broadly?
- What do you consider the most promising up-and-coming area within AD research?
- What are your opinions on local, state, and federal funding for AD research, diagnostics, and care?

III. ALZHEIMER'S ASSOCIATION STAFF
- Background: What is your role and how long have you been with the Association?
- What is the objective of the Association? What is the objective of your specific role within the Association?
- How would you define, or describe, AD for a lay audience?
- How would you define, or describe, MCI for a lay audience?
- How would you like to see the Association develop over the next 10 years? Are there any areas you think need to be explored?
- What initiatives are the Association (or your department) taking to include the individuals with AD (target, dispense, inform programs and policy)?
- What do you perceive as the major barriers to incorporating this voice?
- What is the biggest change you have seen during your time with the Association?
- What do you consider the most effective policy/advocacy initiatives?

- What is the biggest change in aging services that you have seen in your tenure?
- Where would you like to see more AD-related monies allocated?
- What are your thoughts on Alzheimer's disease as a social movement within the U.S.? And globally? What is the Association's role within this movement?

APPENDIX B

Study Design and Methodology

This research project was informed by an inductive method of data collection, sampling, and analysis. Rather than testing existing hypotheses or applying sociological theories to data, this book instead aims to discover theory as grounded in the data itself. As such, the product of this research is a mid-range substantive theory and its generalizability lies in the concepts discovered within the sample studied rather than the larger population from which it was drawn.[1] This is not to suggest that this project has not been informed by larger theoretical perspectives, since all sociological research draws from a framework of how society works. Thus, my inquiry is primarily guided by a symbolic interactionist tradition and social constructionism framework, but I also draw from phenomenology as well. In this endeavor, a qualitative study design utilizing the methods of participant observation, in-depth interviews, focus groups, and website monitoring was devised for purposes of triangulation. Interview and observation data collection began in 2002 and continued through 2009. Website monitoring and accumulation of state-of-the-science findings were ongoing through August, 2015.

Data obtained from eighteen months of participant observation of the diagnostic process (2003–2005) for memory loss included attendance at neuropsychological and medical examinations, informant (i.e., family member) interviews, the team disposition meetings where clinicians met to discuss cases and determine a diagnosis, and the delivery of that diagnosis. Observation also included attendance of various scientific, clinical, and policy conferences related to Alzheimer's and mild cognitive impairment (2003–2014), many of which were sponsored by the Alzheimer's Association. The interview data, including group interviews, were gathered in a semi-structured manner with open-ended guides and lasted from 45 minutes to 3 hours. They were gathered in two waves (2003–2005 and 2008–2009), primarily in the San Francisco Bay Area with additional interviews in Chicagoland. The aim of the focus groups and interviews was to collect detailed accounts of illness experiences from the perspectives of AD-/MCI-diagnosed individuals and of the philosophies and daily practices of clinical staff at the specialty diagnostic centers and the American Alzheimer's Association. The websites of the national branch and various local chapters of the Alzheimer's Association, Alzheimer's Disease International, Dementia Advocacy Support Network International, the Alzheimer's Foundation of America, and, most recently, Dementia Alliance International were routinely monitored to track how Alzheimer's and mild cognitive impairment, and individuals diagnosed with these conditions, were portrayed, the history of the organizations and how they were structured, who the key actors and national spokespeople were, and any efforts underway to incorporate diagnosed individuals.

Sampling

The complete sample (N=153) included four groups of respondents, whom I have entitled potential patients (N=86), potential care partners (N=32), clinicians (N=22), and Association staff (N=12). Convenience and snowball sampling methodologies were used for recruitment.

The target population of the first part of the sample (N=86) included observation of individuals undergoing the diagnostic process (N=46), including follow-up interviews with 28 of them and in-depth interviews with people recently diagnosed with early-stage AD (ESAD)[2] or MCI (N=40),[3] when a person is considered to be high functioning (a diagnostic term typically used to indicate a person who is capable of conversation, responding to direct questions, and has recall). These interviews consisted of six (6) 1½ hour focus groups (N=32) and 2–3 hour in-person interviews (N=8) with people diagnosed in the early stages of AD (N=24) or with Mild Cognitive Impairment (N=16). Observation was conducted at the diagnostic centers of a research-based teaching university and a Veteran's Health Administration Hospital in Northern California. Every participant had been, or was being, medically evaluated and was deemed preclinical or in the early stages of AD (mini-mental state examination [MMSE] scores ranged from 22 to 30). Since the level of cognition rather than the duration of the condition determine the severity, or stage, of Alzheimer's—that is, the person with ESAD/MCI could have had the condition for one week or many years—the range of time since diagnosis varied from weeks (for the 48 I observed being diagnosed) to 4 years (for the 40 respondents I recruited elsewhere). The elapsed time since diagnosis varied because stage refers to a categorization independent of illness duration. All respondents were over 65 years old, and the mean age was 73.5 years. The sample included 48 men (56%) and 38 women (44%), which is clearly not representative of the general population of older adults.[4] All but 12 (9%) were married and resided with a spouse. Of those not married, 9 were widowed (75%) and 3 were single, and all these individuals lived alone at the time of the interview. The respondents who sought medical attention at the two specialty diagnostic centers were predominantly financially well off, married, Caucasians.[5] The focus groups were conducted in pre-existing support groups for people diagnosed with ESAD or MCI at either a) local Alzheimer's Association chapters or b) the psychiatric diagnostic center, which was an Alzheimer's Research Center of California (ARCC). The participants for in-person interviews were recruited from observation at either of the diagnostic centers, pre-existing support groups, or the Alzheimer's Association clinical research registry. The second component of the sample consisted of observation of what clinics called "informant interviews" (N=10), where data were collected from the loved one(s) of the "potential patient" by a clinician to corroborate the evidence gathered from the individuals themselves, and three (3) focus groups (N=22) within pre-existing support groups that met simultaneously with the groups for individuals with ESAD/MCI. This subsection of the sample resulted largely from the requests from the care partners at one of the study sites who were informed of the research I was conducting with the diagnosed individuals and then wanted to participate.

The third segment of the sample entailed observation (N=22) and subsequent in-person interviews (N=8) with clinicians evaluating cognition and rendering diagnoses in the two diagnostic centers. Clinicians observed/interviewed included neurologists, neuro/psychiatrists, nurses, resident MDs, neuro/psychologists, clinical research coordinators, and general clinicians. Demographically, there were 16 male (73%) and 6 female (27%) clinicians; 18 Caucasians (82%), 3 Asian Americans

(14%), and 1 Southeast Asian (4%). Age varied considerably from resident MDs to seasoned clinicians who had been in the field for thirty years.

The final section of the sample (N=12) utilized telephone (N=5) and in-person (N=7) in-depth interviews in 2003–2005 with staff members of the Alzheimer's Association, the national advocacy organization devoted to dementia and the major player in the U.S.-based social movement surrounding Alzheimer's.[6] All respondents had been with the Association for at least a year, with a mean length of employment of 4 years. There were 5 men (42%) and 7 women (58%). These respondents were representatives of the Public Relations, Public Policy, Community Outreach, Education Management, and Program Management departments or were the CEO/Administrator at 8 different chapters, both rural and urban. The Interim President was also interviewed. Potential participants were selected if their job description on the website stated involvement with patient issues, including patient services, patient quality of care or life, patient advocacy, or policy issues concerning patients or if they were referred by a previous respondent. Comprehensive demographic information on age and race were not collected for this part of the sample, although most participants were middle-aged Caucasian women who had personal experiences with Alzheimer's. The larger age range was probably from 30 to 60.

Data Collection

Participant observation occurred during the scheduled medical visits to the two specialty clinics enrolled in the study. Observation was largely restricted to people over 65 years of age who reported complaints consistent with dementia of the Alzheimer's type, although a few cases included individuals less than 65 years old or with other types of dementia. Verbal consent was obtained by the clinician being followed before any potential patient/care partner was observed. Observation of conferences geared toward Alzheimer's/MCI included: the 2002 8th International Conference on Alzheimer's Disease and Related Disorders in Stockholm, Sweden; the 2003 Unlocking the Mysteries of Memory Loss in Washington, D.C.; the 2003 Caring Counts! conference in Sacramento, California; and the 2003 Public Policy Day for Alzheimer's in

Sacramento, California. Audiotapes were also obtained from the 2001 Alzheimer's Disease International in Wellington, New Zealand; the 2003 Public Policy Forum in Washington, D.C.; the 2003 Caregiving Plenary in Washington, D.C.; the 2006 International Conference on Brain-hood in Rio de Janeiro, Brazil; the 1st Early-Stage Forum in Pasadena, California, in 2006; 2007 Alzheimer's Day, Northwestern University Alzheimer's Disease Center; the 18th Alzheimer Europe Conference in Oslo, Norway, in 2008; 2008 Seminar Series, Northwestern University Alzheimer's Disease Center; and the annual Gerontological Society of America meetings 2001 through 2014. At many of these, I presented preliminary findings.

Various Alzheimer's Association websites were also monitored to analyze the projection of AD/MCI, the incorporation of people with these conditions, and the type and level of information made available to the public. Relevant information was printed and analyzed. The focus groups occurred at the regularly scheduled time and place of the support groups for people with early-stage Alzheimer's disease (ESAD) or MCI and lasted roughly 1½ hours. The interviews with diagnosed individuals took place in their homes at a time chosen by them and, when living with a spouse, often included the presence of the partner. Interviews with clinicians occurred in their offices and lasted approximately 45 minutes. Interviews with Association staff were performed both in-person at local chapters and via telephone and lasted approximately 1 hour.

The aim of participant observation was to elicit an understanding of the experiences of memory loss, including nonverbal gestures and reactions to diagnosis; interactions with others, including family members and medical staff; and the encounter between potential patients and neuropsychological testing and clinicians as well as the daily practices of clinicians diagnosing AD/MCI. At the conferences, I presented and collected data on the state-of-the-science. Detailed notes were taken either at the time of observation or dictated into a tape recorder immediately following. Team case disposition meetings were tape recorded. All notes and tapes were transcribed within approximately 2–3 weeks of the date of observation.

Interview data were gathered via a conversational format utilizing open-ended, unstructured guides. General questions for AD-/MCI-

diagnosed respondents included their experiences of cognitive evaluation and diagnosis, how their life and/or identity had changed, if at all,
since diagnosis; how they described, or made sense of, their condition;
their opinions regarding the general public's awareness of, or reaction to,
their condition; what they perceived as their role in informing research
and care; and thoughts on the future. Questions for the clinical staff pertained primarily to the neurobiology/neuropsychiatry of Alzheimer's/
MCI, clarifications on any terminology or situations observed, general
background training, areas of future promise, disease classification, and
most noteworthy changes in the field. Interview guides with Association staff covered job description and duties, the objectives of both the
organization and specific departments, obstacles to these aims, how they
defined AD, what they saw as the role of individuals with AD within
the Association, what was being done, on either an individual or organizational level, to encourage the visibility of diagnosed spokespeople,
and existing barriers thereto. All interviews were taped and transcribed
within approximately 2–3 weeks. An overview memo highlighting main
themes and general impressions was generated immediately following
each interview. Throughout the process, copious memos were written
to record researcher observations and thoughts or to engage existing
theory.

Data Analysis

As a qualitative researcher, all data—including interview and conference
transcripts, field notes, memos, and website/textual materials—were
taped, transcribed, and then analyzed using the constant comparative
method and coding paradigm of grounded theory.[7] Since grounded
theory aims to consolidate information into matrices to generate overarching themes, the ongoing process of taking notes, writing memos,
and (re)reading data lends itself to emergent themes and categories
for simplifying and articulating data. As line-by-line coding occurs,
themes are generated. Thus, theory is inductively derived from the data.
Throughout the process of coding data, analytic questions were repeatedly explored: under what conditions does this happen, and with what
mechanisms, strategies, rhetoric, and with what consequences?[8] This
inductive mode included revision of analysis through presentation of

data to participants for verification, sampling for new participants based on emerging concepts and theories, and comparing findings to those in the literature.

The general principles of phenomenology[9] that highlight the subjective, lived experiences of everyday life and illness experiences, and the daily work performed by clinicians and Association staff, also informed this study. Since all sciences are the products of scientists working together, this study avoided an *ex post facto* critique of knowledge and instead aimed to understand the consciousness of a given epoch. The main influence of this paradigm was the need for reflexivity, describing structures of experience, and the constant reminder that the experience is processual. Therefore, data reflect a snapshot of the daily lives of the people in this study when they were interviewed or observed.

Detailed notes were dictated to ensure that emerging theoretical thoughts and a general overview of the data were recorded immediately following each interview. Therefore, interviews were replayed or reread as soon as possible to encourage incremental development of theory and categorization of ideas and themes. Analysis began with open coding[10] that involved identification of the dimensions and properties of the themes as they emerged. To the extent possible, themes were labeled using the words of the respondents. As more and more themes were discovered, the feeling of saturation eventually resulted (for example, it became clear that all data fit into existing themes or that two concepts could be collapsed into one). Next, I aimed to consolidate themes by using an explanatory matrix to identify core variables, or chose to focus on specific variables for the purposes of presentation (say, sociopsychological aspects) within a particular substantive area. Again, the themes emerging from the data were constantly verified through correspondence with original respondents, input from colleagues, and keeping up to date with the existing literature. These processes were performed as a tool of quality control for ensuring that themes occurred within the data themselves and that they were consistently observed.

Although the themes presented throughout the book may appear to be distinct, it is important to highlight that they are nestled within each other and various other overlapping categories. Further, although the results of this study have been presented in a linear fashion, this is not to suggest that individuals experience these things in any sort of deterministic staged manner. Rather, these data are based on complex interactions among multiple individuals in diverse social worlds. I have chosen in this book to present the data in the way I felt best captures the essence of the joint story of over 150 very different people. Of course, I will not have perfectly represented every respondent, but I hope that most of the diagnosed individuals that I spoke with, at least, feel I have accurately told their story.

APPENDIX C

Study Sites and Procedures

The primary specialty disciplines involved in diagnosing and managing memory loss are neurology and psychiatry. This research was conducted through participant observation of the diagnostic process at one of each type of clinic. Both sites were located within large teaching universities; the psychiatrically oriented center, an Aging Clinical Research Center (ACRC)[1] and an Alzheimer's Research Center of California (ARCC)[2] is also situated within a Department of Veterans Affairs and the neurologically based center is attached to a tertiary teaching hospital. Whereas the neurological center is discipline-based and directly linked to a medical center, the psychiatric center is not a primary care center—it does not prescribe medications, interpret lab results, or have expertise in performing physical/neurological examinations.

While this book demonstrated a surprising amount of overlap in clinical practice and patient experiences of the diagnostic process of memory loss between my study sites, this appendix will outline the distinct settings, techniques, and tools used, and the clinical process at the Brain Clinic and the Health Center.

I. The Brain Clinic

The Brain Clinic[3] is a neurological diagnostic center at a large research university in northern California. It is nestled amongst many other campus buildings and sits directly across from the university hospital. On the eighth floor of one of the campus's tallest buildings, the memory wing of the clinic feels professional and sterile. The hallways are busy and there is a sense of fervor in the air. There are five or six small rooms, each the size of a doctor's office. They are all equipped with the typical items found in a medical setting: a blood pressure cuff, cotton swabs, a sink, an examination table, a desk, and a few spare chairs. There is also one main office with a computer, where clinicians await patients, discuss cases, conduct internet searches, review MRI-scans, or dictate findings. During my time at the clinic, I routinely observed two male attending neurologists, one the dynamic, middle-aged director and the other a kind, likable man with roughly a decade of experience under his belt, and one tall, well-spoken senior neuropsychologist. The five to six neurology residents were mostly white men in their thirties, but I did observe one Indian woman and another Asian male, in that same age cohort. The two neuropsychology staff I routinely observed were both friendly, soft-spoken Caucasian women in their thirties. The clinic had the feel of a professional office building, with people smartly dressed in business clothing and carrying themselves with comportment.

After an average wait of one month, individuals seeking medical attention for their memory loss follow the yellow footprints through the long corridor of offices and sit in the waiting room at the end of the hall overlooking the campus. Few people come alone to these visits. Typically, they have brought a spouse with them and on occasion it is an adult child, a friend, or a sibling. It is not uncommon for there to be more than one person attending these appointments with them.

History and Physical

If the bustling clinic is not running late, the day begins at 9:45 a.m. when the person with suspected memory loss (and loved ones, if present) is brought into one of the rooms by the medical student on rotation that day. This component begins with the History and Physical (H&P), where a resident MD will first take information regarding the individual's past medical history and that of his/her family, observed symptoms and/or changes related to memory, everyday functioning, current medications, and social history.

The patient, and any available family member(s), tells about the "history of the present illness," including the chief complaint (e.g., short-term memory loss), its onset, and length of duration. This component also focuses on other potentially diagnostic behavioral features, such as changes in personality, language or navigational skills, or compulsive behavior. Specific examples of the first symptom, particularly from the family, are strongly encouraged, as are concrete instances (e.g., stories) of memory loss. Next, the past medical history is taken, which covers a general overview as well as incidents of head trauma, loss of consciousness, respiratory insufficiency, hepatic or renal insufficiency, and sleep apnea.

Although the resident MD has presumably already read the medical chart, the doctor (I only observed one female resident in my time there) will ask the patient to list the medications being taken. Beyond standard medications, the focus is on memory and psychoactive medications and their effect. Also discussed are alternative therapies and over-the-counter remedies. The family history includes age and health status (if living) and cause of death (if deceased) of all first degree relatives. Specifically, psychiatric, neurologic, and behavioral, including substance abuse, criminal, or antisocial, problems are explored. The family history is diagrammed in the standard pedigree format. The social history includes background data such as place of birth, education (how much, what field of study, and where), occupations, hobbies, and substance use history. *In addition to being diagnostically useful, the ability of the patient to provide this information is considered an indication of the status of remote memory. As such, this report is in theory an important piece of the puzzle, or one of the medical facts, leading to diagnosis.*

The resident MD will then perform a neurological exam that includes the following items: general appearance and behavior, mental status (apraxia), facial expression or appearance, cranial nerves (vision/ hearing), motor skills (bulk and muscle appearance, tone, pronator drift, and strength), coordination, reflexes, stance (posture, balance), gait, and sensory ability. In an attempt at differential diagnosis, precautions are taken to rule out movement disorders. A general behavioral assessment is also conducted at this time.

The list of things to be covered is standardized and the majority of the thirty observations I made of the H&P were indistinguishable between physicians. Most potential patients tended to be calm during this experience as it is a familiar and routine examination like so many others they have undergone in their lives. Some people, however, do become upset when discussing their experiences of memory loss. From start to finish, this process takes approximately one hour.

When completed, the resident leaves the patient in the room to wait for the neuropsychologist. Unless there is a delay in a previous neuropsych (NP) exam, the neuropsychologist tends to come into the room shortly after the resident departs. The resident MD then dictates the findings, which will be included in the report sent to the referring physician.

Neuropsych

The neuropsychologist introduces him- or more often herself and explains briefly that s/he is there to administer some tests of the person's cognition. Often, the neuropsychologist states that some exercises will be more difficult than others and encourages the person being examined to simply do the best he can or tells her there is no right or wrong. In general, *there is little room for small talk and the clinician is very professional and formulaic in presentation. It is very standardized and gives off a strong impression of research objectivity.*

The main domains tested during this process include: global cognition, orientation, and working memory; semantic, episodic, visual and verbal memory; language and episodic functioning; visuospatial skill; praxis; abstract reasoning/problem solving; and a psychiatric depression screen.

- The tests begin with the administration of the *Folstein, Folstein and McHugh (1975) mini-mental state examination* (MMSE), which is a thirty-item survey including the year, season, month, day of month, day of the week; the name of the place where the test is being conducted, the floor of the building they are on; what city, county, and state they are in; the recall of three items (ball, flag, and tree); the spelling both forward and backward of the word WORLD; a delayed recall of the three items above; the naming of two items pointed to (watch and pencil); repetition of the following phrase: "No ifs, ands, or buts"; following a three-step command ("Listen carefully. I am going to give you a piece of paper. Take the paper in your right hand, fold it in half, and put it on the floor"); following a stimulus command (handed a piece of paper that says "Close your eyes," in which patient is told "Read the words on this page, then do what it says"); writing a complete sentence; and copying intersecting polygons from another piece of paper.
- The *California Verbal Language Test* (CVLT-MS), adapted by the lead

neuropsychologist at the Brain Clinic, involves reading a list of nine words, which can be grouped into three categories, and having the patients repeat as many as they can recall. The test administrator records responses verbatim. This is repeated four times and then a "thirty-second distractor interval" is introduced by asking the person to count backward from a hundred. Typically, the subject is told to stop once s/he has reached seventy-nine, unless s/he had considerable trouble, in which case s/he might have been stopped earlier. Then the patient is asked to recall the nine items from the CVLT list again. The number of intrusions, or words not present on the list, is also recorded as well as the time of day. After ten minutes, the subject is again asked to recall the list after completing other exercises. Next, the cued recall involves the neuropsychologist reading a longer list of words and having the patient say whether or not it was on the original list. Lastly, five minutes after the "yes/no recognition," the person is given a "forced choice recognition" where s/he is given an either/or situation and must choose which of the two words was on the original list.

- *Modified trails* is a timed test which involves drawing lines in numerical order between circled numbers and days of the week on a page (i.e., connecting the dots). The test administrator demonstrates the process drawing from number one to Sunday, to number two, to Monday and then asks the patient to begin. S/he is instructed to "Draw the lines as quickly as you can." The subject is corrected if a mistake is made and directions are repeated if necessary. The total time is recorded (with a cut-off time of 120 seconds), as are the number of correct lines and number of sequencing errors.

- *Design Fluency* is a timed test where the patient is given a page of paper filled with small boxes each with five dots inside. Patients are asked to "Use only four straight lines to connect the dots. Each line must be connected with another line and a dot." "Also," s/he is told, "you don't have to use all the dots and it's okay for the lines to intersect. In each of these squares, make a different design by connecting the dots with four straight lines." This test begins with a miniature sample page, on which the tester demonstrates. After the sample, the administrator repeats: "Now draw as many different designs as you can until I say stop. Remember to use only four straight lines to connect the dots. Work as quickly as you can and make every design different." The number of correct designs (e.g., different and with four straight lines) are recorded, as are the number of repeated designs, rule violations, and repeated rule violations.

- The patient is next handed a piece of paper with a design on the top and is told to copy it below. After drawing this design, the tester says, "Now remember this design, because I'll ask you to draw it again later," and takes it away. The time of day is recorded and there are seventeen possible points for this, including two points for six different details and a bonus point if all six of these tasks were completed perfectly.

- *Calculations* then begin, with the tester pointing to a paper containing the following problem: 214 x 35. The tester says, "Please solve this arithmetic problem." If the subject gets this correct, the remaining problems are skipped. If incorrect, the patient is asked to solve the remaining (more basic) problems, including addition and subtraction. The number of correct responses out of five is recorded.

- *Alternating m and n* involves writing, in cursive, the letters m and n over and over again across a page. The tester first demonstrates the task and then asks the subject to do the same. The goal is to discover "perseverative errors," whereby the patient has lost track of the pattern or used micrographic writing, where the writing gets much smaller or slants considerably in any direction.

- *Delayed Verbal Memory* involves the delayed recall and recognition conditions of the CVLT-MS. If the person has significant difficulty with the recognition portion of the test, the forced choice paradigm (outlined above) is then administered.

- *Comprehension 1* includes the following list of commands: 1a. "Make a fist," 2a. "Point to the ceiling, then to the floor," 3a. "Before touching your chin, point to your eye," 4a. The tester places a piece of paper on the table and says, "Under the paper, put your hand."

- *Echopraxia* is examined by the tester pointing to his or her nose and saying, "Point to your ear" and extending a hand (as if to shake hands) and saying, "Point to the lights."

- *Comprehension 2* includes the following list of questions: 1b. "A lion and a tiger were fighting. If the lion was killed by the tiger, which animal is dead?" 2b. "Do you put your socks on before your shoes?" 3b. "Do two pounds of flour weigh less than one pound?"

- *Repetition* includes the following three items: "Down to earth," "Pry the tin lid off," and "No ifs, ands or buts" (which is not given but used from the MMSE response).

- *Working Memory* includes the tester saying some numbers and asking the patient to repeat them backward. It begins with two-digit numbers and goes up to six-digit spans and there are two sets of these. The total backward span is recorded as the furthest number of digits the patient got twice.
- *Verbal fluency* involves the tester picking one letter of the alphabet and asking the subject to recite as many words as s/he can think of that begin with that letter. Instructions disqualify any names of people or places and the same words with different conjugations. The letter used is "D" and all responses are recorded for 60 seconds. If a patient pauses for 10–15 seconds, the tester asks what other words they can think of that begin with "D" and records these. The responses are recorded in 15-second intervals from 0"–15", 16"–30", 31"–45", and 46"–60". The number of correct D words, repetition of D words, and the number of rule violations are all recorded.

Next the subject is asked to name all the animals s/he can think of, beginning with any letter. And the same intervals are used to record the same information regarding number, repetitions, and rule violations.

- *Visual Memory* includes asking the patient to again draw the figure s/he had copied earlier. The intention is for there to be approximately ten minutes between these drawings. The score is recorded in the same manner as it was the first time. Then the subject is presented with four figures and asked to identify which of them was the one that was originally copied.
- *Conversational Speech* is rated on a scale of 0 (impaired) to 4 (normal) for the following categories: melodic line, phrase length, grammatical form, paraphasic errors, word finding, and comprehension. These are all based on the tester's impression or clinical judgment.
- *Facial Recognition Test* includes a book of faces where the patient is asked to match a specific face with a row of three faces. This is repeated six times.
- *Confrontation Naming* utilizes the Boston Naming Test (BNT) to elicit the name for a given drawing. The drawings include: bed, flower, helicopter, mushroom, camel, seahorse, globe, harmonica, igloo, knocker, pyramid, funnel, asparagus, yoke, and trellis. The appropriate probes are given if

the person cannot recall or does so incorrectly. The first hint, *the stimulus cue*, describes the item (helicopter: "it is used for air travel") or asks a question (mushroom: "Is it a fruit?") and the second, *the phonemic cue*, tells the patient: "It begins with the sound . . ."

- *Abstraction* involves first noting how two given words are alike. "For example, if I said guitar and piano, you could say they were both musical instruments." The given analogies are: dog and lion; table and chair; and anger and joy. Next, the metaphor "That's a loud tie" is read aloud and the patient is asked to interpret it. Lastly, the following three proverbs are read aloud and the patient is asked to interpret each of them: "An old ox plows a straight row," "Shallow brooks are noisy," and "A beard well-lathered is half shaven."

- *Facial Affect Matching* includes a stimulus page with one face on the top and five faces below and the subject is asked to "Indicate which of the five faces shows the same emotion as the face on the top." The emotions include: happiness, surprise, disgust, neutrality, anger, fear, and sadness.

- *Cube* entails copying a cube from a three-dimensional drawing.

- *Praxis* tests the patient's ability to carry out given movements using a specified hand. The buccofacial realm is measured with the command "Show me how you": "Cough" and "Blow out a match." The "intransitive limb" is examined through the command salute. The "transitive limb" is tested with the command "Show me how you": "Brush your teeth" (right hand), "Use a hammer" (left hand), "Saw wood" (left hand), and "Comb your hair" (right hand).

- *Stroop* includes a page of paper with the words red, blue, and green written all over the page in different colors than that which the written word represents (for example, blue is written in red ink). The instructions are: "I want you to tell me the color of ink these words are printed in. Don't read the words." The tester presents the stimulus page and demonstrates the first one and then says, "Begin here and say the color the letters are printed in as quickly as you can without skipping any or making mistakes." The subject continues this task for sixty seconds and the number of correct responses and the "stimulus-bound errors" are recorded.

- *Number Location* involves a sheet of paper with a box that has many numbers circled on it. The patient is then given a blank sheet of paper with a dot on it and asked to identify the number that matches the position of the dot on the paper next to it. This is done ten times.

- *Psychiatric Screening* includes a thirty-item Geriatric Depression Scale (GDS), which is self-administered after all the NP testing has been completed.

This process takes approximately one hour from start to finish.

The neuropsychologist then fills out her "Impressions" of the patient:

1) *The Bedside Screen Error Codes* include overall screen data status: good for research or not for research; factors affecting data: none, data are valid; speech difficulties; visual impairment; hearing impairment; motor difficulties; minimal education; English-as-a-second-language (ESL); lack of effort; or other.

2) A checklist describing the subject is completed, including: "interrupts, refuses to tolerate interruption, ignores professional boundaries, ignores personal boundaries, tests interviewer, makes personal comments, makes requests of interviewer, tends to be tangential, fills in dead space, exhibits unusual calmness or ease, became frustrated with argument avoidance, perseverates, expresses ethical superiority, expresses narcissism, incorporates interviewer into personal stories, seeks alliance with interviewer, displays showmanship, or is angry." These items are ranked on a five-point likert scale from "not at all" to "perfectly."

RN Interview

While the patient undergoes the NP testing, the nurse talks with any available family member(s) or friend(s), called the informant(s), about functional status (how well the patient is doing, if s/he is aware of his or her impairments (e.g., has insight), and so on). The nurse explores the living arrangements the family presently has, the psychosocial stressors, and utilization of community resources.

- The *Neuropsychiatric Inventory* (NPI) is administered, which covers the family's impressions regarding presence and severity of specific behavioral problems, including: "delusions, hallucination, agitation, depression, anxiety, euphoria, apathy, disinhibition, irritability, aberrant motor behavior, night-time behavior, and eating habits."

- The *Clinical Dementia Rating* (CDR) Scale is also administered. This is an instrument used in staging the severity of dementia and rates impairment in six cognitive categories from the family's perspective: memory, orientation, judgment and problem solving, community affairs, home and hobbies, and personal care, each on a five-point scale.

This component takes roughly one hour.

Team Disposition Meeting

After the H&P and the NP/RN interviews have all been conducted, the patient and family are typically given a two-hour lunch break, at which point the team disposition conference takes place. On the weekly intake of new patients, there are generally two teams comprised of a resident MD, a neuropsychologist, and a nurse practitioner who had seen (caregiver) informants from each family. They meet with one of four attending neurologists. In all, there were seven to ten people present per meeting (including myself). The format was standardized as such: the resident MD recalls the presenting symptom(s) and duration, past history, family history, and findings of the neurological and physical examinations. Based on this information, the attending neurologist typically asks each team member to guess an MMSE score.

Next, the neuropsychologist reveals the results of the battery of neuropsych tests outlined above, highlighting areas of difficulty and systematically noting the scores, standard deviations, and pictures or other anecdotal information where relevant. It is not uncommon for either (or both) the resident or NP to speculate on the accuracy of the patient's reporting, typically in terms of whether he or she is a "good/bad historian."

The attending neurologist typically asks the resident MD what s/he thinks is going on and often asks the neuropsychologist specifics about certain tests or if s/he thinks there were any biases unaccounted for in the testing environment. On several occasions, the attending neurologist drew various pictures of the brain on the marker board in the room or asked others to do so if it was their area of expertise. Almost daily, discussions centered on recent findings or empirical suggestions concerning the specifics of the cases being discussed. Often, the general distinctions between conditions and referrals were made to recent literature discussed in their weekly journal club. Without question, the team disposition meetings were a learning environment where the attending neurologist taught—primarily, but certainly not exclusively— the resident MD. In fact, the attending neurologist would often ascertain that everyone (including others on rotation or observers like myself) understood any vague terminology used. In the event that there was anyone new (or with a different paradigm, such as myself) observing, the attending neurologist regularly asked for the person's impression of the situation. Although this meeting was run primarily as a teaching session, it was an open conversation and exchange between the different people present.

There were occasionally divergent opinions regarding etiology, frequently taking the form of neuropsychology on one side and neurology on the other. Disparities regarding the magnitude of impairment (e.g., whether to classify a person as AD/MCI/nothing) were also somewhat customary. *Although this process prevented the outcome from feeling top-down, in most instances the attending neurologist made the ultimate decision unilaterally.* Discussion of follow-up treatment (such as additional labs or tests, medications, and when to return) and research eligibility was standard practice. When MRI scans were available, they would all be displayed on the screen by the resident MD; everyone would stand around while the attending neurologist (and often the resident) would point out the areas of "gray" and "white matter" present on the brain images, the latter of which represent the amyloid plaques characteristic of Alzheimer's. These meetings would cover two cases and often lasted close to three hours. There was always someone, typically the RN, noting the time and reminding the attending neurologist that the family was waiting for him/her.

Diagnosis Delivery

Typically, the nurse or the neuropsych clinician would go to the waiting room and escort the family back to the exam room for the diagnosis. The attending neurologist would either introduce himself or one of the clinicians would introduce him. The diagnosis was rendered in the same small, narrow office where the H&P and NP were conducted and often up to five people in addition to the family and/or patient were present, including the resident MD, the attending neurologist, the neuropsych administrator, and two to three student observers (such as myself, but more commonly medical students). Although the attending neurologist would ask permission for so many people to be in the room, no one refused during my observation and it did not seem a person really could refuse such observation even if it bothered him/her. The attending MD would sit at the desk next to the chairs where the family sat. The observers sat on the exam table and/or leaned against the wall.

The attending neurologist began by telling the family that we had just had a team meeting to go over all the test results and that those findings would now be reported. The most experienced attending neurologists I observed typically asked the patient to tell them what the main problem was rather than assuming they knew it and used a compassionate, respectful tone.

At this point, any pending questions from the team disposition meeting were explored. This took only a few minutes and might involve corroboration from the family, if present. Then the attending neurologist would conduct an abbreviated physical exam to test for any abnormalities that may not have been detected or to verify ones that were. This would typically involve hand-eye coordination, reflexes, vision, and occasionally gait. Within five to ten minutes of arriving, the attending neurologist would begin discussing the findings of the tests, mainly the neuropsych exam and periodically the MRIs.

There was significant variation between the attending neurologists in delivering diagnoses. Although most began with encouraging information or findings, some would start with the clinical name itself, saying, "We think what is going on is Alzheimer's," or "It looks like dementia." In other cases, they never used any label or disease name at all, even in the case of Alzheimer's. A few doctors were very clinical and technical in their presentation of the results, whereas others were basic and easy to understand. Some welcomed questions, while others did not. Some spoke with ease and compassion, allowing each diagnosis of the same condition to fit the patient being diagnosed, and others were far less adept at the task. Some were incredibly kind and reassuring, often touching the patient's knee, while others were abrasive and preoccupied. Many would stress the importance of exercise and nutrition.[4]

The attending neurologist then went over the recommended medications, including vitamin E, and how to take them. Most neurologists would ask if there were any additional questions. After answering any questions, the MD would then tell the patient that a report would be sent to the referring physician. In many cases, the patient would be returning to the clinic for a one- to three-month follow-up. If not, the attending neurologist might never see the patient again. Within twenty to thirty minutes the diagnosis was delivered, signaling the end of a long day, and the family was on their way. The room would clear out and the nurse would come in to get their consent for future research studies, including using their demographic information in the clinic's patient database, and would give them a packet of information concerning community resources they might want to avail themselves of, after which they were free to leave. They would possibly have no further contact with the clinic (until three months later, if at all).

In total, for patients most days began at 9.30–9.45 a.m. and ended around 3–4 p.m.

II. The Health Center

The Health Center[5] is a few miles away from the main campus of a northern California research university, nestled far back behind the many medical buildings within the self-contained Veterans Administration Hospital. The ARCC is on the first floor of an old institutional brick building that feels like a public school or clinical setting. As soon as you walk into the building, there are florescent pink signs saying "University Name/VA Health Center," with arrows pointing in the direction of the office. The same signs may be seen on either side of the door entering the reception area for the clinic. The hallway leading to the reception area is devoid of people and lined with closed office doors. Further down the same hall are the offices of the three to four clinicians who see patients; the other arm of the hall is comprised of researchers, a data manager, and administrative staff. As one enters the door, there is a reception desk (though I rarely saw anyone sitting at it) to greet people.

There are six small offices and two other rooms adjacent to the reception area. In this part of the clinic, there are three clinical research coordinators (also called research assistants, one of whom is responsible for doing in-take with all new patients and another who conducts phone screenings of people seeking services). They are all eager twenty-something women with open office doors. Two of the offices are typically empty and one administrative office is occupied. The main reception area also houses a room with supplies, a copier, and mailboxes, which is directly across from the reception desk. At the other end of the Health Center's hallway is a small room where a neurological exam is sometimes conducted. It is the only room in the entire facility that is set up like a doctor's office or examination room. It has the exam table, desk, and miscellaneous items. There is no sink nearby. I only observed patients being brought in there on two occasions.

The entryway to the reception area has two signs that read: "Quiet please, testing area" and "Please ring bell for assistance." When someone enters the center, the coordinators greet the person, offer him/her coffee, and escort him/her to the room that says, "Patient Waiting Room" above the door. This room seats ten to fifteen people comfortably and is filled with reading materials regarding research and general information on Alzheimer's disease. There is also a small buffet that holds coffee, cream, water, and sometimes snacks. It does not feel like a typical doctor's office waiting room. The coordinator (or receptionist) will then call the designated clinician to inform her that the patient has arrived. The clinician will then typically come to greet the patient and any friends or family present in the waiting room and will direct them back to her office (in my observations, all the clinicians were female).

The clinician's offices vary drastically from the ones in the reception area. They are spacious with quality desks and chairs and bookshelves filled with reference materials. There were three clinicians seeing clients during the time I was observing: the codirector and head clinician, who was a compassionate middle-aged Caucasian woman, and held a M.S. and R.N.C.S.; the staff psychiatrist was a somewhat severe Indian woman in her forties; and a general clinician, a professional, soft-spoken Asian woman also in her forties, who earned her doctorate in Clinical Psychology with a M.S.G. and an M.S.W. There were also two male psychiatrists, one of whom was the director, who I only observed during the weekly team conferences.

Telephone Screen

When calling to schedule an appointment, one of the RAs conducts a phone interview with the individual (typically the care partner/informant but occasionally the person with memory loss). This interview collects background data, such as name and contact information for patient, primary caregiver, and caller as well as details regarding referral source, affiliation, and reason for the appointment. The patient and primary caregiver demographics, veteran status, medical history, and history of complaints are collected at this time. Information regarding a description and onset of symptoms and activities of daily living (ADLs) are specifically probed.

A Typical Day at the Health Center

The sixteen potential patients that I observed arrived shortly before 8 a.m.

8–8:30 a.m.: The first thirty minutes are spent with the in-take Research Assistant (RA) getting consent and background demographic data from both the "informant" and the patient.

The following questions are recorded:

I. Procedural Data
   - A randomized ARCC code/patient ID number
   - Date of first clinic visit
II. Patient Demographic Data
   - Date of birth
   - Zip code of principal place of residence
   - Gender
   - Military status, if applicable
   - Race/ethnicity
     A. Spanish/Hispanic/Latino origin? If yes, specify. If no, what is your race?
   - Current marital status
   - Living arrangement
   - Years of school attended

- Health care coverage
- Reimbursement mechanism for primary health coverage
- Primary payment mechanism for ARCC evaluation

III. Caregiver Data

- patient's primary informal caregiver

Next, the RA goes over the form of consent to participate in research—page by page—with the patient and loved one, if present. In some cases, the patient is given the form to read. Then the RA does an "Evaluation of Decision-Making Capacity for Consent to Act as a Research Subject" checklist to assure that the patient is capable of consenting. This form contains seven questions confirming that the patient understood what the RA had just read. If a yes/no question is not answered correctly, a cue is used that reminds the person of something and then the question is asked again.[6] The RA then answers the following questions on the form: Is the patient alert and able to communicate with the examiner? Does the patient demonstrate adequate decision-making capacity? Finally, the authorization to release medical records or health information form is filled out and signed by the patient, including where results from the evaluation should be sent.

8:30 a.m.: The RA takes the patient to pick up the results of CT/blood work that were conducted prior to coming in for an appointment. If they were not already conducted, the CT scan and blood work are done at this point.

9 a.m.: The informant(s), if present, remains in the waiting room until the clinician brings him/her to her office, where the reason for coming to the clinic is discussed and background information is garnered. The room is an office where the clinician sits behind a large desk with the informant on the other side. The conversation begins with the clinician asking the informant to talk about what has been going on with the patient. After listening to the informant's narrative, the clinician begins asking specific questions about past medical, surgical, and psychiatric history, whether any other conditions are being treated, and current medications.

9:30 a.m.: After returning from the CT/blood work, the same clinician talks with the patient in her office. The clinician begins by asking what has brought the person into the clinic. Depending on perceived level of insight, or acceptance regarding impairment, the patient will discuss experiences of memory loss along a continuum from having no problems to giving specific details and examples of what s/he has noticed. The same information on past medical, surgical, and psychiatric history, other conditions, and current medications is then collected from the patient.

Next, the following tests are administered: *Geriatric Depression Scale* a seventeen-item test asking questions about mood (for example, "Do you feel most people are better off than you?" or "Do you feel worthless?"), *Mini-mental state examination (MMSE)* a thirty-point scale where a lower number signifies more significant cognitive impairment. This test includes questions about the current president of the United States, day of the week, city they are presently in, home address, season, etc. The patient is then asked:

- To repeat the following words: "apple, table, penny."
- To spell the word "world" forward and backward.
- To recall the 3 previous words repeated above.
- To count backward from 100 in increments of 7. They are stopped once (if) they consecutively do so to approximately 65.
- To count down from 20.
- To identify two objects which are pointed to by the administrator: "pencil and watch."
- To repeat the phrase: "No ifs, ands, or buts."
- To follow a three-step command: "Take the paper in your right hand, fold it in half, and leave it on the desk."
- To "read this piece of paper and do what it says" ("Close your eyes").
- To write a full sentence.
- To copy a paper with two intersecting pentagons.

In some cases, the clinician will conduct the neuropsych examination herself (it was not clear to me when/why this was the case but presumably time and training were factors). In the event that the clinician administers the NP, the same tests listed below are utilized and the RA will simply schedule a follow-up with the patient after the NP battery is completed.

10–10:30 a.m.: After talking with the clinician, the patient is escorted back to the waiting room. The RA then brings the patient into her office, while the informant remains in the waiting room. The patient is given the Neuropsych testing by the in-take RA from the morning. This component takes up to an hour and involves the following:

- *Logical Memory I*: Part A involves the test administrator reading a short story (86 words), broken into 25 possible points by themes, and having the patient recall as many details as possible immediately following the story. The RA will circle details as the patient recalls them. Clock time is recorded.

Part B involves a second story with different details but the same scoring and time allotted. The sum of both stories is recorded, out of a possible 50 points. The patient is told at this point to remember this story, as questions will be asked about it later.

- *Animal Fluency Category Task* involves naming as many different animals as possible within a 60 second time period. All responses are recorded, including repeats and non-animals.
- *Trail Making A* involves connecting the dots between numbers that are circled. A sample, beginning with 1 and ending with 8, is performed by the RA and then a new sheet of paper ranging from 1 to 25 is given for the subject to complete.
- *Trail Making B* includes alternating between circled numbers and letters. A sample beginning with 1 and ending with D is performed by the RA and then another sheet ranging from 1-A to L-13 is administered.
- *Boston Naming Test* includes naming the following sketched pictures: bed, tree, pencil, house, whistle, scissors, comb, flower, saw, toothbrush, helicopter, broom, octopus, mushroom, hanger, wheelchair, camel, mask, pretzel, bench, racquet, snail, volcano, seahorse, dart, canoe, globe, wreath, beaver, harmonica, rhinoceros, acorn, igloo, stilts, dominoes, cactus, escalator, harp, hammock, knocker, pelican, stethoscope, pyra-

mid, muzzle, unicorn, funnel, accordion, noose, asparagus, compass, latch, tripod, scroll, tongs, sphinx, yoke, trellis, palette, protractor, and abacus.

If a person has difficulty naming an object, a "stimulus cue" will be given (for example, "It's a utensil" or "It measures angles."). If a person still cannot name an item, a "phonemic" cue is given (for example, [sphinx] "It starts with the sounds *sphy* . . ." or [mushroom] "*ma* . . ."). The number of objects named are recorded as "correct without cue," "latency secs," "in/correct with stimulus cue," and "in/correct with phonemic cue."

- *Block Design* involves assembling blocks with red, white, or combined red and white sides into the given design shown to the patient on a picture that remains in front to him/her. The tester demonstrates with a simple design to be sure the patient understands the directions. The designs get incrementally more complex. This test is timed and scored according to how much time it takes to complete the task. There are a total of nine designs. After three consecutive failures, the test is discontinued.
- *Logical Memory II* involves asking the subject to recall as many details as possible about each of the two stories read (approximately 30 minutes) earlier. Again the patient is scored 25 points per story, for a total of 50 possible points.

There is considerable variation in this process. If the clinician is a psychiatrist (one out of three I observed), then the clinician also conducts a gross neurological exam. If not, this part happens in significantly abbreviated form or not at all:

- Patients are told to hold their hands out in front of them with their fingers apart.
- The cranial nerve is tested: follow without moving your head, ringing a bell, snapping in their ears, shoulders up, tongue up, say "ah," smile.
- Motor skills are tested: reflexes, rigidity (wrist and elbow), tremors.
- Sensation: "Close your eyes and tell me when I touch you," as clinician touches various parts of the patient's face, arms, and legs. Then a point touch (prick) test is conducted. Position sense involves the patient closing his/her eyes and telling the clinician when s/he feels her touching his/her

fingers and toes. Vibration sense uses the vibrating wand and touches the person.

- Cerabellar: involves alternating the turning of one hand in the palm of the other over and over, touching the clinician's finger and then one's nose (including with one's eyes closed), and touching one's heel to one's shin and moving it all the way down the leg.
- Gait: involves observing the patient walk, including heel to toe and pushing the patient slightly while his/her eyes are closed to test balance.

If the clinician does not perform a neurological exam, she might or might not conduct the NP herself (1 of 3). If the clinician is an experienced staff member (codirector), she might do an extremely abbreviated version of the neurological exam (gait, tremors, coordination) but not conduct the NP herself (1 of 3). Further, the sequencing of the tests or the actual items of a given measure are not followed in a standardized manner. As a result, this was often difficult for me to follow. Also, the psychologist utilized a digital timer which beeped for the timed tests whereas the other two test administrators used their watches, which did not make a noise.

Immediately following the testing, the RA schedules an appointment for the "family conference meeting" to give the results. The RA tells them that the team needs to meet for a consensus diagnosis and to discuss any recommendations if appropriate. This appointment is typically made within two to three weeks. At this point, the patient is dismissed and the RA bids farewell to both the subject and the informant.

Most appointments are over by 11 a.m., making for no longer than three hours at the Center.

Consensus Conference

The entire staff, including research assistants, the lead neuropsychiatrist, the head nurse, the one neurologist, and any other neuropsychiatrists, assembled weekly for what they called their consensus conference. They would meet in a small conference room that felt like a classroom and discuss the previous week's patients. The primary staff member who had administered the battery of tests would read a summary report she had written (which she had left in all participants' mail boxes prior to the meeting) and declare the diagnosis she was preparing to inform the family at the family conference. There was little to no discussion, including between the lead practitioner and the RA who had consented, collected background demographic data, and administered the basic scales. I never observed any physical images (they often didn't even have access to the CT scan results at this point) and the scans were rarely even mentioned. This was not a teaching environment per se, and felt far more like a business meeting than a dialogue. I did not witness any dispute (or even discussion per se) over the diagnosis determined by the lead clinician. Each patient/client would be presented within roughly five minutes. The entire weekly session tended to last twenty-five to thirty minutes, depending on how many people were seen that week.

Diagnostic Disclosure: Family Conference

The family conference was, as mentioned, scheduled two to three weeks following the evaluation with the intention of gathering as many interested parties as possible, including family members, friends, and neighbors. While this was the intended aim of the meeting, I only observed a few family members (typically adult children) being called in for the meeting. More often, the spouse would be the only person present with the client.

As the prologue shows, this interaction, despite the intended purpose and framing of the event, was very formulaic and scripted. There was again no dialogue per se between the client and the clinician. The clinician would cover the extensive list of topics below essentially verbatim:

Topic

---

1 Contact the Alzheimer's Association [with contact information listed]

2 Legal/Financial Issues: Obtain Durable Power of Attorney for Finances and for Health Care. Contact the Family Caregiver Alliance [with contact information listed]

3 Attend Support Groups

4 Medical Needs: Obtain primary care physician or continue with primary care physician. Health Center/VA Alzheimer's Disease Research Center of California will send our evaluation to your physician(s), with signed consent from you

5 Medications: Caregiver should be responsible for monitoring medications. Contact physician regarding medications.

6 Obtain Medic-Alert or other ID bracelet

Topic

7 Home Safety: Obtain home assessment. Home safety precautions such as installing rails, shower chair, getting home help, etc. Can patient dial 911 on the phone? Can patient be left home alone?

8 Driving Safety: Patient should not drive until retested by DMV

9 Seek Day Care/Respite Care.

10 Seek Long Term Care: In-home care, Board and Care Facility, Skilled Nursing Facility, or Other.

In addition, the clinician would talk about ongoing research studies offered at the center. There was a keen sense that an ongoing relationship was being established and there was far less emphasis on the medical label itself. Any discussion of medications ended with a recommendation that they speak with their primary care physician about the matter.

While there was in theory far more focus on addressing the psychosocial needs of clients, in practice it felt rehearsed and not tailored to the person in question. The entire interaction typically lasted around fifteen minutes and there was little deviation from the script or tailoring of the interaction. The clinician would then tell the patient to schedule a one-month follow-up appointment with the research assistant.

NOTES

PROLOGUE

1 All parentheticals are my own additions for purposes of clarification.

CHAPTER 1. THE MEANING OF MEMORY LOSS

1 Beach 1987; Dillmann 1990; Forbes and Hirdes 1993; Gubrium 1986; Lock 2013; Ming and Fernandez 2001; Swane 1993.

2 Most notably, Drs. John Hardy and John Mayer, who at the 2011 "Models of Dementia: The Good, the Bad and the Future" meeting were given the opportunity to openly debate the proposal "the amyloid cascade has misled the pharmaceutical industry." But countless critics and bench scientists alike have noted the lack of efficacious medications that currently exist for AD, at any stage. Of course, renowned neurologist Peter Whitehouse is another leading opponent of the Amyloid Cascade Hypothesis, despite being in the lab that discovered the acetyl-choline theory upon which four of the five medications are based. Dr. John Morris also makes similar claims. Neurologists Mark Smith, Rudolph Tanzi, and public health experts Carol Brayne and Daniel Davis have also made important contributions to the debate.

3 Robertson 1990.

4 The diagnostic guidelines released in 2011 will be explicitly discussed in the following chapter.

5 Fox 1989; Fox 2000.

6 Alzheimer's Association 2012, 131.

7 Alzheimer's Disease International 2015.

8 Lock 2013, 12.

9 Norton, Matthews, and Brayne 2013, 4.

10 Lobo et al. 2007; Manton, Gu, and Ukraintseva 2005; Schrijvers et al. 2012.

11 Cummings et al. 1998.

12 Alzheimer's Association 2014b; Hebert et al. 2013.

13 Conrad 2007.

14 Foucault 1988.

15 Armstrong 1995.

16 I term them "potential patients" for this reason.

17 Casper and Berg 1995.

18 Alzheimer's Association 2008.

19 When I use the term AD, I am referring to the medical definition of a progressive, degenerative disease, manifesting primarily in memory loss, which includes functional impairment in daily living (chapter 2 will address this fully). The individuals who were part of this study were all deemed to be in the "early stages" by medical professionals; that is, they had minor memory loss.

20 Until 2011, MCI was believed to be simply a potential precursor of Alzheimer's disease.

21 Lock 2013, 7.

22 Cf., Beard and Neary 2012; Post 1995, 2000; Lock 2013; Whitehouse and Deal 1995; Whitehouse and Gaines 2006; Whitehouse and George 2008; Whitehouse and Moody 2006.

23 To a lesser extent, clinicians also have a good deal of flexibility as to when and if they diagnose, or at least use the words "Alzheimer's disease" with their patients.

24 Milne et al. 2000.

25 Keady and Gilliard 2002.

26 Wilcock, Bucks, and Rockwood 1999.

27 Wright and Lindesay 1995.

28 In this study, I am using the Association as a proxy for the larger social movement.

29 My use of the term MCI interchangeably with AD is not to imply that important qualitative differences between the experiences of being diagnosed with Alzheimer's and mild cognitive impairment do not exist. Rather, for the purposes of understanding personal experiences of early diagnoses, data from individuals diagnosed with AD and MCI will be presented simultaneously. Although I did not find significant differences in terms of subjective experiences of AD/MCI, noteworthy differences may well exist in larger, more representative samples of people diagnosed with MCI.

30 For more details on the study methods and design, see Appendix A.

31 National Institute of Health 2015.

32 For more details on the study sites, see Appendix B.

CHAPTER 2. HISTORY AND TECHNOSCIENCE

1 Mauer, Volk, and Garbaldo 2000.

2 Moller and Graeber 2000.

3 Mauer, Volk, and Garbaldo 2000.

4 George et al. 2012.

5 Although it is unclear when exactly this divide came to be labeled as such, it was common by 1991 (Tanzi and Parson 2000). The term "Baptist" comes from beta-amyloid protein.

6 Grundman 2001, 173.

7 Le Couteur et al. 2013.

8 Oxman and Baynes 1994, 6.

9 Beach 1987.

10 Haber 1984.
11 Fox 1989.
12 Berger and Luckmann 1966; Mattingly and Garro 2000.
13 Berrios 1990; Berrios 2003; Holden 1987.
14 Gubrium 1978.
15 Dillman 2000; George et al. 2012.
16 Beach 1987; Hoff 1991.
17 Holstein 1997.
18 Gellerstedt 1933.
19 Craik 1977; Poon 1985.
20 Kral 1962.
21 Haber 1984.
22 Blessed, Tomlinson, and Roth 1968.
23 Terry and Katzman 1983.
24 Armaducci, Rocca, and Schoenberg 1986; Constantinidis 1978; Newton 1948; Tomlinson, Blessed, and Roth 1970.
25 Cf., Beach 1987; Dillmann 1990; Forbes and Hirdes 1993; Fox 1989; Gubrium 1986; Swane 1993; Von Dras and Blumenthal 1992.
26 Beach 1987; Holstein 1997.
27 Fox 1989; Fox 2000; Lyman 1993.
28 Dillman 2000.
29 Le Couteur et al. 2013.
30 Emery and Oxman 1994; Gottfries et al. 1990.
31 Dillman 1990; Dillman 2000; Fox 1989; Fox 2000; Lock 2013; Whitehouse and George 2008.
32 Blennow, Wallin, and Gottfries 1994.
33 Berrios 1990.
34 Post 2000, 254.
35 Estes and Binney 1989; Kaufman, Shim, and Russ 2004; Lyman 1989.
36 Holstein 1997, 82.
37 Lock, Young, and Cambrosio 2000.
38 Gubrium 1986.
39 Linked to chromosome 14 and 19, respectively. Tanzi and Parson 2000.
40 Less than 2 percent of Alzheimer's cases afflict individuals who are under 65 years of age, according to Golomb et al. 2001. The Alzheimer's Association reports "up to 5% of cases" are younger/early-onset (2014f).
41 Tanzi and Parson 2000.
42 U.S. Congress, Office of Technology Assessment 1987.
43 Alzheimer's Association 2004.
44 Katzman 1976.
45 Barnes and Yaffe 2011; Farlow 2000.
46 Van Duijn 2004.
47 Arai 2014.

48 This is known as Hippocampal Sclerosis (HS); Nag et al. 2015.
49 Keage et al. 2014.
50 Josephs et al. 2015.
51 Uchino et al. 2015.
52 Elias et al. 2000.
53 Cf., American Psychiatric Association 1994; Blackford and La Rue 1989; Crook et al. 1986; Graham et al. 1997; Petersen et al. 1997; World Health Organization 1993 for further discussion.
54 Graham et al. 1997; and Petersen et al. 1997, respectively.
55 Golomb et al. 2001, vii; and Winblad et al. 2004, respectively.
56 Winblad et al. 2004.
57 Artero et al. 2006; Palmer, Fratiglioni, and Winblad 2003; Ritchie and Touchon 2000; Whitehouse and Moody 2006.
58 Corner and Bond 2006; Graham and Ritchie 2006; Ritchie and Touchon 2000.
59 There remains considerable scientific controversy over what, if anything, MCI is pathologically. While many clinicians treat it in practice as early-AD, this has never been empirically proven.
60 Le Couteur et al. 2013, 5125.
61 Elias et al. 2000; and Krasuki et al. 1998, respectively.
62 Dawe, Proctor, and Philpot 1992; and Grundman et al. 1996, respectively.
63 Elias et al. 2000; and Flicker, Ferris, and Reisberg 1991, respectively.
64 Daly et al. 2000; Wolf, Grunwald, and Ecke 1998; and Ritchie, Ledesert, and Touchon 2000, respectively.
65 Wolf, Grunwald, and Ecke 1998.
66 Ganguli et al. 2011; and Mitchell and Shiri-Feshki 2009, respectively.
67 Ganguli et al. 2011.
68 Mitchell and Shiri-Feshki 2009, 252.
69 Ibid.
70 Ibid., 263.
71 Galasko et al. 1994; Jellinger 1996.
72 Petersen 1994, 33.
73 Ritchie and Touchon 2000, 227.
74 Ritchie and Touchon 2000.
75 Albert et al. 2011; Reisberg et al. 2010; Sperling et al. 2011.
76 Reisberg et al. 2010.
77 Schulz 2001.
78 Lock 2013, 18.
79 See Beard and Neary 2012 for more details.
80 Lock 2013.
81 See Lock 2013 for a well-written and thoroughly researched overview of "The Alzheimer's Conundrum," which is beyond the scope of this book.
82 Conrad 2007.
83 Whitehouse and Moody 2006; Whitehouse and Gaines 2006.

84 Le Couteur et al. 2013.
85 Pres. Proclamation 6158; www.loc.gov/loc/brain/proclaim.html.
86 Ibid.
87 U.S. Library of Congress 2004.
88 Czerner 2001, 3–4.
89 Ibid.
90 Kliger 2000.
91 Ibid.; Latour and Woolgar 1986; Lock 2013.
92 Rose 2006; Rose 1998.
93 Dumit 2003.
94 Conrad and Schneider 1980; Merleau-Ponty 1964.
95 Dumit 2003.
96 Armstrong 1984; Arney and Bergen 1984.
97 Rabinow 1992; see also Chambré 2006; Epstein 1996; and Klawiter 1999.
98 Dumit 2003.
99 Oxman and Baynes 1994, 6.
100 Emery and Oxman 1994.
101 Oxman and Baynes 1994, 5.
102 Referred to as "ceiling" and "floor" effects, the sensitivity of these scales is questionable because individuals who are well-educated are often "off the charts" until
progression is quite severe and, conversely, those with lower education levels or
learning disabilities may have always appeared impaired. The bar is too low or too
high, respectively, to accurately measure decline.
103 Cf. Petersen 2004 for the variability among patients.
104 Ivnik et al. 1991; Smith and Ivnik 2003.
105 The debates regarding the validity and reliability of these tests, including differences in terms of gender, education, socioeconomic status, sociocultural ability,
ethnicity, and linguistics, are extensive. Allegedly there are both floor and ceiling
effects even when a "baseline" exists.
106 Activities of daily living, such as cooking, cleaning, bathing, and dressing, and
instrumental activities of daily living, including shopping, managing a checkbook,
and driving.
107 Tanzi and Parson 2000.
108 Niederehe and Oxman 1994; and Mandybur 1990, respectively.
109 Hauw, Duyckaerts, and Delaere 1991.
110 For an in-depth discussion of these areas, see Oxman and Baynes 1994. Additionally, MCI is explicitly addressed in Golomb et al. 2001.
111 Backman et al. 2004, 199.
112 Snowdon 2003; Swartz, Black, and Hyslop 1999.
113 Winblad et al. 2004.
114 Simons and Spiers 2003.
115 Backman et al. 2004.
116 Golomb et al. 2001.

117 Convit et al. 1993; Jack et al. 1997; Jack et al. 2011; Krasuki et al. 1998.
118 Golomb et al. 1993.
119 Wolf et al. 1998.
120 Krasuki et al. 1998.
121 Celsis, Agneil, and Cardebat 1997.
122 Ritchie and Touchon 2000.
123 McKelvey et al. 1999.
124 Golomb et al. 2001.
125 Winblad et al. 2004.
126 See Lock 2013 for a more detailed examination of this topic.
127 Alzheimer's Association 2014f; Golomb et al. 2001.
128 Winblad et al. 2004.
129 Petersen et al. 1995; Saunders et al. 1993.
130 Jonsson et al. 2013.
131 Winblad et al. 2004.
132 As Lock demonstrates, dementia incidence rates cap after about 90 years of age (2013, 17).
133 Tanzi and Parson 2000.
134 Grundman 2001.
135 Winblad et al. 2004, 245.
136 NMDA is N-methyl-D-aspartate. "Scientists have discovered that oxygen deprivation in the brain triggers an abnormal buildup of a signaling chemical called glutamate that kills neurons by overstimulating them. Drugs that block these proteins, called NMDA receptor blockers, can prevent glutamate from harming neurons" (Society for Neuroscience 2005). For more information, see http://web.sfn.org/content/Publications/BrainBriefings/nmda.html.
137 Alzheimer's Association 2014c.
138 Adlard et al. 2014; Alzheimer's Association 2014e; Bun et al. 2014; Gauthier and Schlaefke 2014; La Fata, Weber, and Mohajeri 2014; Marutle et al. 2013; Solfrizzi and Panza 2015.
139 Alzheimer's Association 2014e.
140 Lim et al. 2000.
141 Grundman 2001.
142 Dye et al. 2012; and Lau et al. 2014, respectively.
143 Khalil et al.2012.
144 Garcia and Juncos 2006; McGrowder et al. 2011.
145 Lock 2013.
146 Alzheimer's Association 2014b.
147 George et al. 2012, 1986.
148 Lock 2013, 65.
149 Hyman 1996; see also George et al. 2012, Hardy and Mayer 2011.
150 George et al. 2012.
151 Lock 2013, 232.

152 See Mitchell, Meader, and Pentzek 2011, in Le Couteur et al. 2013.

153 NIH 2015; Alzheimer's Association 2015.

154 Le Couteur et al 2013, 4.

CHAPTER 3. CONSTRUCTING FACTS IN CLINICAL PRACTICE

1 The new diagnostic criteria outlined in chapter 2 may well increase consensus among the memory-related disciplines, or perhaps even GPs and specialists and/ or countries, but this will remain unclear until it can be tested longitudinally in coming decades and it could easily have the opposite effect.

2 Le Couteur et al. 2013, 3.

3 Coombes 2009; Lindesay et al. 2002; Wright and Lindesay 1995.

4 Le Couteur et al. 2013.

5 What sociologists refer to as "institutional logics."

6 Cf., Emile Durkheim on "social facts." I borrow the following usage: "A social fact is any way of acting, whether fixed or not, capable of exerting over the individual an external constraint; or: which is general over the whole of a given society whilst having an existence of its own, independent of its individual manifestations" (1982, 59).

7 Arney and Bergen 1984; Gubrium 1986; Kliger 2000; Latour and Woolgar 1986.

8 Latour and Woolgar 1986, 37.

9 Moreira, May, and Bond 2009, 685.

10 May et al. 2004.

11 Keating and Cambrioso 2003.

12 A detailed description of these differences is outlined in Appendix B on the two study sites.

13 This was not what I expected to find. I thought surely different philosophical and disciplinary beliefs would generate unique experiences for people coming to the centers.

14 Davenport 2011; Holmes and Ponte 2011; Lutfey and McKinlay 2009.

15 Gillett 2004; Holmes and Ponte 2011; Timmermans and Angell 2001.

16 See also Wiener 2000.

17 Holmes and Ponte 2011.

18 Davenport 2011, 874.

19 Heimer 2001.

20 Holmes and Ponte 2011.

21 Lutfey and McKinlay 2009.

22 Holmes and Ponte 2011.

23 See also Davenport 2011; and Holmes and Ponte 2011.

24 Holmes and Ponte 2011, 263.

25 LB: Lewy-body dementia; PD: Parkinson's disease; FTD: Frontotemporal dementia.

26 VaD: Vascular dementia; CBD: Corticobasal degeneration; PSP: Progressive Supranuclear Palsy; MSA: multiple system atrophy.

27 Davenport 2011; Holmes and Ponte 2011.

28 The Director was the only male clinician I met and I only saw him during this meeting. I never observed him seeing patients or around the center when I was there.

29 Lock 2013.
30 Joyce 2008.
31 Dumit 2004.
32 Joyce 2008.
33 Davenport 2011, 873.
34 Keating and Cambrioso 2003.
35 Dumit 2006.
36 Moreira, May, and Bond 2009.
37 Brodaty, Griffin, and Hadzi-Pavlovic 1990; Holroyd, Turnbull, and Wolff 2002; Marzanski 2000; Vassilas and Donaldson 1998.
38 Carpenter and Dave 2004.
39 In the state of California, doctors were required by law to report people diagnosed with dementia to the Department of Motor Vehicles, who would then retest them to see if they were deemed fit to drive. A few respondents said that their licenses were just revoked via a mailed letter after being diagnosed.
40 See Appendix B.
41 Heimer 2001.
42 Estes and Binney 1989; Kaufman 1994b; Werner, Goldstein, and Heinik 2009.
43 Lutfey and McKinlay 2009.
44 Koch and Svendsen 2005.
45 Gillett 2004, 734.
46 May et al. 2004.
47 Davenport 2011; Holmes and Ponte 2011.
48 Davenport 2011, 873.
49 Blaxter 2009, 15.

CHAPTER 4. BEING COGNITIVELY EVALUATED

1 Manthorpe et al. 2013.
2 Armstrong 1984; Crawford 1994; Kaufman 1994a.
3 Beard and Estes 2002.
4 Kontos 2004.
5 Bender and Cheston 1997; Kitwood and Bredin 1993; Sabat and Harre 1992.
6 Cf., Christine Bryden, Jenny Knauss, Gloria Sterin, and Richard Taylor who all spoke out about the perceived injustices of life with dementia.
7 E.g., Becker 1997; Chambré 2006; Epstein 1996; Karp 1996; Shorter 1991; Shorter 1992; Star 1992; Wiener 1981; Young 1995.
8 E.g., Casper 1995; David-Floyd and Dumit 1998; Lock, Young, and Cambrosio 2000; Rapp 1999; Strauss et al. 1997.
9 E.g., Armstrong 1995; Franklin and Lock 2001; Hogle 1999; Kleinman 1999; Latour 1987; Rabinow 1996.
10 Goffman 1959.
11 Beard 2004.
12 Gullette 2011.

13 The only type of Alzheimer's which technically has a familial component is early-onset, when persons are diagnosed younger than 65 years of age. Although this type of AD comprises a very small minority, some claim less than 1 percent of cases and others estimate 10 percent, some study participants did have multiple family members with late-onset, or "typical" AD.

14 Cockerham et al. 1986; Strauss et al. 1997.

15 Berg and Mol 1998; Bowker and Star 1999.

16 Glaser and Strauss 1971.

17 Manthorpe et al. 2013.

18 Booth and Booth 1999.

CHAPTER 5. HEARING "THE A WORD"

1 Glaser and Strauss 1971.

2 Becker 1963.

3 Glaser and Strauss 1971.

4 Beard and Fox 2008.

5 Karp 1996; Hughes 1958; Strauss et al. 1997.

6 Becker 1997; Charmaz 1991; Clarke and James 2003; Frank 1993; Karp 1996; Tishelman and Sachs 1998; Ware 1992; Weitz 1991.

7 Manthrope et al. 2013, e69.

8 Parsons 1951.

9 Dumit 2006.

10 Heimer 2001.

11 Aminzadeh et al. 2007; Robinson et al. 2011.

12 People are initially shocked and ask, "why me?" but they are also largely relieved that there is something to blame, a medical label to ascribe to their condition, and they are not "going crazy."

13 Of course, this is related to a selection bias in my study in that respondents were probably more likely to be "health seekers" than the general public.

14 Beard, Knauss, and Moyer 2009; Harris 2002.

15 Lock 2013.

16 E.g., Glaser and Strauss 1965; Kastenbaum 1969; Sudnow 1967; Sweeting and Gilhooly 1997.

17 Karp 1996; Hughes 1951; Strauss et al. 1997.

18 For example, to access services through the Alzheimer's Association, to qualify for research studies, or to elicit help when necessary.

19 Chambré 2006; DeShazer 2013; Epstein 1996; Klawiter 1999; Kokler 2004; Radley and Bell 2007; Robertson 2000.

20 Clarke et al. 2010; Clarke et al. 2003.

CHAPTER 6. EVERYDAY LIFE WITH DIAGNOSIS

1 Glaser and Strauss 1971.

2 Becker 1963; Hughes 1958.

3 It is important to note that these were all early-stage or preclinical cases of AD, so assumptions that this might be a matter of lack of insight or awareness—so rampant in the medical and mass media framings of Alzheimer's—do not apply here. No one denied that they had AD/MCI.

4 Becker 1997; Hawkins 1993; Jenkins and Barrett 2004; Kleinman 1980; Kleinman 1988; Mattingly and Garro 2000.

5 Kleinman 1988.

6 Frank 1995.

7 Becker 1953; Becker 1963; Goffman 1963; Hughes 1958.

8 Karp 1996.

9 Adams, Pill, and Jones 1997; Beard 2004b; Clarke and James 2003; Gatter 1995; Karp 1996; Steffen 1997; Strauss 1975; Weitz 1991.

10 Charmaz 1991; Goffman 1959; Kaufman 1986; Orona 1990; Strauss 1959.

11 Bury 1982; and Becker 1997, respectively.

12 Denzin 1992.

13 Williams 2000.

14 Carricaburu and Pierret 1995; Faircloth et al. 2004; and Williams 1984, respectively.

15 Strauss 1975.

16 Strauss 1959.

17 Becker 1997.

18 Charmaz 1983.

19 Sveilich 2004.

20 Dumit 2006.

21 McIntosh and McKeganey 2000.

22 Cohen-Mansfield, Golander, and Arnheim 2000; Herskovits 1995; Orona 1990.

23 Beyond the progressive nature of the condition over time, it has been well documented that the level of "functioning" varies throughout different periods of the day for people (this is referred to as "sundowning"; c.f., Dewing 2003; Staedt and Stoppe 2005; Taylor et al. 1997). Since "sundowning" is experienced by many people with memory loss, lucidity fluctuates both in general and from moment to moment.

24 Kaufman 1986.

25 The family members who participated in this research were simultaneously attending "caregiver" support groups for Alzheimer's/mild cognitive impairment in a loved one, typically a spouse.

26 Beard 2004b; Strauss 1959.

27 Le Couteur et al. 2013, 4.

28 Ibid., 3.

29 Beard et al. 2012.

30 Hellstrom, Nolan, and Lundh 2005; and Davies 2011, respectively.

31 Bunn et al. 2012.

32 Gordon 1994.

33 Beard et al. 2012.

34 "A.A. had its beginnings in 1935 in Akron, Ohio, as the outcome of a meeting between Bill W., a New York stockbroker, and Dr. Bob S., a surgeon. Both had been hopeless alcoholics and each had been in contact with a mostly nonalcoholic fellowship that emphasized universal spiritual values in daily living. Under this spiritual influence, Bill had gotten sober and had maintained his recovery by working with other alcoholics. When Dr. Bob and Bill finally met, the doctor found himself face to face with a fellow sufferer who had made good. Bill emphasized that alcoholism was a malady of mind, emotions and body. Although Dr. Bob had not known alcoholism to be a disease, he soon got sober, never to drink again. Both men immediately set to work with alcoholics at Akron's City Hospital. The name Alcoholics Anonymous had not yet been coined but these three men were the first A.A. group. In the fall of 1935, a second group of alcoholics slowly took shape in New York. A third appeared at Cleveland in 1939. It had taken over four years to produce 100 sober alcoholics in the three founding groups. By 1950, 100,000 recovered alcoholics could be found worldwide" http://www.alcoholics-anonymous.org/default/en_about_aa_sub.cfm?subpageid=27andpageid=24

    Formal membership lists are not kept, but it is estimated that over 1 million Americans are involved in AA and over 2 million worldwide.

35 Sullivan and Beard 2014.

36 Goffman 1963.

37 Swora 2001.

38 Beard 2004a; Swora 2001.

39 Becker 1997; Clarke and James 2003; Karp 1996; Weitz 1991.

40 Mauldin 2002.

41 Couch and Wade 2003; DeShazer 2013; Henderson 2000; Shakespeare 1999.

42 Boxer and Cortes-Conde 1997; Davies 1998; Lennox and Ashforth 2002.

43 DeShazer 2013.

44 Boxer and Cortes-Conde 1997.

45 Lennox and Ashforth 2002.

46 Beard 2004b; Karp 1996; Sontag 1977; Strauss 1975.

47 Wiener and Dodd 1993.

48 Butler and Rosenblum 1996; Sandstrom 1990; Sontag 1977; Weitz 1991.

49 For example, joking may not be appropriate in clinical or research settings to the extent it is in support groups and being proactive and optimistic are far more important in the former context, whereas there is room to be serious, depressed, and negative in the latter without having this be viewed as symptomatic of the disease process.

50 Dumit 2006.

51 Charmaz 1991; Karp 1996; Swora 2001; Weitz 1991.

52 Wiener and Dodd 1993.

53 Ferguson 2001.

54 Frankl 1984, 104.

55 Riley 2000.
56 Medlicott 1999.
57 Buckler 1996; Epstein 1996; Frankl 1984; Klawiter 1999; Turner 1996; Robertson 2000.
58 Brownfield, Sorenson, and Thompson 2001.
59 Phelan and Hunt 1998.
60 Lock 2013.
61 The ultimate paradox in AD is that a failure to admit one's deficits is labeled "denial" in clinical practice, something that is an exclusion criterion from many support groups and research projects despite the apparent link between AD symptomology and such experiences. Further, individuals with dementia, particularly in the late stages, are believed to "lack insight" into their memory loss. Although it is sometimes talked about as symptomatic of the condition, its use as criterion for eligibility in research, support groups, or psychotherapy implies that there is also some agency ascribed to such unawareness. See Lopez et al. 1994 or Trouillet, Gély-Nargeot, and Derouesné 2003 for more on the medical focus of this debate.
62 Beard 2004b.
63 Beard, Knauss, and Moyer 2009.

CHAPTER 7. ADVOCATING ALZHEIMER'S
1 Selznick 1949.
2 Chaufan et al. 2012.
3 Meyer and Rowan 1977; and DiMaggio and Powell 1983, respectively.
4 Archibald and Crabtree 2010.
5 Meyer and Rowan 1977.
6 Fox 1989; Fox 2000.
7 Booth and Booth 1999.
8 Beard 2004a.
9 Chambré 2006; Epstein 1996; Klawiter 1999; Robertson 2000.
10 Of course, this was obviously affected by the fact that the loss of life in youth is considered very different from the anticipated death of senior members of society.
11 Chambré 2006; Epstein 1996; Klawiter 1999; Robertson 2000.
12 Rucht 1996.
13 Estes 1979.
14 It is not that the disability or mental health movements have not proposed other models to combat the medical model, namely, the social, but activists from both these movements have been less resistant to modern medical approaches than members of AIDS or breast cancer movements. Consequently, relationships between social movements and medicine vary significantly.
15 Glaser and Strauss 1965; Kastenbaum 1969; Sudnow 1967.
16 Sweeting and Gilhooly 1997.
17 Billis and Glennerster 1998.
18 Cutler 1986; and Gubrium 1986, respectively.

19 Booth and Booth 1999.

20 Cohen 1991; Cottrell and Schulz 1993; Kitwood and Bredin 1992; Sabat and Harre 1992.

21 Bryden 2005; Davis 1989; DeBaggio 2002; Dyer 1996; Henderson 1998; Knauss and Moyer 2006; Friel-McGowin 1993; Rose 1996; Sterin 2002; Taylor 2006.

22 Beard 2004b; Beard and Fox 2008; Clare, Rowlands, and Quin 2008; Corner and Bond 2006; Harris 2002; Herskovitz 1995; Holst and Hallberg 2003; Hulko 2009; MacQuarrie 2005; Phinney and Chesla 2003; Sabat 2001; Wilkinson 2002.

23 Beard, Knauss, and Moyer 2009; Harris and Sterin 1999.

24 Beard and Estes 2002; Bond 1992; Canguilhem 1991.

25 See Clarke and Montini 1993 on implicated actors for the ways in which even those people who are not outwardly interested in seeking a medical diagnosis for their memory loss in particular, but also all members of society in general, are affected by the actions of social movements and their organization.

26 Booth and Booth 1999.

27 The debate over designated (or Request for Proposal) research versus investigator-initiated studies is at the heart of this claim.

28 Alzheimer's Association 2014f.

29 As reported at the 2006 Early Stage Forum in Southern California and the 2008 Early Stage Dementia Town Hall meeting in Chicago, Illinois, in the 2008 "Voices of Alzheimer's Disease: A Summary Report on the Nationwide Town Hall Meetings for People with Early Stage Dementia" (see http://www.alz.org/national/documents/report_townhall.pdf), and anecdotally to me by various members of the original Advisory Board.

30 Alzheimer's Association 2014a.

31 The U.S. Food and Drug Administration (FDA) has approved two classes of drugs to treat the cognitive symptoms of Alzheimer's disease. The first Alzheimer medications to be approved were cholinesterase inhibitors. Three of these drugs are commonly prescribed—donepezil Aricept®, approved in 1996; rivastigmine Exelon®, approved in 2000; and galantamine Reminyl®, approved in 2001. Tacrine Cognex®, the first cholinesterase inhibitor, was approved in 1993 but is rarely prescribed today because of associated side effects, including possible liver damage. The latter three are prescribed in the early and moderate stages while the former, by far the most commonly used, is approved for all stages. The final medication, a regulator of glutamate activity, Memantine Namenda®, was approved in 2003 for use in the moderate to severe stages. Alzheimer's Association. 2014. Medications for Memory Loss. Retrieved 03/6/2014 from http://www.alz.org/alzheimers_disease_standard_prescriptions.asp.

32 E.g., Aneshensel et al. 1995; Gordon, Brenner, and Noddings 1996; Henry and Capitman 1995; Lawton et al. 1991; Noonan and Tennstedt 1997; Zarit et al. 1998.

33 Selznick 1949.

34 Meyer and Rowan 1977.

35 Alzheimer's Association 2014f.

36 DiMaggio and Powell 1983.
37 Clarke 1991; Strauss 1978; Wiener 1981.
38 Beard and Williamson 2011.
39 Meyer and Rowan 1977.
40 Selznick 1949.
41 Clarke et al. 2003.
42 Recall from chapter 2 that the conversion rates from MCI to AD are widely
    variable. Thus, a linear relationship between MCI and AD has to date not been
    scientifically established, although the joint NIA-AA 2011 proposed guidelines
    aim to do precisely that.
43 For example, much of the Association-sponsored media coverage projects cata-
    strophic images of people with AD as completely incapacitated. Most notably, the
    PBS adaptation of David Shenk's 2001 book The Forgetting portrayed familial AD
    and the subsequent devastations despite the indisputable rarity of this condition.
    Stereotypical depictions of "bed-ridden" and stupefied people with AD are ram-
    pant even within the Association itself.
44 Stockdale 1999; and DeShazer 2013, respectively.
45 Importantly, those who make effective spokespersons in the opinion of staff at the
    Association tend not to be the articulate study respondents that I have introduced
    throughout this book, but instead the "tragically" muted young individuals, a
    phenomenon which was shown in chapter 2 to be extremely rare.
46 Lock 2013, 172.
47 Robertson 1990.
48 Gubrium 1986.
49 Alzheimer's Association 2004a.
50 Alzheimer's Association 2014d.
51 Stockdale 1999.
52 This is possibly in part due to the emerging need to expand services to address the
    needs of people with AD.
53 In 2004, the website reported 167 free-standing chapters.
54 Meyer and Rowan 1977.
55 DiMaggio and Powell 1983.
56 Selznick 1949.
57 Billis and Glennerster 1998.
58 Alzheimer's Association 2014f.
59 Beard and Estes 2002.
60 Through, for example, support of coverage such as the PBS documentary "The
    Forgetting" or books like The 36-Hour Day.
61 Lyman 1989; Lyman 1993.
62 Hedgecoe 2003.
63 E.g., Beach 1987; Fox 1989; Herskovits 1995; Ming and Fernandez 2001.
64 Apesoa-Varano, Barker, and Hinton 2011.
65 Stockdale 1999.

66. DiMaggio and Powell 1983.
67. Archibald and Crabtree 2010.
68. Booth and Booth 1999.
69. Post 1995; and Dumit 2004, respectively.
70. Stockdale 1999.
71. Lock 2013.
72. Fox 2000.
73. Rucht 1996.
74. Fox 2000.
75. http://www.dasninternational.org/principles.php.
76. Clare, Rowlands, and Quin 2008, 9.
77. http://www.alzfdn.org/AboutUs/missionstatement.html.
78. Ibid.
79. DAI 2015a.
80. DAI 2015b.
81. ADI 2015.
82. http://www.alzquilt.org/about_quilt.shtml.
83. http://www.youngleadersofafa.org/.
84. http://www.alzfdn.org/2015.
85. Beard and Williamson 2011.
86. Fox 1989; Fox 2000.
87. Stockdale 1999.
88. Alzheimer's Association 2014c, https://www.alz.org/media_17778.asp retrieved March 6, 2014.

CHAPTER 8. FORGET ME NOT

1. NIH 2015. Of course, these are only the projects funded explicitly under the AD Mechanism. One can only assume that the actual numbers of funds allocated under the rubrics of aging, neuroscience, or clinical research would increase that figure exponentially.
2. Le Couteur et al. 2013, 3.
3. Richard and Jenny were both called upon by the Alzheimer's Association to give public talks about their experiences locally and at sponsored conferences. They also published their own unabashed accounts, of *Alzheimer's from the Inside Out* and Alzheimer's as a "manageable disability," respectively.

   Richard, a Ph.D. in psychology, went on to gain global recognition as a leading voice of dementia, including speaking at Alzheimer's Association and Alzheimer's Disease International conferences. He was a founding director of Dementia Alliance International, and was a force within the movement. His mantra was "stand up and speak out!" based on his experiences living with dementia. He worked to design and promote the use of web-based technology to allow people living with dementia to "form enabling support networks with their kindred spirits." He was a prolific writer and would routinely send out emails to his listserv, which I was on, graphically detailing his experiences.

Jenny chose to spend her time at the Chicago Art Institute following a newfound interest in sketching. She also founded an advocacy group named Alzheimer's Spoken Here in 2003 with her husband Don Moyer where she went into Chicagoland schools to talk about her experiences with children. In March 2004, Knauss and two Alzheimer's-diagnosed men were the first diagnosed persons to address a plenary session of the Alzheimer's Association Public Policy Forum. In July 2005, Knauss addressed a plenary session of the Alzheimer's Association Dementia Care Conference. In the fall of 2005, Knauss and Moyer organized a nationwide petition to get the Alzheimer's Association to include diagnosed persons in the planning process. The Alzheimer's Association formed an Early Stage Advisory Group which commenced activity in January 2006 and Knauss served on the first group.

4 Behuniak 2011.
5 It should be noted that both the clinicians and Association staff in this study were generally professional and compassionate individuals with admirable intentions of helping persons with memory loss. The trends reported here are based far more on the structural constraints operating at the various sites and nationally than individual-level clinician or staff dynamics. After all, staff members operate within the environmental ethos of the Association and our environments shape us.
6 Heimer 2001.
7 Hacking 1990; Haraway 1991; Latour 1999.
8 Lock 2013, 53.
9 Wiener 1981; and Broom and Woodward 1996, respectively.
10 Charmaz 1991; Karp 1996; Sontag 1977.
11 Becker 1953; Hughes 1958.
12 Yoshida 1993.
13 Beard and Neary 2012.
14 Whitehouse, Frisoni, and Post 2004; Gaines and Whitehouse 2006; Whitehouse and Moody 2006; Whitehouse and George 2008.
15 Whitehouse and George 2008; Basting 2009; Ballenger et al. 2009; Lock 2013.
16 See Beard 2012; deMedeiros and Basting 2014, 352.
17 Lock 2013, 242.
18 Loe 2011.
19 My colleagues and I on the Healthy Aging Network's Brain Health Initiative found a similar redefinition of dementia and aging well by those diagnosed and their families. Beard et al. 2009.
20 Beard et al. 2012; Beard, Knauss, and Moyer 2009.
21 Gullette 2011.
22 Oliver 2006.

APPENDIX B

1 C.f., Yoshida 1993.

2 When I use the term Alzheimer's disease, I am referring to the biomedical definition of a progressive, degenerative disease, manifesting primarily in memory loss,
which includes *functional impairment* in daily living (chapter 3 addresses this
specifically). My use of the term refers to the condition that affects people over 65
years old and can last up to twenty years. I am not speaking about the rare condition called early-onset Alzheimer's, where individuals are in their third to fifth
decades of life and have a much more rapid decline, typically living only three to
five years. To distinguish it from the former, when I talk about Alzheimer's I am
referring to what is sometimes called late-onset AD, which comprises the vast
majority of Alzheimer's cases. The individuals who were part of this study were all
deemed in the "early stages" by medical professionals, that is, they were believed
to have minor memory loss. In clinical practice, this is designated by a score on
the mini-mental state exam, which is the litmus test for dementia, of 25 [out of a
possible 30] or better.

3 Mild cognitive impairment is believed to be a preclinical stage of Alzheimer's
disease. Despite significant scientific controversy about the condition, the medical
community largely agrees that people with MCI are at heightened risk of developing AD within five years. Consequently, it is increasingly diagnosed in specialty
practice.

4 This is either a finding which requires further investigation or a limitation of my
sample, as one would expect far more women than men to participate due to
demographic trends.

5 There is a glaring omission of cultural diversity, which could also be an indication of which populations have awareness of or access to specialty medicine, or it
could simply be a sample limitation.

6 In this study, I am using the Association as a proxy for the larger social movement.

7 Glaser and Strauss 1967; Strauss and Corbin 1997.

8 Wiener 1981, 19.

9 Schutz 1967.

10 Strauss and Corbin 1990.

APPENDIX C

1 The ACRC was formed to study memory loss associated with aging. The main
purpose of the ACRC is to investigate the complex nature of Alzheimer's disease,
its progression over time, its response to treatments, and problems patients and
caregivers experience in dealing with the changes that occur. They reportedly
utilize a multidisciplinary approach.

2 http://www.dhs.cahwnet.gov/Alzheimers/html/arccprogram.htm.

3 This is a pseudonym.

4 Although not clinically proven to slow progression of Alzheimer's pathology, these recommendations are based on general medical beliefs that "lifestyle" factors such as good eating and exercise habits promote health.

5 This, too, is a pseudonym.

6 This was intended to verify that a potential research subject was capable of understanding the intention of the research and the consent form. Examples included: True or False: "This is a research project, and not routine medical care," or "I understand that I can choose not to participate at any time without harm to me or having it affect my health care."

REFERENCES

Adams, Stephanie, Roisin Pill, and Alan Jones. 1997. Medication, Chronic Illness and Identity: The Perspective of People with Asthma. *Social Science and Medicine* 45:189–201.

Adlard, Paul A., Jacqui Parncutt, Varsh Lal, Simon James, Dominic Hare, Philip Doble, David I. Finkelstein, and Ashley I. Bush. 2014. Metal Chaperones Prevent Zinc-Mediated Cognitive Decline. *Neurobiology of Disease* S0969–9961(14)00383–0. doi: 10.1016/j.nbd.2014.12.012. [Epub ahead of print]

Albert, Marilyn S., Steven T. DeKosky, Dennis Dickson, Bruno Dubois, Howard H. Feldman, Nick C. Fox, Anthony Gamst, David M. Holtzman, William J. Jagust, Ronald C. Petersen, Peter Snyder, Maria C. Carrillo, Bill Theis, and Creighton H. Phelps. 2011. The Diagnosis of Mild Cognitive Impairment due to Alzheimer's Disease: Recommendations from the National Institute of Aging and Alzheimer's Association Working Group. *Alzheimer's and Dementia* 7:270–79.

Alzheimer's Association. 2004a. *About Us: History*. Retrieved 1/31/04 from www.alz.org/AboutUs/History/overview.htm

———. 2004b. *About Us: Overview*. Retrieved 1/31/04 from http://www.alz.org/AboutUs/overview.htm

———. 2004c. *About Us: Timeline*. Retrieved 1/31/04 from www.alz.org/AboutUs/History/overview.htm

———. 2004d. *Statistics about Alzheimer's Disease*. Retrieved 1/31/04 from http://www.alz.org/AboutAD/Statistics.asp

———. 2008. 2008 Alzheimer's Disease Facts and Figures. *Alzheimer's and Dementia: The International Journal of Social Research and Practice* 4:110–33. doi: 10.1016/j.jalz.2008.02.005

———. 2012. 2012 Alzheimer's Disease Facts and Figures. *Alzheimer's and Dementia* 8(2):131–68. doi:10.1016/j.jalz.2012.02.001.

———. 2014a. *About Us*. Retrieved 3/6/14 from https://www.alz.org/about_us_about_us_.asp#research

———. 2014b. 2014 Alzheimer's Disease Facts and Figures. *Alzheimer's and Dementia* 10(2):e47–e92.

———. 2014c. *Current Alzheimer's Treatments*. Retrieved 06/8/14 from http://www.alz.org/research/science/alzheimers_disease_treatments.asp

———. 2014d. *A Future without Alzheimer's*. Retrieved 06/14/14 from http://www.alz.org/research/

———. 2014e. *Medications for Memory Loss*. Retrieved 06/10/2014 from http://www.alz.org/alzheimers_disease_standard_prescriptions.asp

———. 2014f. *Younger/Early Onset Alzheimer's and Dementia.* Retrieved 06/10/14 from http://www.alz.org/alzheimers_disease_early_onset.asp

———. 2015. *Our Commitment to Accelerate Global Research: We Fund.* Retrieved 03/23/15 from http://www.alz.org/research/funding/alzheimers_our_commitment. asp#wefund

Alzheimer's Disease International (ADI). 2015. *World Alzheimer Report 2015: The Global Impact of Dementia.* Retrieved 8/21/15 from http://www.alz.co.uk/research/world-report-2015

American Psychiatric Association. 1994. *Diagnostic and Statistical Manual of Mental Disorders DSM-IV,* 4th edition. Washington, D.C.: American Psychiatric Association.

Aminzadeh, Faranak, Anna Byszewski, Frank J. Molnar, and Marg Eisner. 2007. Emotional Impact of Dementia Diagnosis: Exploring Persons with Dementia and Caregivers' Perspectives. *Aging and Mental Health* 11(3):281–90.

Andreasen, Nancy C. 2004. *Brave New Brain: Conquering Mental Illness in the Era of the Genome.* Oxford: Oxford University Press.

Aneshensel, Carol S., Leonard I. Pearlin, Joseph T. Mullan, and Steven H. Zarit. 1995. *Profiles in Caregiving: The Unexpected Career.* New York: Academic Press.

Apesoa-Varano Ester C., Judith C. Barker, and Ladson Hinton. 2011. Curing and Caring: The Work of Primary Care Physicians with Dementia Patients. *Qualitative Health Research* 21(11):1469–83.

Arai, Tetsuaki. 2014. Significance and Limitation of the Pathological Classification of TDP-43 Proteinopathy. *Neuropathology* 34(6):578–88.

Archibald, Matthew E., and Charity Crabtree. 2010. Health Social Movements in the United States: An Overview. *Sociology Compass* 4/5:334–43.

Armaducci, Luigi, Walter A. Rocca, and Bruce S. Schoenberg. 1986. Origin of the Distinction between Alzheimer's Disease and Senile Dementia: How History Can Clarify Nosology. *Neurology* 36(5):1497–99.

Armstrong, David A. 1984. *Political Anatomy of the Body: Medical Knowledge in Britain in the Twentieth Century.* Cambridge, U.K.: Cambridge University Press.

———. 1995. The Rise of Surveillance Medicine. *Sociology of Health and Illness* 17(3):393–404.

Arney, William R., and Bernard J. Bergen. 1984. *Medicine and the Management of Living: Taming the Last Great Beast.* Chicago: Chicago University Press.

Artero, Sylvaine, Ronald Petersen, Jacques Touchon, and Karen Ritchie. 2006. Revised Criteria for Mild Cognitive Impairment: Validation within a Longitudinal Population Study. *Dementia and Geriatric Cognitive Disorders* 22:465–70.

Backman, Lars, Sari Jones, Anna-Karin Berger, Erika Jonsson Laukka, and Brent J. Small. 2004. Multiple Cognitive Deficits during the Transition to Alzheimer's Disease. *Journal of Internal Medicine* 256:195–204.

Ballenger, Jesse F. 2000. "Beyond the Characteristic Plaques and Tangles: Mid-Twentieth Century American Psychiatry and the Fight against Senility." Pp. 83–103 in *Concepts of Alzheimer Disease: Biological, Clinical and Cultural Perspectives, edited* by P. Whitehouse, K. Maurer, and J. F. Ballenger. Baltimore: Johns Hopkins University Press.

Ballenger, Jesse F., Peter J. Whitehouse, Constantine G. Lyketsos, Peter V. Rabins, and Jason H. T. Karlawish. 2009. *Treating Dementia: Do We Have a Pill for It?* Baltimore: Johns Hopkins University Press.

Barnes, Deborah E., and Kristine Yaffe. 2011. The Projected Impact of Risk Factor Reduction on Alzheimer's Disease Prevalence. *Lancet Neurology* 10(9):819–28.

Basting, Anne D. 2009. *Forget Memory: Creating Better Lives for People with Dementia.* Baltimore: Johns Hopkins University Press.

Beach, Thomas G. 1987. The History of Alzheimer's Disease: Three Debates. *Journal of the History of Medicine and Allied Sciences* 42:327–49.

Beach, Wayne A. 2001. Diagnosing "Lay Diagnosis." *Text* 21:13–18.

Beard, Renée L. 2004a. Advocating Voice: Organisational, Historical, and Social Milieu of the Alzheimer's Disease Movement. *Sociology of Health and Illness* 26(6):797–819.

———. 2004b. In Their Voices: Identity Preservation and Experiences of Alzheimer's Disease. *Journal of Aging Studies* 18:415–28.

———. 2012. Art Therapies and Dementia Care: A Systematic Review. *Dementia: The International Journal of Social Research and Practice* 11(5):633–56.

Beard, Renée L., and Carroll L. Estes. 2002. "Medicalization of Aging." Pp. 883–86 in *Macmillan Encyclopedia of Aging,* edited by D. J. Ekerdt. London: Macmillan.

Beard, Renée L., David J. Fetterman, Bei Wu, and Lucinda L. Bryant. 2009. The Two Voices of Alzheimer's: Attitudes toward Brain Health by Diagnosed Individuals and Support Persons. *Gerontologist* 49(S1):S40–S49.

Beard, Renée L., and Patrick Fox. 2008. Resisting Social Disenfranchisement: Negotiating Collective Identities and Everyday Life with Memory Loss. *Social Science and Medicine* 66(7):1509–20.

Beard, Renée L., Jenny Knauss, and Don Moyer. 2009. Managing Disability and Enjoying Life: How We Reframe Dementia through Personal Narratives. *Journal of Aging Studies* 23(4):227–35.

Beard, Renée L., and Tara M. Neary. 2012. Making Sense of Nonsense: Experiences of Mild Cognitive Impairment. *Sociology of Health and Illness* 35(1):130–46.

Beard, Renée L., Sasha Sakhtah, Vanessa Imse, and James E. Galvin. 2012. Negotiating the Joint Career: Couples Adapting to Alzheimer's and Aging in Place. *Journal of Aging Research.* Special Issue on "Aging in Place in Late Life." doi:10.1155/2012/797023

Beard, Renée L., and John B. Williamson. 2004. Generational Equity and Generational Interdependence: Framing of the Debate over Health and Social Security Policy in the United States. *Indian Journal of Gerontology* 18(3&4):348–62.

———. 2011. Symbolic Politics, Social Policy, and the Senior Rights Movement. *Journal of Aging Studies* 25(1):22–33.

Becker, Gay. 1997. *Disrupted Lives: How People Create Meaning in a Chaotic World.* Berkeley: University of California Press.

Becker, Gay, and Sharon R. Kaufman. 1995. Managing an Uncertain Illness Trajectory in Old Age: Patients' and Physicians' Views of Stroke. *Medical Anthropology Quarterly* 9(2):165–87.

Becker, Howard. 1953. Becoming a Marihuana User. *American Journal of Sociology* (November):235–42.

———. 1963. *Outsiders*. New York: Macmillan.

Behuniak, Susan M. 2011. The Living Dead? The Construction of People with Alzheimer's Disease as Zombies. *Ageing and Society* 31:70–92.

Bendelow, Gillian A., and Simon J. Williams. 1995. Transcending the Dualisms: Towards a Sociology of Pain. *Sociology of Health and Illness* 17(2):139–65.

Bender, Michael, and Richard Cheston. 1997. Inhabitants of a Lost Kingdom: A Model of the Subjective Experiences of Dementia. *Ageing and Society* 17:513–32.

Bennett, David A., Robert S. Wilson, Julie A. Schneider, Denis A. Evans, Laurel A. Beckett, Neelum T. Aggarwal, Lisa L. Barnes, Jacob H. Fox, and Jean-Francois Bach. 2002. Natural History of Mild Cognitive Impairment in Older Persons. *Neurology* 59:198–205.

Berg, Marc, and Ann Marie Mol, eds. 1998. *Differences in Medicine: Unraveling Practices, Techniques, and Bodies*. Durham, N.C.: Duke University Press.

Berger, Peter L., and Thomas Luckmann. 1966. *The Social Construction of Reality*. New York: Doubleday & Company.

Berrios, German E. 1990. "Memory and the Cognitive Paradigm of Dementia during the 19th Century: A Conceptual History." Pp. 194–211 in *Lectures on the History of Psychiatry*, edited by R. M. Murray and T. H. Turner. London: Gaskell/Royal College of Psychiatrists.

———. 2003. The Insanities of the Third Age: A Conceptual History of Paraphrenia. *Journal of Nutrition, Health and Aging* 7(6):394–99.

Billis, David, and Howard Glennerster. 1998. Human Services and the Voluntary Sector: Towards a Theory of Comparative Advantage. *Journal of Social Policy* 27(1):79–98.

Binney, Elizabeth A., Carroll L. Estes, and Stanley R. Ingman. 1990. Medicalization, Public Policy and the Elderly: Social Services in Jeopardy? *Social Science and Medicine* 30(7):761–71.

Blackford, Richard C., and Asenath La Rue. 1989. Criteria for Diagnosing Age-Associated Memory Impairment: Proposed Improvement from the Field. *Developmental Neuropsychology* 5:295–306.

Blackmore, Susan. 2004. *Consciousness: An Introduction*. New York: Oxford University Press.

Blaxter, Mildred. 2009. The Case of the Vanishing Patient? Image and Experience. *Sociology of Health and Illness* 31(5):1–17.

Blennow, Kaj, Anders Wallin, and C. G. Gottfries. 1994. "Clinical Subgroups of Alzheimer Disease." Pp. 95–107 in *Dementia: Presentations, Differential Diagnosis, and Nosology*, edited by V. O. B. Emery and T. E. Oxman. Baltimore: Johns Hopkins University Press.

Blessed, G., B. E. Tomlinson, and Martin Roth. 1968. The Association between Quantitative Measures of Dementia and of Senile Change in the Cerebral Grey Matter of Elderly Subjects. *British Journal of Psychiatry* 114:797–811.

Blumer, Howard. 1969. *Symbolic Interactionism: Perspective and Method*. Englewood Cliffs, N.J.: Prentice-Hall.

Bond, John. 1992. The Medicalization of Dementia. *Journal of Aging Studies* 6(4):397–403.

Booth, Thomas, and W. Booth. 1999. Parents Together: Action Research and Advocacy Support for Patients with Learning Disabilities. *Health and Social Care in the Community* 7(6):464–74.

Bowen, James, Linda Teri, Walter Kukull, Wayne McCormick, Susan M. McCurry, and Eric B. Larson. 1997. Progression to Dementia in Patients with Isolated Memory Loss. *Lancet* 349:763–65.

Bowker, Geoffrey C., and Susan L. Star. 1999. *Sorting Things Out: Classification and Its Consequences*. Cambridge, Mass.: MIT Press.

Boxer, Diana, and Florencia Cortés-Conde. 1997. From Bonding to Biting: Conversational Joking and Identity Display. *Journal of Pragmatics* 27(3):275–94.

Bozoki, Andrea, Bruno Giordani, Judith L. Heidebrink, Stanley Berent, and Norman L. Foster. 2001. Mild Cognitive Impairments Predict Dementia in Nondemented Elderly Patients with Memory Loss. *Archives of Neurology* 58:411–16.

Brodaty, Henry, Dianne Griffin, and Dusan Hadzi-Pavlovic. 1990. A Survey of Dementia Carers: Doctors' Communications, Problem Behaviours, and Institutional Care. *Australian and New Zealand Journal of Psychiatry* 24:362–70.

Broom, Dorothy H., and Roslyn V. Woodward. 1996. Medicalization Reconsidered: Toward a Collaborative Approach to Care. *Sociology of Health and Illness* 18:357–78.

Brownfield, David, Ann Marie Sorenson, and Kevin M. Thompson. 2001. Gang Membership, Race, and Social Class: A Test of the Group Hazard and Master Status Hypotheses. *Deviant Behavior: An Interdisciplinary Journal* 22:73–89.

Bryden, Christine. 2005 *Dancing with Dementia: My Story of Living Positively with Dementia*. London: Jessica Kingsley Publishers.

Buckler, Steven. 1996. Historical Narrative, Identity and the Holocaust. *History of the Human Sciences* 9(4):1–20.

Bulow, Pia H. 2004. Sharing Experiences of Contested Illness by Storytelling. *Discourse and Society* 15(1):33–53.

Bun, Shogyoku, Chiaki Ikejima, Jiro Kida, Atsuko Yoshimura, Adam Jon Lebowitz, Tatsuyuki Kakuma, and Takashi Asada. 2014. A Combination of Supplements May Reduce the Risk of Alzheimer's Disease in Elderly Japanese with Normal Cognition. *Journal of Alzheimers Disease* 45(1): 15–25. doi: 10.3233/JAD-142232

Bunn, Frances, Claire Goodman, Katie Sworn, Greta Rait, Carol Brayne, Louise Robinson, Elaine McNeilly, and Steve Iliffe. 2012. Psychosocial Factors that Shape Patient and Carer Experiences of Dementia Diagnosis and Treatment: A Systematic Review of the Qualitative Studies. *PLoS Med* 9:e1001331.

Bury, Michael. 1982. Chronic Illness as Biographical Disruption. *Sociology of Health and Illness* 4(2):167–82.

Bush, Ashley I., Warren H. Pettingell, G. D. P. M. Multhaup, Marc d Paradis, Jean-Paul Vonsattel, James F. Gusella, Konrad Beyreuther, Colin L. Masters, and Rudolph E. Tanzi. 1994. Rapid Induction of Alzheimer's AB Amyloid Formation by Zinc. *Science* 265:1464–67.

Butler, Sandy, and Barbara Rosenblum. 1996. *Cancer in Two Voices*. 2nd edition. Denver, Colo.: Spinsters Ink Books.

Byszewski, Anna M., Frank J. Molnar, Faranak Aminzadeh, Marg Eisner, Fauzia Gardezi, and Raewyn Bassett. 2007. Dementia Diagnosis Disclosure: A Study of Patient and Caregiver Perspectives. *Alzheimer Disease and Associated Disorders* 21:107–14.

Canguilhem, Georges. 1991. *On the Normal and the Pathological*. New York: Zone Books.

Carpenter, B., and J. Dave. 2004. Disclosing a Dementia Diagnosis: A Review of Opinion and Practice, and a Proposed Research Agenda. *Gerontologist* 44(2):149–58.

Carricaburu, Daniele, and Janine Pierret. 1995. From Biographical Disruption to Biographical Reinforcements: The Case of HIV Positive Men. *Sociology of Health and Illness* 17(1):65–88.

Casper, Monica J. 1995. "Fetal Cyborgs and Technomoms on the Reproductive Frontier: Which Way to the Carnival?" Pp. 183–202 in *The Cyborg Handbook*, edited by C. H. Gray. London: Routledge.

———. 1998. *The Making of the Unborn Patient: A Social Anatomy of Fetal Surgery*. New Brunswick, N.J.: Rutgers University Press.

Casper, Monica J., and Michael Berg. 1995. Introduction to Special Issue on Constructivist Perspectives on Medical Work: Medical Practice in Science and Technology Studies. *Science, Technology, and Human Values* 20:395–407.

Castleman, Michael, Dolores Gallagher-Thompson, and Matthew Naythons. 1999. *There's Still a Person in There: The Complete Guide to Treating and Coping with Alzheimer's*. New York: G. P. Putnam's Sons.

Celsis, P., A. Agneil, and D. Cardebat. 1997. Age Related Cognitive Decline: A Clinical Entity? A Longitudinal Study of Cerebral Blood Flow and Memory Performance. *Journal of Neurology, Neurosurgery and Psychiatry* 62:601–08.

Census. 2013. *Neurology* 80(19):1778–83.

Chambré, Susan. 2006. *Fighting for Our Lives: New York's AIDS Community and the Politics of Disease*. New Brunswick, N.J.: Rutgers University Press.

Charmaz, Kathy. 1983. Loss of Self: A Fundamental Form of Suffering in the Chronically Ill. *Sociology of Health and Illness* 5(2):168–95.

———. 1990. "Discovering" Chronic Illness: Using Grounded Theory. *Social Science and Medicine* 30(11):1161–72.

———. 1991. *Good Days, Bad Days: The Self in Chronic Illness and Time*. New Brunswick, N.J.: Rutgers University Press.

Charmaz, Kathy, and Virginia Olesen. 1997. Ethnographic Research in Medical Sociology: Its Foci and Distinctive Contributions. *Sociological Methods and Research* 25(4):452–94.

Chaufan, Claudia, Brooke Hollister, Jennifer Nazareno, and Patrick Fox. 2012. Medical Ideology as a Double-Edged Sword: The Politics of Cure and Care in the Making of Alzheimer's Disease. *Social Science and Medicine* 74:788–95.

Cheston, Richard, and Michael Bender. 1999. *Understanding Dementia: The Man with the Worried Eyes*. London: Jessica Kingsley Publishers.

Ciambrone, Desirée. 2001. Illness and Other Assaults on Self: The Relative Impact of HIV/AIDS on Women's Lives. *Sociology of Health and Illness* 23(4):517–40.

Clare, Linda, Rebecca Rowlands, and Julia M. Quin. 2008. Collective Strength: The Impact of Developing a Shared Social Identity in Early-Stage Dementia. *Dementia: International Journal of Social Research and Practice* 7(1) 9–30.

Clarke, Adele. 1991. "Social Worlds/Arenas Theory as Organizational Theory." Pp. 119–158 in *Social Organization and Social Process: Essays in Honor of Anselm Strauss*, edited by D. R. Maines. New York: Aldine de Gruyter.

Clarke, Adele, Laura Mamo, Jennifer R. Fosket, Jennifer R. Fishman, and Janet K. Shim. 2010. *Biomedicalization: Technoscience, Health, and Illness in the U.S.* Durham, N.C.: Duke University Press.

Clarke, Adele, and Theresa Montini. 1993. The Many Faces of RU 486: Tales of Situated Knowledges and Technological Contestations. *Science, Technology and Human Values* 18:42–78.

Clarke, Adele, Janet K. Shim, Laura Mamo, Jennifer R. Fosket, and Jennifer R. Fishman. 2003. Biomedicalization: Technoscientific Transformations of Health, Illness, and U.S. Biomedicine. *American Sociological Review* 68(2):161–94.

Clarke, Juanne N., and Susan James. 2003. The Radicalized Self: The Impact on the Self of the Contested Nature of the Diagnosis of Chronic Fatigue Syndrome. *Social Science and Medicine* 57(8):1387–95.

Cockerham, W. C., Lueschen, G., Kunz, G., and Spaeth, J. L. 1986. Social Stratification and Self-Management of Health. *Journal of Health and Social Behavior* 27(1):1–14.

Cohen, Donna. 1991. The Subjective Experiences of Alzheimer's Disease: The Anatomy of an Illness as Perceived by Patients and Families. *American Journal of Alzheimer's Care and Related Disease and Research* (May–June):6–11.

Cohen-Mansfield, Jiska, Hava Golander, and Glyorah Arnheim. 2000. Self-Identity in Older Persons Suffering from Dementia: Preliminary Results. *Social Science and Medicine* 51:381–94.

Connell, Cathleen M., Linda Boise, John C. Stuckey, Sara B. Holmes, and Margaret L. Hudson. 2004. Attitudes toward the Diagnosis and Disclosure of Dementia among Family Caregivers and Primary Care Physicians. *Gerontologist* 44(4):500–07.

Conrad, Peter. 2000. "Medicalization, Genetics, and Human Problems." Pp. 322–333 in *Handbook of Medical Sociology*, edited by P. Conrad, C. E. Bird, and A. M. Fremont. Upper Saddle River, N.J.: Prentice Hall.

———. 2007. *The Medicalization of Society: On the Transformation of Human Conditions into Treatable Disorders*. Baltimore: Johns Hopkins University Press.

Conrad, Peter, and Jonathan Schneider. 1980. *Deviance and Medicalization: From Badness to Sickness*. St. Louis: C. W. Mosby.

Constantinidis, Jean. 1978. "Is Alzheimer's Disease a Major Form of Senile Dementia? Clinical, Anatomical, and Genetic Data." Pp. 15–25 in *Alzheimer's Disease: Senile Dementia and Related Disorders*, edited by R. Katzman, R. Terry, and K. Bick. New York: Raven Press.

Convit, Antonio, Mony J. De Leon, James Golomb, A. E. George, C. Y. Tarshish, M. Bobinski, W. Tsui, S. De Santi, J. Wegiel, and H. Wisniewski. 1993. Hippocampal Atrophy in Early Alzheimer's Disease: Anatomic Specificity and Validation. *Psychiatry Quarterly* 64(4):371–87.

Coombes, Rebecca. 2009. Evidence Lacking for Memory Clinics to Tackle Dementia, Say Critics. *British Medical Journal* 338:b550.

Corbin, Juliet M., and Anselm Strauss. 1998. *Basics of Qualitative Research: Techniques and Procedures for Developing Grounded Theory*. New York: Sage Publications.

Corner, Lynne, and John Bond. 2006. The Impact of the Label of Mild Cognitive Impairment on Individual's Sense of Self. *Philosophy, Psychiatry, and Psychology* 13(1):3–12.

Cottrell, Victoria, and Richard Schulz. 1993. The Perspective of the Patient with Alzheimer's Disease: A Neglected Dimension of Dementia Research. *Gerontologist* 32:205–11.

Couch, Stephen R., and Barbara A. Wade. 2003. "I Want to Barbecue bin Laden": Humor after 9/11. *International Journal of Mass Emergencies and Disasters* 21(3):67–86.

Craik, Fergus I. M. 1977. "Age Differences in Human Memory." Pp. 384–414 in *Handbook of the Psychology of Aging*, edited by J. E. Birren and K. W. Shaie. New York: Van Nostrand Reinhold.

Crawford, Robert. 1994. The Boundaries of the Self and the Unhealthy Other: Reflections on Health, Culture and AIDS. *Social Science and Medicine* 38(10):1347–65.

Crook, Thomas, Raymond T. Bartus, Steven H. Ferris, Peter Whitehouse, Gene D. Cohen, and Samuel Gershon. 1986. Age-Associated Memory Impairment: Proposed Diagnostic Criteria and Measures of Clinical Change—Report of a National Institute of Mental Health Work Group. *Developments in Neuropsychiatry* 2:361–76.

Cummings, Jeffrey L., P. A. Cyrus, F. Bieber, J. Mas, J. Orazem, and B. Gulanski. 1998. Metrifonate Treatment of the Cognitive Deficits of Alzheimer's Disease: Metrifonate Study Group. *Neurology* 50(May):1214–21.

Cutler, Neal. 1986. "Public Response: The National Politics of Alzheimer's Disease." Pp. 161–89 in *The Dementias: Policy and Management*, edited by M. Gilhooly, S. Zarit, and J. Birrens. Englewood Cliffs, N.J.: Prentice Hall.

Czerner, Thomas B. 2001. *What Makes You Tick? The Brain in Plain English*. New York: John Wiley & Sons.

Daley, Tamara C. 2004. From Symptom Recognition to Diagnosis: Children with Autism in Urban India. *Social Science and Medicine* 58(7):1323–35.

Daly, Ella, Deborah Zaitchik, Maura Copeland, Jeremy Schmahmann, Jeanette Gunther, and Marilyn Albert. 2000. Predicting Conversion to Alzheimer Disease Using Standardized Clinical Information. *Archives of Neurology* 57(5): 675–80.

Davenport, Nancy H. M. 2011. Medical Residents' Use of Narrative Templates in Story-telling and Diagnosis. *Social Science and Medicine* 73:873–81.

Davies, Christie. 1998. Jewish Identity and Survival in Contemporary Society: The Evidence from Jewish Humor. *Sociological Papers* 6:123–44.

Davies, Judie C. 2011. Preserving the "Us Identity" through Marriage Commitment while Living with Early-Stage Dementia. *Dementia: International Journal of Social Research and Practice* 10(2):217–34.

Davis-Floyd, Robbie, and Joseph Dumit. 1998. *Cyborg Babies: From Techno-Sex to Techno-Tots*. New York: Routledge.

Davis, Daniel H. J. 2004. Dementia: Sociological and Philosophical Constructions. *Social Science and Medicine* 58:369–78.

Davis, Robert. 1989. *My Journey into Alzheimer's Disease*. Carol Stream, Ill.: Tyndale House Publishers.

Dawe, Bridget, Andrew Proctor, and Michael Philpot. 1992. Concepts of Mild Cognitive Impairment in the Elderly and Their Relationships to Dementia: A Review. *International Journal of Geriatric Psychiatry* 7:473–79.

DeBaggio, Thomas. 2002. *Losing My Mind: An Intimate Look at Life with Alzheimer's*. New York: Free Press.

de Medeiros, Kate, and Anne Basting. 2014. "Shall I Compare Thee to a Dose of Done-pezil?" Cultural Arts Interventions in Dementia Care Research. *Gerontologist* 54(3) 344–53.

Dementia Alliance International (DAI). 2015a. *Homepage*. Retrieved 8/21/15 from http://www.dementiaallianceinternational.org/

———. 2015b. Mission. Retrieved 8/21/15 from http://www.dementiaallianceinterna-tional.org/about-us/mission/

———. 2015c. *Our Vision*. Retrieved 8/21/15 from http://www.dementiaallianceinterna-tional.org/about-us/vision/

Denzin, Neal. 1992. *Symbolic Interactionism and Cultural Studies: The Politics of Inter-pretation*. Oxford: Blackwell Press.

DeShazer, Mary K. 2013. *Mammographies: The Cultural Discourses of Breast Cancer Narratives*. Ann Arbor, Mich.: University of Michigan Press.

Dewar, Anne L., and Elizabeth A. Lee. 2000. Bearing Illness and Injury. *Western Jour-nal of Nursing Research* 22(8):912–26.

Dewing, Jan. 2003. Sundowning in Older People with Dementia: Evidence Base, Nurs-ing Assessment and Interventions. *Nursing Older People* 15(8):24–31.

Dillman, R. J. M. 1990. "Medical Knowledge and the Concept of Disease." Pp. 1–32 in *Alzheimer's Disease: The Concepts of Disease and the Construction of Medical Knowledge*. Amsterdam: Thesis Publishers.

———. 2000. "Alzheimer's Disease: Epistemological Lessons from History?" Pp. 129–57 in *Concepts of Alzheimer's Disease: Biological, Clinical and Cultural Perspectives*, edited by P. J. Whitehouse, K. Maurer, and J. F. Ballenger. Baltimore: Johns Hopkins University Press.

DiMaggio, Paul, and Walter W. Powell. 1983. The Iron Cage Revisited. *American Socio-logical Review* 48:147–60.

Dippel, Raye Lynne, and J. Thomas Hutton, eds. 1991. *Caring for the Alzheimer Patient: A Practical Guide*, 2nd edition. New York: Prometheus Books.

Dumit, Joseph. 2003. Is It Me or My Brain? Depression and Neuroscientific Facts. *Journal of Medical Humanities* 24(1/2):35–47.

———. 2004. *Picturing Personhood: Brain Scans and Biomedical Identity*. Princeton, N.J.: Princeton University Press.

———. 2006. Illnesses You Have to Fight to Get: Facts as Forces in Uncertain, Emergent Illnesses. *Social Science and Medicine* 62(3): 577–90.

Durkheim, Emile. 1982. *The Rules of the Sociological Method*, edited by S. Lukes, translated by W. D. Halls. New York: Free Press.

Dye, Richelin V., Karen J. Miller, Elyse J. Singer, and Andrew J. Levine. 2012. Hormone Replacement Therapy and Risk for Neurodegenerative Diseases. *International Journal of Alzheimer's Disease*, Article ID 258454, 18 pages. doi:10.1155/2012/258454

Dyer, Joyce. 1996. *In a Tangled Wood*. Dallas: Southern Methodist University Press.

Edvardsson, David, Deirdre Fetherstonhaugh, and Rhonda Nay. 2010. Promoting a Continuation of Self and Normality: Person-Centered Care as Described by People with Dementia, Their Family Members and Aged Care Staff. *Journal of Clinical Nursing* 19:2611–18.

Edwards, Carla D., Amber McClave, and Yvonne J. Combs. 2000. Breast Cancer: An Examination of the Social Correlates Relationship to Diagnosis and Treatment. *Research in the Sociology of Health Care* 18:35–51.

Elias, Merrill F., Alexa Beiser, Philip A. Wolf, Rhoda Au, Roberta F. White, and Ralph B. D'Agostino. 2000. The Preclinical Phase of Alzheimer Disease: A 22-Year Prospective Study of the Framingham Cohort. *Archives of Neurology* 57(6):808–13.

Emery, V. Olga B., and Thomas E. Oxman, eds. 1994. *Dementia: Presentations, Differential Diagnosis, and Nosology*. Baltimore: Johns Hopkins University Press.

Epstein, Stephen. 1996. *Impure Science: AIDS, Activism, and the Politics of Knowledge*. Berkeley: University of California Press.

Estes, Carroll L. 1979. *The Aging Enterprise: A Critical Examination of Social Policies and Services for the Aged*. San Francisco: Jossey-Bass.

Estes, Carroll L., and Elizabeth Binney. 1989. The Biomedicalization of Aging: Dangers and Dilemmas. *Gerontologist* 29:587–96.

Evans, Denis A., H. Harris Funkenstein, Marilyn S. Alpert, Paul A. Scherr, Nancy R. Cook, Marilyn J. Chown, Liesi E. Hebert, Charles H. Hennekens, and James O. Taylor. 1989. Prevalence of Alzheimer's Disease in a Community Population of Older Persons. Higher than Previously Reported. *Journal of American Medical Association* 262(18):2251–56.

Faircloth, Christopher A., Craig Boylstein, Maude Rittman, Mary E. Young, and Jaber Gubrium. 2004. Sudden Illness and Biographical Flow in Narratives of Stroke Recovery. *Sociology of Health and Illness* 26(2):242–61.

Farlow, Martin, Ravi Anand, John Messina Jr., Richard Hartman, and Jeffrey Veach. 2000. A 52-Week Study of the Efficacy of Rivastigmine in Patients with Mild to Moderately Severe Alzheimer's Disease. *European Neurology* 44(4):236–41.

Fazio, Sam, Dorothy Seman, and Jane Stansell, eds. 1999. *Rethinking Alzheimer's Care.* Baltimore: Health Professions Press.

Featherstone, Mike, and Mike Hepworth. 1991. "The Mask of Ageing and the Postmodern Life Course." Pp. 371–89 in *The Body: Social Process and Cultural Theory*, edited by M. Featherstone, M. Hepworth, and B. S. Turner. London: Sage Publications.

Feil, Nancy. 1993. *The Validation Breakthrough: Simple Techniques for Communicating with People with "Alzheimer's-Type Dementia."* Baltimore: Health Professions Press.

Ferguson, Susan J. 2001. *Shifting the Center: Understanding Contemporary Families.* London: McGraw-Hill.

Figert, Anne. 1995. The Three Faces of PMS: The Professional, Gendered and Scientific Structuring of a Psychiatric Disorder. *Social Problems* 42(1):56–73.

Flicker, Charles, Steven H. Ferris, and Barry Reisberg. 1991. Mild Cognitive Impairment in the Elderly: Predictors of Dementia. *Neurology* 41:1006–09.

Forbes, William F., and John P. Hirdes. 1993. The Relationship between Aging and Disease: Geriatric Ideology and Myths of Senility. *Journal of American Geriatrics Society* 41:1267–71.

Forss, Anette, Carol Tishelman, Catarina Widmark, and Lisbeth Sachs. 2004. Women's Experiences of Cervical Cellular Changes: An Unintentional Transition from Health to Liminality? *Sociology of Health and Illness* 26(3):306–25.

Foucault, Michel. 1980. *Power/Knowledge: Selected Interviews and Other Writings 1972–1977*, edited by C. Gordon. New York: Pantheon Books.

———. 1988. *Technologies of the Self: A Seminar with Michel Foucault.* Amherst: University of Massachusetts Press.

Fox, Patrick J. 1989. From Senility to Alzheimer's Disease: The Rise of the Alzheimer's Disease Movement. *Milbank Quarterly* 67(1):58–102.

———. 2000. "The Role of the Concept of Alzheimer's Disease in the Development of the Alzheimer's Association in the United States." Pp. 209–33 in *Concepts of Alzheimer's Disease: Biological, Clinical and Cultural Perspectives*, edited by P. J. Whitehouse, K. Maurer, and J. F. Ballenger. Baltimore: Johns Hopkins University Press.

Fox, Patrick J., Susan E. Kelly, and Sara L. Tobin. 1999. Defining Dementia: Social and Historical Background of Alzheimer's Disease. *Genetic Testing* 3(1):13–19.

Frank, Arthur. 1993. The Rhetoric of Self-Change: Illness Experience as Narrative. *Sociological Quarterly* 34:39–52.

———. 1995. *The Wounded Storyteller: Body, Illness, and Ethics.* Chicago: University of Chicago Press.

Frankl, Viktor E. 1984. *Man's Search for Meaning.* London: Washington Square Press.

Franklin, Sarah, and Margaret Lock. eds. 2001. *Remaking Life & Death: Toward an Anthropology of the Biosciences.* Santa Fe: School of American Research Press.

Friel-McGowin, Diane. 1993. *Living in the Labyrinth: A Personal Journey through the Maze of Alzheimer's*. New York: Dell Publishing.

Gaines, Atwood D., and Peter J. Whitehouse. 2006. Building a Mystery: Alzheimer's Disease, Mild Cognitive Impairment, and Beyond. *Philosophy, Psychiatry, and Psychology* 13(1):61–74.

Galasko, Douglas, Lawrence A. Hansen, Robert Katzman, Wigbert Wiederholt, Eliezer Masliah, Robert Terry, L. Robert Hill, Phyllis Lessin, and Leon J. Thal.1994. Clinical Neuropathological Correlations in Alzheimer's Disease and Related Dementias. *Archives of Neurology* 51:888–95.

Ganguli, Mary, Beth E. Snitz, Judith A. Saxton, Chung-Chou H. Chang, Ching-Wen Lee, Joni Vander Bilt, Tiffany F. Hughes, David A. Loewenstein, Frederick W. Unverzagt, and Ronald C. Petersen. 2011. Outcomes of Mild Cognitive Impairment Depend on Definition: A Population Study. *Archives of Neurology* 68(6):761–67.

García, Néstor H., and Luis I. Juncos. 2006. The Association between Inflammatory Markers and Hypertension. A Call for Anti-Inflammatory Strategies? *TheScientificWorldJOURNAL* 6:1262–73 doi:10.1100/tsw.2006.190

Gatter, Philip N. 1995. Anthropology, HIV and Contingent Identities. *Social Science and Medicine* 41:1523–33.

Gauthier, Serge, and Sandra Schlaefke. 2014. Efficacy and Tolerability of Ginkgo Biloba Extract EGb 761® in Dementia: A Systematic Review and Meta-Analysis of Randomized Placebo-Controlled Trials. *Clinical Interventions in Aging* 9:2065–77.

Gellerstedt, Nils. 1933. Zur Kenntnis der Hirnveranderungen bei der normalen Altersinvolution. *Upsala Lakareforenings Forhandlingar* 38:193–408.

George, Daniel R., Peter J. Whitehouse, Simon D'Alton, and Jesse Ballenger. 2012. The Art of Medicine: Through the Amyloid Gateway. *Lancet* 380:1986–87.

Gillett, Grant. 2004. Clinical Medicine and the Quest for Certainty. *Social Science and Medicine* 58:718–38.

Glaser, Barney G., and Anselm L. Strauss. 1965. *Awareness of Dying*. Chicago: Aldine de Gruyter.

———. 1967. *Discovery of Grounded Theory: Strategies for Qualitative Research*. Chicago: Aldine de Gruyter.

———. 1971. *Status Passage: A Formal Theory*. Chicago: Aldine Publishing.

Goffman, Erving. 1959. *The Presentation of Self in Everyday Life*. New York: Anchor Books.

———. 1963. *Stigma: Notes on the Management of Spoiled Identity*. Englewood Cliffs, N.J.: Prentice-Hall.

Goldsmith, Malcolm. 1996. *Hearing the Voice of People with Dementia: Opportunities and Obstacles*. London: Jessica Kingsley Publishers.

Golomb, James, Mony J. de Leon, Alan Kluger, Ajax E. George, Chaim Tarshish, and Steven H. Ferris. 1993. Hippocampal Atrophy in Normal Aging: An Association with Recent Memory Impairment. *Archives of Neurology* 50:967–73.

Golomb, James, Alan Kluger, and Steven H. Ferris. 2000. Mild Cognitive Impairment: Identifying and Treating the Earliest Stages of Alzheimer's. *Neuroscience News* 3:46–53.

Golomb, James, Alan Kluger, Peter Garrard, and Steven H. Ferris. 2001. *Clinician's Manual on Mild Cognitive Impairment.* London: Science Press.

Gordon, Michael R. 1994. In Poignant Public Letter, Reagan Reveals That He Has Alzheimer's. *New York Times* November 6. Retrieved 06/8/14 from: http://www.nytimes.com/1994/11/06/us/in-poignant-public-letter-reagan-reveals-that-he-has-alzheimer-s.html

Gordon, Susan, Patricia Benner, and Nel Noddings. 1996. *Caregiving: Readings in Knowledge, Practice, Ethics, and Politics.* Philadelphia: University of Pennsylvania Press.

Gottfries, C.-G., Kai Blennow, B. Regland, and Anders Wallin. 1990. "Alzheimer's Disease—One, Two or Several?" Pp. 342–56 in *Alzheimer's Disease: Epidemiology, Neuropathology, Neurochemistry, and Clinics*, edited by K. Maurer, P. Riederer, and H. Beckman. New York: Springer-Verlag.

Gouras, Gunnar K., Huaxi Xu, Rachel S. Gross, Jeffrey P. Greenfield, Bing Hai, Rong Wang, and Paul Greengard. 2000. Testosterone Reduces Neuronal Secretion of Alzheimer's Beta-Amyloid Peptides. *Proceedings of the National Academy of Sciences (USA)* 97:1202–05.

Graham, Janice E., and Karen Ritchie. 2006. Mild Cognitive Impairment: Ethical Considerations for Nosological Flexibility in Human Kinds. *Philosophy, Psychiatry, and Psychology* 13(1):31–43.

Graham, Janice E., Kenneth Rockwood, B. Lynn Beattie, Robin Eastwood, Serge Gauthier, Holly Tuokko, and Ian McDowell. 1997. Prevalence and Severity of Cognitive Impairment with and without Dementia in an Elderly Population. *Lancet* 349:1793–96.

Grundman, Michael. 2001. Current Therapeutic Advances in Alzheimer's Disease. *Research and Practice in Alzheimer's Disease* 5:172–77.

Grundman, Michael, Ronald C. Petersen, John Morris, Steven H. Ferris, Mary Sano, Martin R. Farlow, Rachel S. Doody, and Leon J Thal. 1996. Rate of Dementia of the Alzheimer's Type (DAT) in Subjects with Mild Cognitive Impairment. *Neurology* 46:A403.

Gubrium, Jaber F. 1978. Notes on the Social Organization of Senility. *Urban Life* 7:23–44.

———. 1986. *Oldtimers and Alzheimer's: The Descriptive Organization of Senility* London: JAI Press.

Gullette, Margret M. 2011. *Agewise: Fighting the New Ageism in America.* Chicago: University of Chicago Press.

Haber, Carole. 1984. From Senescence to Senility: The Transformation of Senile Old Age in the Nineteenth Century. *International Journal of Aging and Human Development* 19:41–45.

Hacking, Ian. 1990. *The Taming of Chance*. Cambridge, U.K.: Cambridge University Press.

Hanson, Barbara G. 1991. Parts, Players, and "Patienting": The Social Construction of Senility. *Family Systems Medicine* 9:267–74.

———. 1997. Who's Seeing Whom? General Systems Theory and Constructivist Implications for Senile Dementia Intervention. *Journal of Aging Studies* 11(1):15–25.

Haraway, Donna. 1991. *Simians, Cyborgs, and Women: The Reinvention of Nature*. New York: Routledge.

Harding, Nancy, and Colin Palfrey. 1997. *The Social Construction of Dementia: Confused Professionals?* London: Jessica Kingsley Publishers.

Hardy, John A., and John Mayer. 2011. The Amyloid Cascade Hypothesis Has Misled the Pharmaceutical Industry. *Biochemical Society Transactions* 39(4): 920–23.

Harris, Phyllis Braudy. 2002. *The Person with Alzheimer's Disease: Pathways to Understanding the Experience*. Baltimore: Johns Hopkins University Press.

Harris, Phyllis Braudy, and Gloria J. Sterin. 1999. Insider's Perspective: Defining and Preserving the Self of Dementia. *Journal of Mental Health and Aging* 5(3):241–56.

Hauw, Jean-Jacques, Charles Duyckaerts, and Pia Delaére. 1991. "Alzheimer's Disease." Pp. 113–47 in *The Pathology of the Aging Human Nervous System*, edited by S. Duckett. Philadelphia: Lea & Febiger.

Hawkins, Anne H. 1993. *Reconstructing Illness: Studies in Pathography*. West Lafayette, Ind.: Purdue University Press.

Hebert Liesi E., Jennifer Weuve, Paul A. Scherr, and Denis A. Evans. 2013. Alzheimer Disease in the United States (2010–2050) Estimated Using the 2010 Census. *Neurology* 80(19): 1778–83.

Hedgecoe, Adam M. 2003. Expansion of Uncertainty: Cystic Fibrosis, Classification and Genetics. *Sociology of Health and Illness* 25(1):50–70.

Heimer, Carol A. 2001. Cases and Biographies: An Essay on Routinization and the Nature of Comparison. *Annual Review of Sociology* 27:47–76.

Hellstrom, Ingrid, Mike Nolan, and Ulla Lundh. 2005. "We Do Things Together": A Case Study of "Couplehood" in Dementia. *Dementia: International Journal of Social Research and Practice* 4(1):7–22.

Henderson, Cary. 1998. *Partial View: An Alzheimer's Journal*. Dallas: Southern Methodist University Press.

Henderson, Debra A. 2000. "It's My Underwear Day and I'm Watching Golf": Humor, Impression Management, and Marital Interaction in the Intermarried Couple. *Sociological Imagination* 37(4):257–82.

Henry, Mary Ellen, and John A. Capitman. 1995. Finding Satisfaction in Adult Day Care: Analysis of a National Demonstration of Dementia Care and Respite Services. *Journal of Applied Gerontology* 14(3):302–20.

Hermans, Hubert J. M. 2003. Clinical Diagnosis as a Multiplicity of Self-Positions: Challenging Social Representations Theory. *Culture and Psychology* 9(4):407–14.

Herskovits, Elizabeth. 1995. Struggling over Subjectivity: Debates about the "Self" and Alzheimer's Disease. *Medical Anthropology Quarterly* 9(2):146–64.

Hilton, B. Ann. 1996. Getting Back to Normal: The Family Experience during Early Stage Breast Cancer. *Oncology Nursing Forum* 23:605–14.

Hoff, P. 1991. "Alzheimer in His Time." Pp. 29–124 in *Eponymists in Medicine: Alzheimer and the Dementias*, edited by G. E. Berrios and H. L. Freeman. London: Royal Society of Medicines Services Limited.

Hogle, Linda F. 1999. *Recovering the Nation's Body: Cultural Memory, Medicine, and the Politics of Redemption.* New Brunswick, N.J.: Rutgers University Press.

Holden, Neil L. 1987. Late Paraphrenia or the Paraphrenias? *British Journal of Psychiatry* 150:635–39.

Holmes, Maya, and Seth M. Ponte. 2011. En-case-ing the Patient: Disciplining Uncertainty in Medical Student Patient Presentations. *Culture, Medicine, and Psychiatry* 35:163–82.

Holroyd, Suzanne, Quentin Turnbull, and Andrew M. Wolff. 2002. What Are Patients and Their Families Told about the Diagnosis of Dementia? Results of a Family Survey. *International Journal of Geriatric Psychiatry* 17:218–21.

Holst, Göran, and Ingalill R. Hallberg. 2003. Exploring the Meaning of Everyday Life for Those Suffering from Dementia. *American Journal of Alzheimer's Disease and Other Dementias* 18(6):359–65.

Holstein, Martha. 1997. Alzheimer's Disease and Senile Dementia, 1885–1920: An Interpretive History of Disease Negotiation. *Journal of Aging Studies* 11(1):1–13.

Horton-Salway, Mary. 2002. Bio-Psycho-Social Reasoning in GPs' Case Narratives: The Discursive Construction of ME Patients' Identities. *Health: An Interdisciplinary Journal for the Social Study of Health, Illness and Medicine* 6(4):401–21.

Horwitz, Allan V. 2002. *Creating Mental Illness.* Chicago: University of Chicago Press.

Hughes, Everett C. 1958. *Men and Their Work.* Glencoe: Free Press.

———. 1962. Good People and Dirty Work. *Social Problems* 10(1):3–10.

———. 1997. Careers. *Qualitative Sociology* 20(3):389–97.

Hulko, Wendy. 2009. From "Not a Big Deal" to "Hellish": Experiences of Older People with Dementia. *Journal of Aging Studies* 23:131–44.

Humphrey, Nicholas. 1992. *A History of the Mind: Evolution and the Birth of Consciousness.* New York: Springer-Verlag.

Husband, H. J. 1999. The Psychological Consequences of Learning a Diagnosis of Dementia: Three Case Examples. *Aging and Mental Health* 3:179–83.

Hyman, Bradley T. 1996. Alzheimer's Disease or Alzheimer's Diseases? Clues from Molecular Epidemiology. *Annals of Neurology* 40(2):135–36.

Ivnik, Robert J., Glenn E. Smith, Eric G. Tangalos, Ronald C. Petersen, Emre Kokmen, and Leonard T. Kurland. 1991. Wechsler Memory Scale: IQ-Dependent Norms for Persons Aged 65 to 97 Years. *Psychological Assessment: A Journal of Consulting and Clinical Psychology* 3(2):156–61.

Jack, Clifford R. Jr., Marilyn S. Albert, David S. Knopman, Guy S. McKhann, Reisa A. Sperling, Maria C. Carrillo, Bill Theis, and Creighton H. Phelps. 2011. Introduction to the Recommendations from the National Institute on Aging and the Alzheimer's Association Workgroups on Diagnostic Guidelines for Alzheimer's Disease. *Alzheimer's and Dementia* 7:257–62.

Jack, Clifford R. Jr., Ronald C. Petersen, Yue Cheng Xu. Stephen C. Waring, Peter C. O'Brien, Eric G. Tangalos, Glenn E. Smith, Robert J. Ivnik, and Emre Kokmen. 1997. Medial Temporal Atrophy on MRI in Normal Aging and Very Mild Alzheimer's Disease. *Neurology* 49:786–94.

Jellinger, Kurt A. 1996. Diagnostic Accuracy of Alzheimer's Disease and Related Dementias. *Acta Neuropathology* 91:219–20.

Jenkins, Janis Hunter, and Robert John Barrett, eds. 2004. *Schizophrenia, Culture, and Subjectivity: The Edge of Experience*. Cambridge, U.K.: Cambridge University Press.

Johnson, Keith A., Kendall Jones, B. Leonard Holman, J. Alex Becker, Paul A. Spiers, Andrew Satlin, and Marilyn S. Albert. 1998. Preclinical Prediction of Alzheimer's Disease Using SPECT. *Neurology* 50:1563–72.

Jonsson, Thorlakur, Hreinn Stefansson, Stacy Steinberg, Ingileif Jonsdottir, Palmi V. Jonsson, Jon Snaedal, Sigurbjorn Bjornsson, Johanna Huttenlocher, Allan I. Levey, James J. Lah, Dan Rujescu, Harald Hampel, Ina Giegling, Ole A. Andreassen, Knut Engedal, Ingun Ulstein, Srdjan Djurovic, Carla Ibrahim-Verbaas, Albert Hofman, M. Arfan Ikram, Cornelia M van Duijn, Unnur Thorsteinsdottir, Augustine Kong, and Kari Stefansson. 2013. Variant of *TREM2* Associated with the Risk of Alzheimer's Disease. *New England Journal of Medicine* 368:107–16.

Josephs, Keith A., Jennifer L. Whitwell, Nirubol Tosakulwong, Stephen D. Weigand, Melissa E. Murray, Amanda M. Serie, Leonard Petrucelli, Matthew L. Senjem, Robert J. Ivnik, Joseph E. Parisi, Ronald C. Petersen, and Dennis W. Dickson. 2015. TDP-43 and Pathological Subtype of Alzheimer's Disease Impact Clinical Features. *Annals of Neurology*. Accepted Article, doi: 10.1002/ana.24493

Joyce, Kelly A. 2008. *Magnetic Appeal: MRI and the Myth of Transparency*. Ithaca, N.Y.: Cornell University Press.

Kalmijn, Sandra, Lenore J. Launer, Alewijn Ott, Jacqueline C. M. Witteman, Albert Hoffman, and Monique M. B. Breteler. 1997. Dietary Fat Intake and the Risk of Incident Dementia in the Rotterdam Study. *Annals of Neurology* 42(5):776–82.

Karp, David A. 1994. Living with Depression: Illness and Identity Turning Points. *Qualitative Health Research* 4(1):6–30.

———. 1996. *Speaking of Sadness: Depression, Disconnection, and the Meanings of Illness*. New York: Oxford University Press.

Kastenbaum, Robert J. 1969. "Psychological Death." In *Death and Dying: Current Issues in the Treatment of the Dying Person*, edited by L. Pearson. Ohio: Case Western Reserve University Press.

Katz, Stephen. 1996. *Disciplining Old Age: The Formation of Gerontological Knowledge*. Charlottesville: University Press of Virginia.

Katzman, Robert. 1976. The Prevalence and Malignancy of Alzheimer's Disease: A Major Killer. *Archives of Neurology* 33:217–18.

Kaufman, Sharon R. 1986. *The Ageless Self: Sources of Meaning in Later Life*. Wisconsin: University of Wisconsin Press.

———. 1994a. Old Age, Disease, and the Discourse on Risk: Geriatric Assessment in U.S. Health Care. *Medical Anthropology Quarterly* 8(4):430–47.

———. 1994b. The Social Construction of Frailty: An Anthropological Perspective. *Journal of Aging Studies* 8(1):45–58.

Kaufman, Sharon R., Janet K. Shim, and Ann J. Russ. 2004. Revisiting the Biomedicalization of Aging: Clinical Trends and Ethical Challenges. *Gerontologist* 44(6):731–38.

Keady, John, and Jane Gilliard. 2002. "Testing Times: The Experience of Neuropsychological Assessment for People with Suspected Alzheimer's Disease." Pp. 3–28 in *The Person with Alzheimer's Disease: Pathways to Understanding the Experience*, edited by P. Braudy Harris. Baltimore: Johns Hopkins University Press.

Keage, Hannah A. D., Sally Hunter, Fiona E. Matthews, Paul G. Ince, John Hodges, Suvi R. K. Hokkanen, J. Robin Highley, Tom Dening, and Carol Brayne. 2014. TDP-43 Pathology in the Population: Prevalence and Associations with Dementia and Age. *Journal of Alzheimer's Disease*. 42(2): 641–50.

Keating, Peter, and Alberto Cambrosio. 2003. *Biomedical Platforms: Realigning the Normal and the Pathological in Late-Twentieth-Century Medicine*. Cambridge, Mass.: MIT Press.

Kelly, Michael P., and Hilary Dickinson. 1997. The Narrative Self in Autobiographical Accounts of Illness. *Sociological Review* 45(2):254–78.

Kenen, Regina, Audrey Ardern-Jones, and Rosalind Eeles. 2003. Living with Chronic Risk: Healthy Women with a Family History of Breast/Ovarian Cancer. *Health, Risk and Society* 5(3):315–31.

Khalil, Abdelouahed, Hicham Berrougui, Graham Pawelec, and Tamas Fulop. 2012. Impairment of the ABCA1 and SR-BI-Mediated Cholesterol Efflux Pathways and HDL Anti-Inflammatory Activity in Alzheimer's Disease. *Mechanisms of Ageing and Development* 133(1):20–29.

Kitwood, Thomas, and Kathleen Bredin. 1992. Towards a Theory of Dementia Care: Personhood and Well-Being. *Ageing and Society* 12:268–87.

———. 1993. Person and Process in Dementia. *International Journal of Geriatric Psychiatry* 8:541–45.

Klawiter, Maren. 1999. Racing for the Cure, Walking Women, and Toxic Touring: Mapping Cultures of Action within the Bay Area Terrain of Breast Cancer. *Social Problems* 46(1):104–26.

Kleinman, Arthur. 1980. *Patients and Healers in the Context of Culture: An Exploration of the Borderland between Anthropology, Medicine, and Psychiatry*. Berkeley: University of California Press.

———. 1988. *The Illness Narratives: Suffering, Healing, and the Human Condition*. New York: Basic Books.

———. 1999. *Experience and Its Moral Modes: Culture, Human Conditions, and Disorder*. The Tanner Lectures on Human Values 20:355–420.

Kliger, Robin A. 2000. The Making and Unmaking of a Modern Memory: An Anthropological Account of the Repressed Memory Controversy. Berkeley: University of California Doctoral Dissertations.

Kluger, Alan, Steven H. Ferris, James Golomb, Mary S. Mittleman, and Barry Reisberg. 1999. Neuropsychological Prediction of Decline to Dementia in Nondemented Elderly. *Journal of Geriatric Psychiatry and Neurology* 12:168–79.

Knauss, Jenny, and Don Moyer. 2006. The Role of Advocacy in Our Adventure with Alzheimer's. *Dementia: International Journal of Social Research and Practice* 5(1):67–72.

Koch, Lene, and Mette N. Svendsen. 2005. Providing Solutions—Defining Problems: The Imperative of Disease Prevention in Genetic Counseling. *Social Science and Medicine* 60:823–32.

Kohut, Sylvester, Jeraldine Kohut, and Joseph J. Fleishman. 1987. *Reality Orientation for the Elderly.* Oradell, N.J.: Medical Economics Books.

Kokler, Emily S. 2004. Framing as a Cultural Resource in Health Social Movements: Funding Activism and the Breast Cancer Movement in the U.S., 1990–1993. *Sociology of Health and Illness* 26(6):820–44.

Kontos, Pia C. 2004. Ethnographic Reflections on Selfhood, Embodiment and Alzheimer's Disease. *Ageing and Society* 24:829–49.

Kral, Vojtech A. 1962. Senescent Forgetfulness: Benign and Malignant. *Canadian Medical Association Journal* 86:257–60.

Kramer, Larry. 1989. *Reports of the Holocaust.* New York: St. Martin's Press.

Kramer, Peter D. 1993. *Listening to Prozac: A Psychiatrist Explores Antidepressant Drugs and the Remaking of the Self.* New York: Viking.

Krasuki, Jack S., Gene E. Alexander, Barry Horwitz, Eileen M. Daly, Declan G. M. Murphy, Stanley I. Rapoport, and Mark B. Schapiro. 1998. Volumes of Medial Temporal Lobe Structures in Patients with Alzheimer's Disease and Mild Cognitive Impairment (and in Healthy Controls). *Biological Psychiatry* 43:60–68.

Kroll-Smith, Stephen, and H. Hugh Floyd. 1997 *Bodies in Protest: Environmental Illness and the Struggle over Medical Knowledge.* New York: NYU Press.

La Fata, Giorgio, Peter Weber, and M. Hasan Mohajeri. 2014. Effects of Vitamin E on Cognitive Performance during Ageing and in Alzheimer's Disease. *Nutrients* 6(12):5453–72.

Larson, Eric B., Marie-Florence Shadlen, Wayne C. McCormick, James D. Bowen, Linda Teri, and Walter A. Kukull. 2004. Survival after Initial Diagnosis of Alzheimer Disease. *Annals of Internal Medicine* 6(April):501–09.

Latour, Bruno. 1987. *Science in Action: How to Follow Scientists and Engineers through Society.* Cambridge, Mass.: Harvard University Press.

———. 1999. *Pandora's Hope: Essays on the Reality of Science Studies.* Cambridge, Mass.: Harvard University Press.

Latour, Bruno, and Steve Woolgar. 1986/1979. *Laboratory Life: The Social Construction of Scientific Facts.* Princeton, N.J.: Princeton University Press.

Lau, Chi-Fai, Yuen-Shan Ho, Clara Hiu-Ling Hung, Suthicha Wuwongse, Chun-Hei Poon, Kin Chiu, Xifei Yang, Leung-Wing Chu, and Raymond Chuen-Chung Chang. 2014. Protective Effects of Testosterone on Presynaptic Terminals against Oligomeric -Amyloid Peptide in Primary Culture of Hippocampal Neurons. *BioMedical Research International*, Article ID 103906, 12 pages. doi. org/10.1155/2014/103906

Lauritzen, Sonja O. 2004. Lay Voices on Allergic Conditions in Children: Parents' Narratives and the Negotiation of a Diagnosis. *Social Science and Medicine* 58(7):1299–1308.

Lawton, Julia. 2003. Lay Experiences of Health and Illness: Past Research and Future Agendas. *Sociology of Health and Illness* 25(3):23–40.

Lawton, M. Powell, Miriam Moss, Morton H. Kleban, Allen Glicksman, and Michael Rovine. 1991. A Two-Factor Model of Caregiving Appraisal and Psychological Well-Being. *Journal of Gerontology: Psychological Sciences* 46:81–89.

Le Couteur, David G., Jenny Doust, Helen Creasey, and Carol Brayne. 2013. Political Drive to Screen for Pre-Dementia: Not Evidence Based and Ignores the Harms of Diagnosis. *British Medical Journal* 347(7925):f5125.

Ledoux, Joseph. 2003. *Synaptic Self: How Our Brains Become Who We Are*. London: Penguin Books.

Lennox, Jenepher T., and Blake E. Ashforth. 2002. From "I" to "We": The Role of Putdown Humor and Identity in the Development of a Temporary Group. *Human Relations* 55(1):55–88.

Levi, Ron. 2000. The Mutuality of Risk and Community: The Adjudication of Community Notification Statutes. *Economy and Society* 29(4):578–601.

Levy-Reiner, Sherry, ed. 1999. *The Adaptable Brain: Decade of the Brain*. Clooingdale, Pa.: Diane Publishing Company.

Lim, Giselle P., Fusheng Yang, Teresa Chu, P. Chen, W. Beech, B. Teter, T. Tran, O. Ubeda, K. Hsiao Ashe, S. A. Frautschy, and Greg M. Cole. 2000. Ibuprofen Suppresses Plaque Pathology and Inflammation in a Mouse Model for Alzheimer's Disease. *Journal of Neuroscience* 20(15):5709–14.

Lindesay, James, Mangesh Marudkar, Erik van Diepen, and Gordon Wilcock. 2002. The Second Leicester Survey of Memory Clinics in the British Isles. *International Journal of Geriatric Psychiatry* 17(1), 41–47.

Lobo Antonio, Pedro Saz, Guillermo Marcos, José-Luis Dia, Concepcion De-la-Camara, Tirso Ventura, José Angel Montañes, Antonio Lobo-Escolar, and Sergio Aznar. 2007. Prevalence of Dementia in a Southern European Population in Two Different Time Periods: The ZARADEMP Project. *Acta Psychiatrica Scandinavica* 116(4):299–307.

Lock, Margaret. 1993. *Encounters with Aging: Mythologies of Menopause in Japan and North America*. Berkeley, Calif.: University of California Press.

———. 2000. "Accounting for Disease and Distress: Morals of the Normal and Abnormal." Pp. 259–76 in *Handbook of Social Studies in Health and Medicine*, edited by R. Fitzgerald, G. L. Albrecht, and S. C. Scrimshaw. Thousand Oaks, Calif.: Sage Publications.

———. 2013. *The Alzheimer Conundrum: Entanglements of Dementia and Aging*. Princeton, N.J.: Princeton University Press.

Lock, Margaret, Allan Young, and Alberto Cambrosio, eds. 2000. *Living and Working with the New Medical Technologies: Intersections of Inquiry.* Cambridge, U.K.: Cambridge University Press.

Loe, Meika. 2011. *Aging Our Way: Lessons for Living from 85 and Beyond.* Oxford, U.K.: Oxford University Press.

Lopez, Oscar L., James T. Becker, Denise Somsak, Mary Amanda Dew, and Steven T. DeKosky. 1994. Awareness of Cognitive Deficits and Anosognosia in Probable Alzheimer's Disease. *European Neurology* 34(5):277–82.

Lutfey, Karen E., and John B. McKinlay. 2009. What Happens along the Diagnostic Pathway to CHD Treatment? Qualitative Results concerning Cognitive Processes. *Sociology of Health and Illness* 31(7):1077–92.

Lyman, Karen. 1989. Bringing the Social Back In: A Critique of the Biomedicalization of Dementia. *Gerontologist* 29(5):597–605.

———. 1993. *Day In, Day Out with Alzheimer's.* Philadelphia: Temple University Press.

Mace, Nancy L., and Paul V. Rabins. 2001/1987. *The 36-Hour Day: A Family Guide to Caring for Persons with Alzheimer Disease, Related Dementing Illnesses, and Memory Loss in Later Life.* New York: Warner Books.

MacQuarrie, Colleen R. 2005. Experiences in Early Stage AD: Understanding the Paradox of Acceptance and Denial. *Aging and Mental Health* 9(5):430–41.

Mandybur, Thaddeus I. 1990. The Distribution of Alzheimer's Neurofibrillary Tangles and Gliosis in Chronic Subacute Sclerosing Panencephalitis. *Acta Neuropathologica* 80:307–10.

Mannings, Nick. 2000. Psychiatric Diagnosis under Conditions of Uncertainty: Personality Disorder, Science and Professional Legitimacy. *Sociology of Health and Illness* 22(5):621–39.

Manthorpe, Jill, Kritika Samsi, Sarah Campbell, Clare Abley, John Keady, John Bond, Sue Watts, Louise Robinson, James Warner, and Steve Iliffe. 2013. From Forgetfulness to Dementia: Clinical and Commissioning Implications of Diagnostic Experiences. *British Journal of General Practice* 63(606):e69-e75.

Manton Kenneth G., XiLiang Gu, and Svetlana Ukraintseva. 2005. Declining Prevalence of Dementia in the U.S. Elderly Population. *Advances in Gerontology* 16:30–37.

Marcus, Gary. 2004. *The Birth of the Mind: How a Tiny Number of Genes Creates the Complexities of Human Thought.* New York: Basic Books.

Marutle, Amelia, Per-Göran Gillberg, Assar Bergfors, Wenfeng Yu, Ruiqing Ni, Inger Nennesmo, Larysa Voytenko, and Agneta Nordberg. 2013. 3H-Deprenyl and 3H-PIB Autoradiography Show Different Laminar Distributions of Astroglia and Fibrillar β-Amyloid in Alzheimer Brain. *Journal of Neuroinflammation* 10(1):90.

Marzanski, Marek. 2000. On Telling the Truth to Patients with Dementia. *Western Journal of Medicine* 173:318–23.

Mattingly, Cheryl, and Linda C. Garro, eds. 2000. *Narrative and the Cultural Construction of Illness and Healing.* Berkeley: University of California Press.

Mauer, Konrad, Stephan Volk, and Hector Gerbaldo. 2000. "Auguste D.: The History of Alois Alzheimer's First Case." Pp. 5–29 in *Concepts of Alzheimer's Disease: Biologi-*

cal, Clinical and Cultural Perspectives, edited by P. J. Whitehouse, K. Maurer, and J. F. Ballenger. Baltimore: Johns Hopkins University Press.

Mauldin, R. Kirk. 2002. The Role of Humor in the Social Construction of Gendered and Ethnic Stereotypes. *Race, Gender and Class* 9(3):76–95.

May, Carl, Gayle Allison, Alison Chapple, Carolyn Chew-Graham, Clare Dixon, Linda Gask, Ruth Graham, Anne Rogers, and Martin Roland. 2004. Framing the Doctor-Patient Relationship in Chronic Illness: A Comparative Study of General Practitioners; Accounts. *Sociology of Health and Illness* 26(2):135–58.

McAllister, Thomas W., and Richard Powers. 1994. "Approaches to the Treatment of Dementing Illness." Pp. 355–83 in *Dementia: Presentations, Differential Diagnosis, and Nosology*, edited by V. O. B. Emery and T. E. Oxman. Baltimore: Johns Hopkins University Press.

McGrowder, Donovan, Cliff Riley, Errol Y. St. A. Morrison, and Lorenzo Gordon. 2011. The Role of High-Density Lipoproteins in Reducing the Risk of Vascular Diseases, Neurogenerative Disorders, and Cancer. *Cholesterol*. Article ID 496925, 9 pages. doi:10.1155/2011/496925

McIntosh, James, and Neil McKeganey. 2000. Addicts' Narratives of Recovery from Drug Use: Constructing a Non-Addict Identity. *Social Science and Medicine* 50:1501–10.

McKelvey, Robert, Howard Bergman, John Stern, C. Rush, G. Zahirney, and H. Chertkow. 1999. Lack of Prognostic Significance of SPECT Abnormalities in Elderly Subjects with a Mild Memory Loss. *Canadian Journal of Neurological Sciences* 26:23–28.

Medlicott, Diana. 1999. Surviving in the Time Machine: Suicidal Prisoners and the Pains of Prison Time. *Time and Society* 8(2):211–30.

Merleau-Ponty, Maurice. 1965. *The Role of the Body-Subject in Interpersonal Relations*. Pittsburgh, Pa.: Duquesne University Press.

Meyer, John W., and Brian Rowan. 1977. Institutionalized Organizations: Formal Structures as Myths and Ceremony. *American Journal of Sociology* 83:340–63.

Miller, Baila, Michael Glasser, and Susan Rubin. 1992. A Paradox of Medicalization: Physicians, Families and Alzheimer's Disease. *Journal of Aging Studies* 6:135–48.

Mills, C. Wright. 1959. *The Sociological Imagination*. London: Oxford University Press.

Mills, Maria A. 1997. Narrative Identity and Dementia: A Study of Emotion and Narrative in Older People with Dementia. *Ageing and Society* 17:673–98.

Milne, Alisoun Janice, H. H. Woolford, J. Mason, and Eleni Hatzidimitriadou. 2000. Early Diagnosis of Dementia by GPs: An Exploratory Study of Attitudes. *Aging and Mental Health* 4:292–300.

Ming, Chen, and Hugo L. Fernandez. 2001. Alzheimer Movement Re-Examined 25 Years Later: Is It a "Disease" or a Senile Condition in Medical Nature? *Frontiers in Bioscience* 6:e30–40.

Mitchell, Alex J., Nicholas Meader, and Michael Pentzek. 2011. Clinical Recognition of Dementia and Cognitive Impairment in Primary Care: A Meta-Analysis of Physician Accuracy. *Acta Psychiatrica Scandinavica* 124(3):165–83.

Mitchell, Alex J., and Mojtaba Shiri-Feshki. 2009. Rate of Progression of Mild Cognitive Impairment to Dementia—Meta-Analysis of 41 Robust Inception Cohort Studies. *Acta Psychiatrica Scandinavica* 119(4):252–65.

Moller, H-J., and M. B. Graeber. 2000. "Johann F: The Historical Relevance of the Case for the Concept of Alzheimer Disease." Pp. 30–46 in *Concepts of Alzheimer Disease: Biological, Clinical, and Cultural Perspectives*, edited by P. J. Whitehouse, K. Maurer, and J. F. Ballenger. Baltimore: Johns Hopkins University Press.

Moore, Dawn, and Mariana Valverde. 2000. Maidens at Risk: "Date Rape Drugs" and the Formation of Hybrid Risk Knowledges. *Economy and Society* 29(4):514–31.

Moreira, Tiago, Carl May, and John Bond. 2009. Regulatory Objectivity in Action: Mild Cognitive Impairment and the Collective Production of Uncertainty. *Social Studies of Science* 39(5):665–90.

Morris, John C., and J. L. Price. 2001. Pathologic Correlates of Nondemented Aging, Mild Cognitive Impairment, and Early-Stage Alzheimer's Disease. *Journal of Molecular Neuroscience* 17:101–18.

Mrackova, Alzbeta. 2004. The Interaction of a Doctor and a Patient When Giving Unwelcome News. *Sociologia—Slovak Sociological Review* 36(1):57–84.

Nag, Sukriti, Lei Yu, Ana W. Capuano, Robert S. Wilson, Sue E. Leurgans, David A. Bennett, and Julie A. Schneider. 2015. Hippocampal Sclerosis and TDP-43 Pathology in Aging and Alzheimer Disease. *Annals of Neurology*. Accepted Article, doi: 10.1002/ana.24388.

National Institutes of Health (NIH). 2015. Estimates of Funding for Various Research, Condition, and Disease Categories (RCDC). Retrieved 3/23/15 from: http://report.nih.gov/categorical_spending.aspx

Nelkin, Dorothy, and M. Susan Lindee. 1995. Elvis' DNA: The Gene as a Cultural Icon. *Humanist* 55(3):10–19.

Nettleton, Sarah, Lisa O'Malley, Ian Watt, and Philip Duffey. 2004. Enigmatic Illness: Narratives of Patients Who Live with Medically Unexplained Symptoms. *Social Theory and Health* 2(1):47–66.

Newton, R. D. 1948. Identity of Alzheimer's Disease and Senile Dementia and Their Relationship to Senility. *Journal of Mental Science* 94:225–49.

Niederehe, G. T., and Thomas E Oxman. 1994. "The Dementias: Construct and Nosologic Validity." Pp. 19–45 in *Dementia: Presentations, Differential Diagnosis, and Nosology*, edited by V. O. B. Emery and T. E. Oxman. Baltimore: Johns Hopkins University Press.

Noonan, Ann E., and Sharon Tennstedt. 1997. Meaning in Caregiving and Its Contribution to Caregiver Well-Being. *Gerontologist* 37(6):785–94.

Norton, Sam, Fiona W. Matthews, and Carol Brayne. 2013. A Commentary on Studies Presenting Projections of the Future Prevalence of Dementia. *BMC Public Health* 13:1–5. http://www.biomedcentral.com/1471-2458/13/1.

Notkola, I-L., Raimo Sulkava, Juha Pekkanen, Timo Erkinjuntti, Christian Ehnholm, Paula Kivinen, Jaakko Tuomilehto, and Aulikki Nissinen. 1998. Serum Total Cholesterol, Apolipoprotein E Epsilon 4 Allele, and Alzheimer's Disease. *Neuroepidemiology* 17(1):14–20.

Novas, Carlos, and Nikolas Rose. 2000. Genetic Risk and the Birth of the Somatic Individual. *Economy and Society* 29(4):485–513.

Oberg, Pamela. 1996. The Absent Body—A Social Gerontological Paradox. *Ageing and Society* 16:701–19.

O'Grady, Aoife, Pascoe Pleasence, Nigel J. Balmer, Alexy Buck, and Hazel Genn. 2004. Disability, Social Exclusion and the Consequential Experience of Justiciable Problems. *Disability and Society* 19(3):259–71.

Oliver, J. Eric. 2006. *Fat Politics: The Real Story Behind America's Obesity Epidemic.* Cambridge, U.K.: Oxford University Press.

Orona, Celia J. 1990. Temporality and Identity Loss due to Alzheimer's Disease. *Social Science and Medicine* 30(11):1247–56.

Oxman, Thomas E., and K. Baynes. 1994. "Boundaries between Normal Aging and Dementia." Pp. 3–18 in *Dementia: Presentations, Differential Diagnosis, and Nosology,* edited by V. O. B. Emery and T. E. Oxman. Baltimore: Johns Hopkins University Press.

Palmer, Katie, Laura Fratiglioni, and Bengt Winblad. 2003. What Is Mild Cognitive Impairment? Variations in Definitions and Evolution of Nondemented Persons with Cognitive Impairment. *Acta Neurologica Scandinavica* 107(s179):14–20.

Parsons, Talcott. 1951. *The Social System.* Glencoe, Ill.: Free Press.

Perakyla, Anssi. 2002. Agency and Authority: Extended Responses to Diagnostic Statements in Primary Care Encounters. *Research on Language and Social Interaction* 35(2):219–47.

Petersen, Ronald C. 2004. Mild Cognitive Impairment as a Diagnostic Entity. *Journal of Internal Medicine* 256:183–94.

Petersen, Ronald C., Glenn E. Smith, Robert J. Ivnik, Emre Kokmen, and Eric G. Tangalos. 1994. Memory Function in Very Early Alzheimer's Disease. *Neurology* 44:867–72.

Petersen, Ronald C., Glenn E. Smith, Robert J. Ivnik, Eric G. Tangalos, Daniel J. Schaid, Stephen N. Thibodeau, Emre Kokmen, Stephen C. Waring, and Leonard T. Kurland. 1995. Apolipoprotein E Status as a Predictor of the Development of Alzheimer's Disease in Memory-Impaired Individuals. *Journal of the American Medical Association* 273:1274–78.

Petersen, Ronald C., Glenn E. Smith, Stephen C. Waring, Robert J. Ivnik, Emre Kokmen, and Eric G. Tangalos. 1997. Aging, Memory and Mild Cognitive Impairment. *International Psychogeriatrics* 9:65–69.

Petersen, Ronald C., Glenn E. Smith, Stephen C. Waring. Robert J. Ivnik, Eric G. Tangalos, and Emre Kokmen. 1999. Mild Cognitive Impairment: Clinical Characterization and Outcome. *Archives of Neurology* 56:303–08.

Phelan, Michael P., and Scott A. Hunt. 1998. Prison Gang Members' Tattoos as Identity Work: The Visual Communication of Moral Careers. *Symbolic Interaction* 21(3):277–98.

Phinney, Alison, and Catherine A. Chesla. 2003. The Lived Body of Dementia. *Journal of Aging Studies* 17:283–99.

Pinker, Steven. 1997. *How the Mind Works*. New York: Norton.

———. 2001. *The Blank Slate*. New York: Viking.

Poon, Leon W. 1985. "Differences in Human Memory with Aging: Nature, Causes, and Clinical Implications." Pp. 427–62 in *Handbook of the Psychology of Aging*, edited by K. W. Shaie. New York: Van Nostrand Reinhold.

Popay, Jennie, Gareth Williams, Carol Thomas, and Tony Gatrell. 1998. Theorising Inequalities in Health: The Place of Lay Knowledge. *Sociology of Health and Illness* 20(5):619–44.

Post, Stephen G. 1994. Genetics, Ethics, and Alzheimer Disease. *Journal of the American Geriatrics Society* 42(7):782–86.

———. 1995. *The Moral Challenge of Alzheimer's Disease*. Baltimore: Johns Hopkins University Press.

———. 2000. "Concepts of Alzheimer's Disease in a Hypercognitive Society." Pp. 245–56 in *Concepts of Alzheimer's Disease: Biological, Clinical and Cultural Perspectives*, edited by P. J. Whitehouse, K. Maurer, and J. F. Ballenger. Baltimore: Johns Hopkins University Press.

Price, John L., and John C. Morris. 1999. Tangles and Plaques in Nondemented Aging and "Preclinical" Alzheimer's Disease. *Annals of Neurology* 45:358–68.

Prussing, Erica, Elisa J. Sobo, Elizabeth Walker, and Paul S. Kurtin. 2005. Between "Desperation" and Disability Rights: A Narrative Analysis of Complementary/Alternative Medicine Use by Parents for Children with Down Syndrome. *Social Science and Medicine* 60:587–98.

Rabinow, Paul. 1992. "Artificiality and Enlightenment: From Sociobiology to Biosociality." Pp. 234–52 in *Incorporations*, edited by J. Crary and S. Kwinter. New York: Zone.

———. 1996. *Essays on the Anthropology of Reason*. Princeton, N.J.: Princeton University Press.

Radley, Alan, and Susan E. Bell. 2007. Artworks, Collective Experience and Claims for Social Justice: The Case of Women Living with Breast Cancer. *Sociology of Health and Illness* 29(3):366–90.

Rapp, Rayna. 1999. *Testing Women, Testing Fetuses: The Social Impact of Amniocentesis in America*. New York: Routledge.

Reisberg Barry, Melanie B. Shulman, Carol Torossian, Ling Leng, and Wei Zhu. 2010. Outcome over Seven Years of Healthy Adults with and without Subjective Cognitive Impairment. *Alzheimers and Dementia* 6(1):11–24.

Rier, David A. 2000. The Missing Voice of the Critically Ill: A Medical Sociologist's First-Person Account. *Sociology of Health and Illness* 22(1):68–93.

Riley, John. 2000. Sensemaking in Prison: Inmate Identity as a Working Understanding. *Justice Quarterly* 17(2):359–76.

Rinken, Sebastian. 1997. The Event of Diagnosis. Diagnosis of HIV/AIDS as a Crisis of Self-Description. *Soziale Systeme* 3(1):101–21.

Ritchie, Karen, Bernard Lédesert, and Jacques Touchon. 2000. Subclinical Cognitive Impairment: Epidemiology and Clinical Characteristics. *Comprehensive Psychiatry* 41:61–65.

Ritchie, Karen, and Jacques Touchon. 2000. Mild Cognitive Impairment: Conceptual Basis and Current Nosological Status. *Lancet* 355:225–28.

Robertson, Ann. 1990. The Politics of Alzheimer's Disease: A Case Study in Apocalyptic Demography. *International Journal of Health Services* 20(3):429–42.

———. 2000. Embodying Risk, Embodying Political Rationality: Women's Accounts of Risks for Breast Cancer. *Health, Risk and Society* 2(2):219–35.

Robinson, Louise, Alan Gemski, Clare Abley, and John Bond. 2011. The Transition to Dementia—Individual and Family Experiences of Receiving a Diagnosis: A Review. *International Psychogeriatrics* 23(7):1026–43.

Romas, Stavra N., Ming-Xin Tang, Lars Berlung, and Richard Mayeux. 1999. APOE Genotype, Plasma Lipids, Lipoproteins, and AD in Community Elderly. *Neurology* 53(3):517–21.

Rose, Larry. 1996. *Show Me the Way to Go Home.* San Francisco: Elder Books.

Rose, Nikolas. 1998. *Inventing Our Selves: Psychology, Power, and Personhood.* Cambridge, U.K.: Cambridge University Press.

———. 2006. *The Politics of Life Itself: Biomedicine, Power, and Subjectivity in the Twenty-First Century.* Princeton, N.J.: Princeton University Press.

Rose, Steven. 2005. *The Future of the Brain: The Promise and Perils of Tomorrow's Neuroscience.* Oxford, U.K.: Oxford University Press.

Roth, Nancy L., and M. S. Nelson. 1997. HIV Diagnosis Rituals and Identity Narratives. *AIDS Care* 9(2):161–79.

Rubin, Eugene H., Martha Storandt, J. Philip Miller, Dorothy A. Kinscherf, Elizabeth A. Grant, John C. Morris, and Leonard Berg. 1998. A Prospective Study of Cognitive Function and Onset of Dementia in Cognitively Healthy Elders. *Archives of Neurology* 55:395–401.

Rucht, Dieter. 1996. "The Impact of National Contexts on Social Movement Structures: A Cross-Movement and Cross-National Comparison." Pp. 185–204 in *Comparative Perspectives on Social Movements,* edited by D. McAdam, J. McCarthy, and M. Zald. New York: Cambridge University Press.

Sabat, Steven R., and Ron Harre. 1992. The Construction and Deconstruction of Self in Alzheimer's Disease. *Ageing and Society* 12(4):443–61.

———. 2001. *The Experience of Alzheimer's Disease: Life through a Tangled Veil.* Oxford: Blackwell Publishers.

Sandstrom, Kent L. 1990. Confronting Deadly Disease: The Drama of Identity Construction among Gay Men with AIDS. *Journal of Contemporary Ethnography* 19(3):271–94.

Sano, Mary, Christopher Ernesto, Ronald G. Thomas, Melville R. Klauber, Kimberly Schafer, Michael Grundman, Peter Woodbury, John Growdon, Carl W. Cotman, Eric Pfeiffer, Lon S. Schneider, and Leon J. Thal. 1997. A Controlled Trial of Selegiline, Alpha-Tocopherol, or Both as Treatment for Alzheimer's Disease.

The Alzheimer's Disease Cooperative Study. *New England Journal of Medicine* 336:1216–22.

Saunders, Ann M., Warren J. Strittmatter, Don E. Schmechel, P. H. St. George-Hyslop, Pericak-Vance, S. H. Joo, B. L. Rosi, J. F. Gusella, D. R. Crapper-MacLachlan, M. J. Alberts, C. Hulette, B. Crain, D. Goldgaber, and A. D. Roses. 1993. Association of Apolipoprotein E Allele e4 with Late-Onset Familial and Sporadic Alzheimer's Disease. *Neurology* 43:1467–72.

Schenk, Dale B., Robin Barbour, Whitney Dunn, Grace Gordo, Henry Grajeda, Teresa Guido, Kang Hu, Jiping Huang, Kelly Johnson-Wood, Karen Khan, Dora Kholodenko, Mike Lee, Zhenmei Liao, Ivan Lieberburg, Ruth Motter, Linda Mutter, Ferdie Soriano, George Shopp, Nicki Vasquez, Christopher Vandevert, Shannan Walker, Mark Wogulis, Ted Yednock, Dora Games, and Peter Seubert. 1999. Immunization with Amyloid-Beta Attenuates Alzheimer-Disease-Like Pathology in the PDAPP Mouse. *Nature* 400:173–77.

Schenk, Dale B., Peter Seubert, Ivan Lieberburg, and Jan Wallace. 2000. B-Peptide Immunization: A Possible New Treatment for Alzheimer's Disease. *Archives of Neurology* 57(7):934–36.

Schrijvers, Elisabeth M. C., Benjamin F. J. Verhaaren, Peter J. Koudstaal, Albert Hofman, M. Arfan Ikram, and Monique M. B. Breteler. 2012. Is Dementia Incidence Declining? Trends in Dementia Incidence since 1990 in the Rotterdam Study. *Neurology* 78(19):1456–63.

Schulz, Richard. 2001. Some Critical Issues in Caregiver Intervention Research. *Aging and Mental Health* 5:S112–15.

Schutz, Alfred. 1967. *The Phenomenology of the Social World.* Evanston, Ill.: Northwestern University Press.

Selznick, Philip. 1949. *TVA and the Grass Roots: A Study in the Sociology of Formal Organization.* Berkeley, Calif.: University of California Press.

Shakespeare, Thomas. 1999. Joking a Part. *Body and Society* 5(4):47–52.

Shorter, Edward. 1991. Historical Changes in the Subjective Experiences of Alzheimer's Disease: The Role of Anxiety. *American Journal of Alzheimer's Care and Related Disorders and Research* May:35–39.

———. 1992. *From Paralysis to Fatigue: A History of Psychosomatic Illness in the Modern Era.* New York: Free Press.

Simons, Jon S., and Hugo J. Spiers. 2003. Prefrontal and Medial Temporal Lobe Interactions in Long-Term Memory. *Nature Reviews Neuroscience* 4:637–48.

Small, Brent J., Laura Fratiglioni, Matti Viitanan, Bengt Winblad, and Lars Backman. 2001. The Course of Preclinical Cognitive Deficits in Alzheimer's Disease. *Research and Practice in Alzheimer's Disease* 5:29–34.

Small, Gary W., Peter V. Rabins, Patricia P. Barry, Neil S. Buckholtz, Steven T. DeKosky, Steven H. Ferris, Sanford I. Finkel, Lisa P. Gwyther, Zaven S. Khachaturian, Barry D. Lebowitz, Thomas D. McRae, John C. Morris, Frances Oakley, Lon S. Schneider, Joel E. Streim, Trey Sunderland, Linda A. Teri, and Larry E. Tune. 1997. Diagnosis and Treatment of Alzheimer Disease and Related Disorders. *Journal of the American Medical Association* 278(16):1363–71.

Smith, André P. 2003. Medicalizing Intersubjectivity: Diagnostic Practices and the Self in Alzheimer's Disease. *Dissertation Abstracts International, A: The Humanities and Social Sciences* 63(7):2717-A.

Smith, Glenn E., and Robert J. Ivnik. 2003. "Normative Neuropsychology." Pp. 63–88 in *Mild Cognitive Impairment: Aging to Alzheimer's Disease*, edited by R. C. Petersen. New York: Oxford University Press.

Snowdon, David A. 2003. Healthy Ageing and Dementia: Findings from the Nun Study. *Annals of Internal Medicine* 139:450–54.

Society of Neuroscience. 2005. *NMDA Receptor Blockers*. Retrieved 3/15/05 from http://web.sfn.org/content/Publications/BrainBriefings/nmda.html.

Solfrizzi, Vincenzo, and Francesco Panza. 2015. Plant-Based Nutraceutical Interventions against Cognitive Impairment and Dementia: Meta-Analytic Evidence of Efficacy of a Standardized Gingko Biloba Extract. *Journal of Alzheimers Disease* 43(2):605–11. doi: 10.3233/JAD-141887.

Sontag, Susan. 1977. *Illness as Metaphor*. New York: Random House.

Sperling, Reisa A., Paul S. Aisen, Laurel A. Beckett, David A. Bennett, Suzanne Craft, Anne M. Fagan, Takeshi Iwatsubo, Clifford R. Jack, Jeffrey Kaye, Thomas J. Montine, Denise C. Park, Eric M. Reiman, Christopher C. Rowe, Eric Siemers, Yaakov Stern, Kristine Yaffe, Maria C. Carrillo, Bill Thies, Marcelle Morrison-Bogorad, Molly V. Wagster, and Creighton H. Phelps. 2011. Toward Defining the Preclinical Stages of Alzheimer's Disease: Recommendations from the National Institute of Aging and Alzheimer's Association Working Group. *Alzheimer's and Dementia* 7:280–92.

Staedt, Jürgen, and Gabriela Stoppe. 2005. Treatment of Rest-Activity Disorders in Dementia and Special Focus on Sundowning. *International Journal of Geriatric Psychiatry* 20(6):507–11.

Stafford, Pamela B. 1991. "The Social Construction of Alzheimer's Disease. Biosemiotics: The Semiotic Web." Pp. 393–406 in *Biosemiotics: The Semiotic Web*, edited by T. A. Seboek and J. Umiker-Sebeok. Berlin: Mouton de Gruyter.

Star, Susan L. 1992. "The Skin, the Skull, and the Self: Toward a Sociology of the Brain." Pp. 204–28 in *So Human a Brain: Knowledge and Values in the Neurosciences*, edited by A. Harrington. Boston: Birkhauser.

Steffen, Vibeke. 1997. Life Stories and Shared Experience. *Social Science and Medicine* 45:99–111.

Steffens, David C., Maria C. Norton, Brenda L. Plassman, JoAnn T. Tschanz, B. W. Wyse, Kathleen A. Welsh-Bohmer, J. C. Anthony, and John C. S. Breitner. 1999. Enhanced Cognitive Performance with Estrogen Use in Nondemented Community-Dwelling Older Women. *Journal of the American Geriatrics Society* 47(10):1171–75.

Sterin, G. 2002. Essay on a Word: A Lived Experience of Alzheimer's Disease. *Dementia: International Journal of Social Research and Practice* 1(1):7–10.

Stockdale, Alan. 1999. Waiting for the Cure: Mapping the Social Relations of Human Gene Therapy Research. *Sociology of Health and Illness* 21(5):579–96.

Strauss, Anselm L. 1959. *Mirrors and Masks: The Search for Identity.* New York: Free Press.

———. 1975. *Chronic Illness and the Quality of Life.* St. Louis: C. V. Mosby.

———. 1978. A Social Worlds Perspective. *Studies in Symbolic Interaction* 1:119–28.

Strauss, Anselm L., Susan Fagerhaugh, B. Suczek, and Carolyn Wiener. 1997. *Social Organization of Medical Work.* New Brunswick, N.J.: Transaction Publishers.

Sudnow, David. 1967. *Passing On: The Social Organization of Dying.* Englewood Cliffs, N.J.: Prentice Hall.

Sullivan, Susan Crawford, and Renée L. Beard. 2014. Faith and Forgetfulness: The Role of Spiritual Identity in Preservation of Self with Alzheimer's. *Journal of Religion, Spirituality and Aging* 26(1):65–91.

Sveilich, Carole. 2004. *Just Fine: Unmasking Concealed Chronic Illness and Pain.* New York: Avid Reader Press.

Swane, Christine E. 1993. Senile: Demented or Old? A Conceptual Difference. *Nord Nytt* 49 (February):97–107.

Swartz, R. H., S. E. Black, and P. St-George Hyslop. 1999. Apolopoprotein E and Alzheimer's Disease: A Genetic, Molecular, and Neuroimaging Review. *Canadian Journal of Neurological Sciences* 26(2):77–88.

Sweeting, Helen, and Mary Gilhooly. 1997. Dementia and the Phenomenon of Social Death. *Sociology of Health and Illness* 19(1):93–117.

Swora, Maria G. 2001. Personhood and Disease in Alcoholics Anonymous: A Perspective from the Anthropology of Religious Healing. *Mental Health, Religion and Culture* 4(1):1–21.

Tanzi, Rudolph E., and Ann B. Parson. 2000. *Decoding Darkness: The Search for the Genetic Causes of Alzheimer's Disease.* Cambridge, Mass.: Perseus Publishing.

Taylor, Joy L., Leah Friedman, Javaid Sheikh, and Jerome A. Yesavage. 1997. Assessment and Management of "Sundowning" Phenomena. *Seminars in Clinical Neuropsychiatry* 2(2):113–22.

Taylor, Richard. 2006. *Alzheimer's from the Inside Out.* Baltimore, Md.: Health Professions Press.

Terry, Robert, and Robert Katzman. 1983. *The Neurology of Aging.* Philadelphia: F. A. Davis Co.

Thorne, Sally, Barbara Paterson, Sonia Acorn, Connie Canam, Gloria Joachim, and Carol Jillings. 2002. Chronic Illness Experience: Insights from a Metastudy. *Qualitative Health Research* 12(4):437–52.

Tierney, M. C., J. P. Szalai, W. G. Snow, R. H. Fisher, T. Tsuda, H. Chi, D. R. McLachlan, and PH St George-Hyslop. 1996. A Prospective Study of the Clinical Utility of ApoE Genotype in the Prediction of Outcome in Patients with Memory Impairment. *Neurology* 46:149–54.

Timmermans, Stephen, and Alison Angell. 2001. Evidence-Based Medicine, Clinical Uncertainty, and Learning to Doctor. *Journal of Health and Social Behavior* 42(2):342–59.

Tishelman, Carol, and Lisbeth Sachs. 1998. The Diagnostic Process and the Boundaries of Normal. *Qualitative Health Research* 8(1):48–60.

Tobin, Sheldon S. 1999. The Deselfing Alzheimer's Disease and Preserving the Self When Nearing the End. In *Preservation of the Self in the Oldest Years: With Implications for Practice.* New York: Springer Publishing.

Tomlinson, B. E., G. Blessed, and Martin Roth. 1970. Observations on the Brains of Demented Old People. *Journal of Neurological Sciences* 11(3):205–42.

Trouillet, Raphaël, Marie-Christine Gély-Nargeot, and Christian Derouesné. 2003. Unawareness of Deficits in Alzheimer's Disease: A Multidimentional Approach. *Psychology and Neuropsychiatry* 1(2):99–110.

Turner, Bryan S. 1992. *Regulating Bodies: Essays in Medical Sociology.* London: Routledge.

Turner, Charles. 1996. Holocaust Memories and History. *History of the Human Sciences* 9(4):45–63.

U.S. Congress, Office of Technology Assessment. 1987. *Losing a Million Minds: Confronting the Tragedy of Alzheimer's Disease and Other Dementias.* Washington, D.C.: U.S. Government Printing Office.

U.S. Library of Congress. 2004. *Project on the Decade of the Brain.* National Institute of Mental Health. Washington, D.C.: U.S. Government Printing Office.

Uchino, Akiko, Masaki Takao, Hiroyuki Hatsuta, Hiroyuki Sumikura, Yuta Nakano, Yuko Saito, Kazutoshi Nishiyama, and Shigeo Murayama. 2015. TDP-43 Accumulation in the Aging Human Brain. *Journal of Neuropathology and Experimental Neurology* 74(6):599–600.

Usita, Paula, Ira E. Hyman, and Keith Herman. 1998. Narrative Intentions: Listening to Life Stories in Alzheimer's Disease. *Journal of Aging Studies* 12(2):185–97.

Vassilas, Christopher A., and Julia Donaldson. 1998. Telling the Truth: What Do General Practitioners Say to Patients with Dementia or Terminal Cancer? *British Journal of General Practice* 48:1081–82.

Vittoria, Anne K. 1998. Preserving Selves: Identity Work and Dementia. *Research on Aging* 21(1):91–136.

———. 1999. "Our Own Little Language": Naming and the Social Construction of Alzheimer's Disease. *Symbolic Interaction* 22(4):361–84.

Von Dras, D. Dean, and Herman T. Blumenthal. 1992. Dementia of the Aged: Disease or Atypical Accelerated Aging? *Journal of the American Geriatrics Society* 40:285–94.

Ware, Norma C. 1992. Suffering and the Social Construction of Illness: The Delegitimation of Illness Experience in Chronic Fatigue Syndrome. *Medical Anthropology Quarterly* 6(4):347–61.

Weiner, Howard L., Cynthia A. Lemere, Ruth Maron, Edward T. Spooner, Trelawney J. Grenfell, Chica Mori, Shohreh Issazadeh, Wayne W. Hancock, and Dennis J. Selkoe. 2000. Nasal Administration of Amyloid-Beta Peptide Decreases Cerebral Amyloid Burden in a Mouse Model of Alzheimer's Disease. *Annals of Neurology* 48(4):567–79.

Weitz, Rose. 1991. *Life with AIDS*. New Brunswick, N.J.: Rutgers University Press.

Werner, Anne, and Kirsti Malterud. 2003. It Is Hard Work Behaving as a Credible Patient: Encounters between Women with Chronic Pain and Their Doctors. *Social Science and Medicine* 57(8):1409–19.

Werner, Perla, Dovrat Goldstein, and Jeremia Heinik. 2009. The Process and Organizational Characteristics of Memory Clinics in Israel in 2007. *Archives of Gerontology and Geriatrics* 49:e115–e20.

Whitehouse, Peter J. 2000. "History and Future of Alzheimer's Disease." Pp. 291–305 in *Concepts of Alzheimer's Disease: Biological, Clinical and Cultural Perspectives*, edited by P. J. Whitehouse, K. Maurer, and J. F. Ballenger. Baltimore: Johns Hopkins University Press.

Whitehouse, Peter J., and William E. Deal. 1995. Situated beyond Modernity: Lessons for Alzheimer's Disease Research. *Journal of American Geriatric Society* 43:1314–15.

Whitehouse, Peter J., Giovanni B. Frisoni, and Stephen Post. 2004. Breaking the Diagnosis of Dementia. *Lancet Neurology* 3(2):124–28.

Whitehouse, Peter J., and Daniel George. 2008. *The Myth of Alzheimer's: What You Aren't Being Told about Today's Most Dreaded Diagnosis*. New York: St. Martin's Press.

Whitehouse, Peter J., Konrad Maurer, and Jesse F. Ballenger, eds. 2000. *Concepts of Alzheimer's Disease: Biological, Clinical and Cultural Perspectives*. Baltimore: Johns Hopkins University Press.

Whitehouse, Peter J., and Harry R. Moody. 2006. Mild Cognitive Impairment. *Dementia: International Journal of Social Research and Practice* 5(1):11–25.

Wiener Carolyn L. 1981. *The Politics of Alcoholism: Building an Arena around a Social Problem*. New Brunswick, N.J.: Transaction Books.

———. 2000. *The Elusive Quest: Accountability in Hospitals*. New York: Aldine de Gruyter.

Wiener Carolyn L., and Dodd M. J. 1993. Coping amid Uncertainty: An Illness Trajectory Perspective. *Scholarly Inquiries in Nursing Practice* 7(1):17–31.

Wilcock, Gordon K., Bucks, R. S., and Rockwood, K., eds. 1999. *Diagnosis and Management of Dementia: A Manual for Memory Disorders Teams*. Oxford, U.K.: Oxford University Press.

Wilkinson, Heather, ed. 2002. *The Perspectives of People with Dementia: Research Methods and Motivations*. London: Jessica Kingsley Publishers.

Wilkinson, Heather, and Andrew J. Milne. 2003. Sharing a Diagnosis of Dementia— Learning from the Patient Perspective. *Aging and Mental Health* 7:300–07.

Williams, Garreth H. 1984. The Genesis of Chronic Illness: Narrative Reconstruction. *Sociology of Health and Illness* 6:175–200.

Williams, Simone J. 2000. Chronic Illness as Biographical Disruption or Biographical Disruption as Chronic Illness? Reflections on a Core Concept. *Sociology of Health and Illness* 22(1):40–67.

Williams, Simone J., and Gillian A. Bendelow. 1996. The "Emotional" Body. *Body and Society* 2(3):125–39.

————. 1998. *The Lived Body: Sociological Themes, Embodied Issues.* New York: Routledge.

Winance, Myriam. 2003. The Two-Faced Experience of People Suffering from Neuro-muscular Diseases: Retraction and Extension. *Sciences Sociales et Santé* 21(2):5–31.

Winblad, Bengt, Katie Palmer, M. Kivipelto, V. Jelic, and Lisa Fratiglioni V. Jelic, L. Fratiglioni, L.-O. Wahlund, A. Nordberg, L. Bäckman, M. Albert, O. Almkvist, H. Arai, H. Basun, K. Blennow, M. De Leon, C. DeCarli, T. Erkinjuntti, E. Giacobini, C. Graff, J. Hardy, C. Jack, A. Jorm, K. Ritchie, C. Van Duijn, P. Visser, and R.C. Petersen. 2004. Mild Cognitive Impairment—Beyond Controversies, Towards a Consensus: Report to the International Working Groups on Mild Cognitive Impairment. *Journal of Internal Medicine* 256:240–46.

Wolf, Henrike, Marlene Grunwald, Gustave Martin Ecke, Dyrk Zedlick, Simone Bettin, Claudia Dannenberg, Jurgen Dietrich, Klaus Eschrich, Thomas Arendt, and Hermann-Josef Gertz. 1998. The Prognosis of Mild Cognitive Impairment in the Elderly. *Journal of Neural Transmission* 54:31–50.

World Health Organization. 1993. *The ICD-10 Classification of Mental and Behavioural Disorders: Diagnostic Criteria for Research.* Geneva: World Health Organization.

Wright, Neil, and James Lindesay. 1995. A Survey of Memory Clinics in the British Isles. *International Journal of Geriatric Psychiatry* 10:379–85.

Yoshida, Karen K. 1993. Reshaping of Self: A Pendular Reconstruction of Self and Identity among Adults with Traumatic Spinal Cord Injury. *Sociology of Health and Illness* 15(2):217–45.

Young, Allan. 1995. *The Harmony of Illusions: Inventing Post-Traumatic Stress Disorder.* Princeton, N.J.: Princeton University Press.

Zarit, Steven, Mary A. P. Stephens, Aloen Townsend, and Rickey Greene. 1998. Stress Reduction for Family Caregivers: Effects of Adult Day Care Use. *Journal of Gerontology: Social Sciences* 53B(5):s267–77.

Zavestoski, Steve, Phil Brown, Sabrina McCormick, Brian Mayer, Maryhelen D'Ottavi, and Jaime C. Lucove. 2004. Patient Activism and the Struggle for Diagnosis: Gulf War Illnesses and Other Medically Unexplained Physical Symptoms in the U.S. *Social Science and Medicine* 58(1):161–75.

INDEX

ABOUT THE AUTHOR

Renée L. Beard is Associate Professor of Sociology at the College of the Holy Cross. She teaches classes on medical sociology, aging, and illness narratives. She lives in Cambridge, Massachusetts, with her husband and two sons.

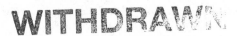